SEXUALLY TRANSMITTED DISEASES

SOURCEBOOK

EIGHTH EDITION

Health Reference Series

SEXUALLY TRANSMITTED DISEASES
SOURCEBOOK
EIGHTH EDITION

Basic Consumer Health Information about Sexual Health and Screening, Diagnosis, Treatment, and Prevention of Common Sexually Transmitted Diseases (STDs) such as Chancroid, Chlamydia, Gonorrhea, Herpes, Hepatitis, Human Immunodeficiency Virus/Acquired Immunodeficiency Syndrome (HIV/AIDS), Human Papillomavirus (HPV), Syphilis, and Trichomoniasis

Along with Facts about Risk Factors and Complications, Tips for Discussing STDs with Doctors, a Glossary of Related Terms, and Resources for Additional Help and Information

OMNIGRAPHICS
An imprint of Infobase

Bibliographic Note

Because this page cannot legibly accommodate all the copyright notices, the Bibliographic Note portion of the Preface constitutes an extension of the copyright notice.

* * *

OMNIGRAPHICS

An imprint of Infobase
132 W. 31st St.
New York, NY 10001
www.infobase.com
James Chambers, *Editorial Director*

* * *

Library of Congress Cataloging-in-Publication Data

Names: Chambers, James (Editor), editor. | Omnigraphics, Inc., issuing body.

Title: Sexually transmitted diseases sourcebook: basic consumer health information about sexual health and the screening, diagnosis, treatment, and prevention of common sexually transmitted diseases (STDs), including chancroid, chlamydia, gonorrhea, herpes, hepatitis, human immunodeficiency virus/acquired immunodeficiency syndrome (HIV/AIDS), human papillomavirus (HPV), syphilis, and trichomoniasis; along with facts about risk factors and complications, tips for discussing sexually transmitted diseases with partners, a glossary of related terms, and resources for additional help and information / edited by James Chambers.

Description: Eighth edition. | New York, NY: Omnigraphics, an imprint of Infobase, [2023] | Series: Health reference series | Includes bibliographical references and index. | Summary: "Provides basic consumer health information about risk factors, symptoms, diagnosis, and treatment of sexually transmitted diseases and related complications, along with facts about prevention strategies. Includes index, glossary of related terms, and other resources"-- Provided by publisher.

Identifiers: LCCN 2023030069 (print) | LCCN 2023030070 (ebook) | ISBN 9780780820821 (library binding) | ISBN 9780780820838 (ebook)

Subjects: LCSH: Sexually transmitted diseases--Popular works.

Classification: LCC RC200.2.S387 2023 (print) | LCC RC200.2 (ebook) | DDC 616.95/1--dc23/eng/20230705

LC record available at https://lccn.loc.gov/2023030069
LC ebook record available at https://lccn.loc.gov/2023030070

Table of Contents

Part 2. Types of Sexually Transmitted Diseases

Part 3. Health Complications That May Co-occur with Sexually Transmitted Diseases

Part 7. Additional Help and Information

Preface

ABOUT THIS BOOK

Sexually transmitted diseases (STDs), as the name indicates, are primarily transmitted through sexual contact involving the genitals and other body parts. In some cases, these diseases can also be transmitted through non-sexual means, such as blood transfusions and the sharing of needles. While STDs can affect people of all ages, they are more prevalent among sexually active young individuals. Today, diagnosing, treating, and preventing potentially life-threatening STDs represent some of the most significant challenges in public health. STDs have significant health consequences if they are not diagnosed and treated.

Sexually Transmitted Diseases Sourcebook, Eighth Edition provides essential information about sexual health and the screening, diagnosis, treatment, and prevention of common STDs, including chancroid, chlamydia, gonorrhea, herpes, hepatitis, human immunodeficiency virus (HIV), acquired immunodeficiency syndrome (AIDS), human papillomavirus (HPV), syphilis, and trichomoniasis. It discusses trends in STD rates and developments in STD vaccine research and provides tips on talking to doctors, a glossary of related terms, and resources for additional help and information.

HOW TO USE THIS BOOK

This book is divided into parts and chapters. Parts focus on broad areas of interest. Chapters are devoted to single topics within a part.

Part 1: Introduction to Sexually Transmitted Diseases covers the basics of sexual and reproductive health, identifies the parts of both the female and male reproductive systems, and discusses trends in sexually transmitted diseases (STDs). It also examines the implications of these infections on women, men, children, teenagers, as well as specific demographics, including pregnant women and individuals involved in same-gender relationships.

The part concludes with statistical data outlining racial disparities and the disproportionate impact of STDs on minority populations.

Part 2: Types of Sexually Transmitted Diseases identifies the symptoms, diagnoses, and treatments of common types of STDs, including chancroid, chlamydia, donovanosis, gonorrhea, herpes, hepatitis, human papillomavirus (HPV), lymphogranuloma venereum (LGV), syphilis, and trichomoniasis. The part also includes information on how human immunodeficiency virus (HIV) causes acquired immunodeficiency syndrome (AIDS), outlining the disease's transmission, testing methodologies, and strategies for managing life with HIV while navigating the financial aspects of medical care.

Part 3: Health Complications That May Co-occur with Sexually Transmitted Diseases provides information about infections and syndromes that may develop after sexual contact, such as bacterial vaginosis, cytomegalovirus, yeast infection, intestinal infections, molluscum contagiosum, pubic lice, and scabies. The part also provides information about conditions related to STDs that can cause long-term health complications, including urethritis and cervicitis, epididymitis, neurosyphilis, pelvic inflammatory disease (PID), infertility, and pregnancy complications.

Part 4: Sexually Transmitted Diseases: Testing and Treatment offers information about how medical professionals test patients for STDs and addresses common issues associated with STD testing, such as maintaining confidentiality and discussing STDs with health-care providers. It discusses antibiotic resistance and prophylactic antibiotics for the prevention of STDs. Information about partner services, expedited partner therapy, and complementary and alternative therapies for STDs is also included.

Part 5: Sexually Transmitted Diseases: Risks and Prevention discusses sexual behaviors that increase the likelihood of STD transmission, such as choosing high-risk partners, having multiple sex partners, and nonsexual factors that raise STD risk, including illegal substance use and douching. The part concludes with methods for preventing STDs: employing safer sex practices and barrier methods such as condoms and dental dams; utilizing post-exposure medication; avoiding mother-to-child transmission during pregnancy; and embracing the use of STD vaccines and microbicides.

Part 6: Living with Sexually Transmitted Diseases explores effective strategies for addressing sensitive topics like disclosing one's HIV status, establishing partner communication and agreements, and combating the social stigma associated with HIV. It also offers insights into managing the physical and mental aspects of living with HIV.

Part 7: Additional Help and Information provides a glossary of important terms related to STDs and a directory of organizations that offer information to people with STDs or their sexual partners.

BIBLIOGRAPHIC NOTE

This volume contains documents and excerpts from publications issued by the following U.S. government agencies: Centers for Disease Control and Prevention (CDC); Centers for Medicare & Medicaid Services (CMS); *Eunice Kennedy Shriver* National Institute of Child Health and Human Development (NICHD); Genetic and Rare Diseases Information Center (GARD); girlshealth.gov; HIV.gov; MedlinePlus; National Institute of Allergy and Infectious Diseases (NIAID); National Institute of Neurological Disorders and Stroke (NINDS); National Institute on Drug Abuse (NIDA); National Institutes of Health (NIH); Office of Disease Prevention and Health Promotion (ODPHP); Office of Research on Women's Health (ORWH); Office on Women's Health (OWH); Surveillance, Epidemiology, and End Results (SEER) Program; and U.S. Department of Veterans Affairs (VA).

It also contains original material produced by Infobase and reviewed by medical consultants.

ABOUT THE *HEALTH REFERENCE SERIES*

The *Health Reference Series* is designed to provide basic medical information for patients, families, caregivers, and the general public. Each volume provides comprehensive coverage on a particular topic. This is especially important for people who may be dealing with a newly diagnosed disease or a chronic disorder in themselves or in a family member. People looking for preventive guidance, information about disease warning signs, medical statistics, and risk factors for health problems will also find answers to their questions in the *Health Reference Series*. The *Series*, however, is not intended to serve as a tool for diagnosing illness, in prescribing treatments, or as a substitute for the physician–patient relationship. All people concerned about medical symptoms or the possibility of disease are encouraged to seek professional care from an appropriate health-care provider.

A NOTE ABOUT SPELLING AND STYLE

Health Reference Series editors use *Stedman's Medical Dictionary* as an authority for questions related to the spelling of medical terms and *The Chicago Manual of Style* for questions related to grammatical structures, punctuation, and other editorial concerns. Consistent adherence is not always possible, however, because the individual volumes within the *Series* include many documents from a wide variety of different producers, and the editor's primary goal is to present material from each source as accurately as is possible. This sometimes means that information in different chapters or sections may follow other guidelines and alternate spelling authorities. For example, occasionally a copyright holder may require that eponymous terms be shown in possessive forms (Crohn's disease vs. Crohn disease) or that British spelling norms be retained (leukaemia vs. leukemia).

MEDICAL REVIEW

Infobase contracts with a team of qualified, senior medical professionals who serve as medical consultants for the *Health Reference Series*. As necessary, medical consultants review reprinted and originally written material for currency and accuracy. Citations including the phrase "Reviewed (month, year)" indicate material reviewed by this team. Medical consultation services are provided to the *Health Reference Series* editors by:

Dr. Vijayalakshmi, MBBS, DGO, MD
Dr. Senthil Selvan, MBBS, DCH, MD
Dr. K. Sivanandham, MBBS, DCH, MS (Research), PhD

HEALTH REFERENCE SERIES UPDATE POLICY

The inaugural book in the *Health Reference Series* was the first edition of *Cancer Sourcebook* published in 1989. Since then, the *Series* has been enthusiastically received by librarians and in the medical community. In order to maintain the standard of providing high-quality health information for the layperson, the editorial staff felt it was necessary to implement a policy of updating volumes when warranted.

Medical researchers have been making tremendous strides, and it is the purpose of the *Health Reference Series* to stay current with the most recent advances. Each decision to update a volume is made on an individual basis.

Some of the considerations include how much new information is available and the feedback we receive from people who use the books. If there is a topic you would like to see added to the update list, or an area of medical concern you feel has not been adequately addressed, please write to: custserv@infobaselearning.com.

Part 1 | Introduction to Sexually Transmitted Diseases

Chapter 1 | An Overview of Sexual Health and the Reproductive System

Chapter Contents

Section 1.1 | Defining Sexual and Reproductive Health

The World Health Organization (WHO) defines sexual health as a state of physical, emotional, mental, and social well-being in relation to sexuality; it is not merely the absence of disease, dysfunction, or infirmity. Sexual health requires a positive and respectful approach to sexuality and sexual relationships, as well as the possibility of having pleasurable and safe sexual experiences, free of coercion, discrimination, and violence.[1]

REPRODUCTIVE AND SEXUAL HEALTH ACROSS THE LIFE STAGES

Reproductive and sexual health is an important part of an individual's overall health, particularly during childbearing years.

Infants

Babies of mothers who do not get prenatal care are three times more likely to have a low birth weight and five times more likely to die than those born to mothers who do get prenatal care.

Adolescents

- Sexually transmitted diseases (STDs) are a risk to adolescents' health and fertility. Nearly half of new sexually transmitted infections are among young people aged 15–24.
- Adolescents who become pregnant are much less likely to complete their education. About 50 percent of teen mothers get a high school diploma by the age of 22, compared with 90 percent of teen girls who do not give birth. Only 50 percent of teen fathers who have children before the age of 18 finish high school or get their general equivalency diploma (GED) by the age of 22.

---

[1] "Sexual Health," Centers for Disease Control and Prevention (CDC), June 25, 2019. Available online. URL: www.cdc.gov/sexualhealth/Default.html. Accessed July 7, 2023.

Older Adults

People aged 50 and over account for decreasing numbers of new human immunodeficiency virus (HIV) diagnoses, and older adults may not consider themselves to be at risk of HIV infection. However, many older adults are sexually active, including those living with HIV, and may have the same HIV risk factors as younger people. Consider the following:

- People aged 50 and over accounted for 17 percent of the new HIV diagnoses in 2015 in the United States.
- Forty-five percent of Americans living with diagnosed HIV are over the age of 50.
- Older women may be especially at risk for HIV infection due to age-related thinning and dryness of vaginal tissue.
- Some older adults, compared with those who are younger, may be less knowledgeable about HIV and, therefore, less likely to protect themselves. Many do not perceive themselves as at risk for HIV, do not use condoms, and are less likely than young people to get tested for HIV or to discuss sexual habits or drug use with their doctor.
- Older people in the United States are more likely than younger people to have late-stage HIV infection at the time of diagnosis.[2]

WOMEN'S REPRODUCTIVE HEALTH

A woman's reproductive system is a delicate and complex system in the body. It is important to take steps to protect it from infections and injury and prevent problems—including some long-term health problems. Taking care of yourself and making healthy choices can help protect you and your loved ones. Protecting your reproductive system also means having control of your health, if and when you become pregnant.

---

[2] Office of Disease Prevention and Health Promotion (ODPHP), "Reproductive and Sexual Health," U.S. Department of Health and Human Services (HHS), February 26, 2022. Available online. URL: www.healthypeople.gov/2020/leading-health-indicators/2020-lhi-topics/Reproductive-and-Sexual-Health/determinants. Accessed July 7, 2023.

FACTORS IMPACTING WOMEN'S REPRODUCTIVE HEALTH
Contraception (Birth Control)

There are several safe and highly effective methods of birth control available to prevent unintended pregnancy. These include intrauterine contraception, hormonal and barrier methods, and permanent birth control (sterilization). Using effective birth control methods can greatly reduce the chances of having an unintended pregnancy. The Division of Reproductive Health of the Centers for Disease Control and Prevention (CDC) has a long history of conducting epidemiologic studies on the safety and effectiveness of contraceptive methods. Results from these studies have informed contraceptive practices.

Depression

Depression is common. Often, trying to get pregnant, being pregnant, or the birth of a baby can increase the risk for depression. Also, many women do not know that depression sometimes happens with other events, such as losing a baby or having trouble getting pregnant. Women may also feel depressed for many other reasons—some may not even know why.

Heart Defects and Women's Reproductive Health

Get informed about contraception, preconception health, and pregnancy for people living with heart defects. If you are living with a heart defect, you may need specialized medical care to manage your reproductive health and heart health.

Hysterectomy

Hysterectomy is the surgical removal of a woman's uterus. The uterus is the place where a baby grows when a woman is pregnant. Sometimes, the cervix, ovaries, and fallopian tubes are also removed. Hysterectomies are very common—one out of three women in the United States has had one by the age of 60.

Female Genital Mutilation/Cutting

Female genital mutilation or cutting (FGM/C) is defined by the WHO as "all procedures involving partial or total removal of the external female genitalia or other injury to the female genital organs for nonmedical reasons." These procedures could mean piercing, cutting, removing, or sewing closed all or part of a girl's or woman's external genitals.

Infertility

Infertility means not being able to get pregnant after one year of trying. If a woman is 35 or older, infertility is based on six months of trying to become pregnant. Women who can get pregnant but are unable to stay pregnant may also be considered infertile. About 10 percent of women (6.1 million) in the United States aged 15–44 have difficulty getting pregnant or staying pregnant.

Menopause

Menopause is a normal change in a woman's life when her period stops. A woman has reached menopause when she has not had a period for 12 months in a row. This often happens between 45 and 55 years of age. Menopause happens because the woman's ovary stops producing the hormones estrogen and progesterone.[3]

MEN'S REPRODUCTIVE HEALTH

Reproductive health is an important component of men's overall health and well-being. Too often, males have been overlooked in discussions of reproductive health, especially when reproductive issues such as contraception and infertility have been perceived as female-related. Every day, men, their partners, and health-care providers can protect their reproductive health by ensuring effective contraception, avoiding STDs, and preserving fertility.

Common issues in male reproductive health include:

- contraception
- avoiding STDs
- infertility/fertility

---

[3] "Women's Reproductive Health," Centers for Disease Control and Prevention (CDC), May 3, 2022. Available online. URL: www.cdc.gov/reproductivehealth/womensrh/index.htm. Accessed July 7, 2023.

Men should consult with their health-care provider to discuss which contraceptive method is best for the couple, based on over-all health, age, frequency of sexual activity, number of partners, desire to have children in the future, and a family history of certain diseases. Contraceptive methods work best when they are used correctly and consistently. Using contraception incorrectly or inconsistently increases the risk of pregnancy and in some cases also increases the risk of STDs.

It is important to discuss the risk factors for STDs with a health-care provider and ask about getting tested. It is possible to have an STD and not know it because many STDs do not cause symptoms. Men with STDs need to ask a health-care provider about treatment to address symptoms, reduce the progression of STDs, and decrease or eliminate the risk of transmitting an STD to their partner.

If you and your partner are interested in having children but have difficulty conceiving, it is important for both the male and the female partner to consult with a health-care provider to assess fertility. Over one-third of infertility cases are caused by male reproductive issues, alone or in combination with female reproductive issues. However, treatments are available to address many of the causes of male infertility.[4]

Section 1.2 | Female Reproductive System

The major function of the reproductive system is to ensure the survival of the species. An individual may live a long, healthy, and happy life without producing offspring, but if the species is to continue, at least some individuals must produce offspring. Within the context of producing offspring, the reproductive system has four functions:
- to produce egg and sperm cells
- to transport and sustain these cells

---

[4] "About Men's Reproductive Health," *Eunice Kennedy Shriver* National Institute of Child Health and Human Development (NICHD), November 18, 2021. Available online. URL: www.nichd.nih.gov/health/topics/menshealth/conditioninfo. Accessed July 7, 2023.

- to nurture the developing offspring
- to produce hormones

These functions are divided between the primary and secondary, or accessory, reproductive organs.

- Primary reproductive organs, or gonads, consist of the ovaries and testes that are responsible for producing egg and sperm cells with gametes and hormones. These hormones function in the maturation of the reproductive system, the development of sexual characteristics, and the regulation of the normal physiology of the reproductive system.
- All other organs, ducts, and glands in the reproductive system are considered secondary, or accessory, reproductive organs. These structures transport and sustain the gametes and nurture the developing offspring.[5]

HOW THE FEMALE REPRODUCTIVE SYSTEM WORKS

The female reproductive system (see Figure 1.1) is all the parts of your body that help reproduce or have babies. Consider these two fabulous facts:

- A female body likely has hundreds and thousands of eggs that could grow into a baby, and they have them from the time they are born.
- Right inside each female is a perfect place for those eggs to meet with the sperm and grow into a whole human being.

What Is Inside the Female Reproductive System?

- **The ovaries.** These are two small organs. Before puberty, it is as if the ovaries are asleep. During puberty, they "wake up." The ovaries start making more estrogen and other hormones, which cause body changes. One important body change is

---

[5] Surveillance, Epidemiology and End Results Program (SEER), "Introduction to the Reproductive System," National Cancer Institute (NCI), November 29, 2011. Available online. URL: https://training.seer.cancer.gov/anatomy/reproductive. Accessed June 14, 2023.

that these hormones cause you to start getting your period, which is called "menstruating." Once a month, the ovaries release one egg (ovum). This is called "ovulation."

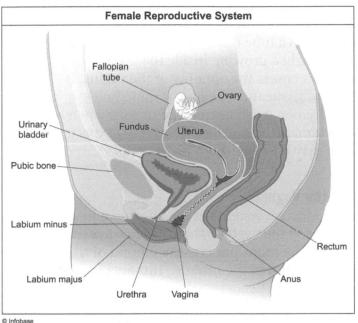

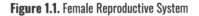

© Infobase

Figure 1.1. Female Reproductive System

Infobase

- **The fallopian tubes.** They connect the ovaries to the uterus. The released egg moves along a fallopian tube.
- **The uterus or womb.** This is where a baby would grow. It takes several days for the egg to get to the uterus. As the egg travels, estrogen makes the lining of the uterus (called the "endometrium") thick with blood and fluid. This makes the uterus a good place for a baby to grow. One can become pregnant if a female has sex with a male without birth control and his sperm joins the egg (called "fertilization") on its way to the uterus. If the egg does not get fertilized, it will be shed along with the lining of the uterus during the

next period (menses). But do not look for the egg—it is too small to see! The blood and fluid that leave the body during the period pass through the cervix and vagina.

- **The cervix.** This is a narrow entryway between the vagina and the uterus. The cervix is flexible, so it can expand to let a baby pass through during childbirth.
- **The vagina.** This is a tube that can grow wider to deliver a baby that has finished growing inside the uterus.
- **The hymen.** This covers the opening of the vagina. It is a thin piece of tissue that has one or more holes in it. Sometimes, a hymen may be stretched or torn when a female uses a tampon or during a first sexual experience. If it does tear, it may bleed a little.

What Is Outside the Vagina?

The external reproductive system lies outside the vagina. The vulva covers the entrance to the vagina. The vulva has five parts:

- **Mons pubis**. The mons pubis is the mound of tissue and skin above the legs, in the middle. This area becomes covered with hair when a female goes through puberty.
- **Labia**. The labia are the two sets of skin folds (often called "lips") on either side of the opening of the vagina. The labia majora are the outer lips, and the labia minora are the inner lips. It is normal for the labia to look different from each other.
- **Clitoris**. The clitoris is a small, sensitive bump at the bottom of the mons pubis that is covered by the labia minora.
- **Urinary opening**. The urinary opening, below the clitoris, is where the urine (pee) leaves the body.
- **Vaginal opening**. The vaginal opening is the entry to the vagina and is found below the urinary opening.

These are the basics of the female reproductive system.[6]

---

[6] girlshealth.gov, "How the Female Reproductive System Works," Office on Women's Health (OWH), April 15, 2014. Available online. URL: www.girlshealth.gov/body/reproductive/system.html. Accessed June 14, 2023.

FEMALE SEXUAL RESPONSE AND HORMONE CONTROL

The female sexual response includes arousal and orgasm. A woman may become pregnant without having an orgasm. Follicle-stimulating hormone (FSH), luteinizing hormone (LH), estrogen, and progesterone have major roles in regulating the functions of the female reproductive system.

At puberty, when the ovaries and uterus respond to certain stimuli, this causes the hypothalamus to secrete a gonadotropin-releasing hormone. This hormone enters the blood and goes to the anterior pituitary gland, where it stimulates the secretion of FSH and LH. These hormones, in turn, affect the ovaries and uterus, and the monthly cycles begin. A woman's reproductive cycle lasts from menarche to menopause.

Menopause occurs when a woman's reproductive cycles stop. This period is marked by decreased levels of ovarian hormones and increased levels of pituitary FSH and LH. The changing hormone levels are responsible for the symptoms associated with menopause.[7]

Section 1.3 | Male Reproductive System

The male reproductive system, like that of the female, consists of those organs whose function is to produce a new individual that is to accomplish reproduction. As shown in Figure 1.2, the reproductive system consists of a pair of testes and a network of excretory ducts (epididymis, ductus deferens (vas deferens), and ejaculatory ducts), seminal vesicles, the prostate, the bulbourethral glands, and the penis.

TESTES

The male gonads, testes or testicles, begin their development high in the abdominal cavity, near the kidneys. During the last two

---

[7] Surveillance, Epidemiology and End Results Program (SEER), "Female Sexual Response and Hormone Control," National Cancer Institute (NCI), September 7, 2016. Available online. URL: https://training.seer.cancer.gov/anatomy/reproductive/female/response.html. Accessed June 14, 2023.

months before birth, or shortly after birth, they descend through the inguinal canal into the scrotum, a pouch that extends below the abdomen, posterior to the penis.

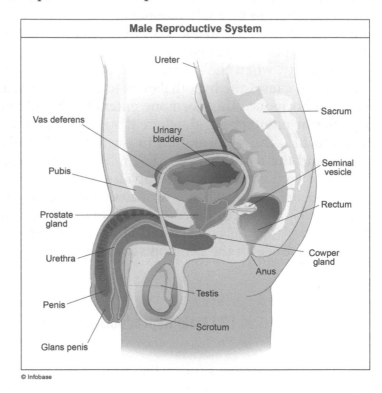

Figure 1.2. Male Reproductive System

Infobase

SCROTUM

The scrotum consists of the skin and subcutaneous tissue. A vertical septum, or partition, of subcutaneous tissue in the center divides it into two parts, each containing one testis. Smooth muscle fibers, called the "dartos muscle," in the subcutaneous tissue contract to give the scrotum its wrinkled appearance. When these fibers are relaxed, the scrotum is smooth. Another muscle, the cremaster muscle, consists of skeletal muscle fibers and controls the position of the scrotum and testes.

Structure

Each testis is an oval structure. A tough, white fibrous connective tissue capsule, the tunica albuginea, surrounds each testis and extends inward to form septa that partition the organ into lobules. There are about 250 lobules in each testis. Each lobule contains one to four highly coiled seminiferous tubules that converge to form a single straight tubule, which leads into the rete testis. Short efferent ducts exit the testes. Interstitial cells (cells of Leydig), which produce male sex hormones, are located between the seminiferous tubules within a lobule.

Spermatogenesis

Sperm are produced by spermatogenesis within the seminiferous tubules. A transverse section of a seminiferous tubule shows that it is packed with cells in various stages of development. Interspersed with these cells, there are large cells that extend from the periphery of the tubule to the lumen. These large cells are the supporting, or sustentacular, cells (Sertoli cells), which support and nourish the other cells.

Early in embryonic development, primordial germ cells enter the testes and differentiate into spermatogonia, immature cells that remain dormant until puberty. Spermatogonia are diploid cells, each with 46 chromosomes (23 pairs), located around the periphery of the seminiferous tubules. At puberty, hormones stimulate these cells to begin dividing by mitosis. Some of the daughter cells produced by mitosis remain at the periphery as spermatogonia. Others are pushed toward the lumen, undergo some changes, and become primary spermatocytes. Because they are produced by mitosis, primary spermatocytes, such as spermatogonia, are diploid and have 46 chromosomes.

Each primary spermatocyte goes through the first meiotic division, meiosis I, to produce two secondary spermatocytes, each with 23 chromosomes (haploid). Just prior to this division, the genetic material is replicated so that each chromosome consists of two strands, called "chromatids," that are joined by a centromere. During meiosis I, one chromosome, consisting of two chromatids, goes to each secondary spermatocyte. In the second meiotic

15

division, meiosis II, each secondary spermatocyte divides to produce two spermatids. There is no replication of genetic material in this division, but the centromere divides so that a single-stranded chromatid goes to each cell. As a result of the two meiotic divisions, each primary spermatocyte produces four spermatids. During spermatogenesis, there are two cellular divisions but only one replication of deoxyribonucleic acid (DNA) so that each spermatid has 23 chromosomes (haploid), one from each pair in the original primary spermatocyte. Each successive stage in spermatogenesis is pushed toward the center of the tubule so that the more immature cells are at the periphery and the more differentiated cells are nearer the center.

Spermatogenesis (and oogenesis in the female) differs from mitosis because the resulting cells have only half the number of chromosomes as the original cell. When the sperm cell nucleus unites with an egg cell nucleus, the full number of chromosomes is restored. If sperm and egg cells were produced by mitosis, then each successive generation would have twice the number of chromosomes as the preceding one.

The final step in the development of sperm is called "spermiogenesis." In this process, the spermatids formed from spermatogenesis become mature spermatozoa, or sperm. The mature sperm cell has a head, midpiece, and tail. The head, also called the "nuclear region," contains 23 chromosomes surrounded by a nuclear membrane. The tip of the head is covered by an acrosome, which contains enzymes that help the sperm penetrate the female gamete. The midpiece, metabolic region, contains mitochondria that provide adenosine triphosphate (ATP). The tail, or locomotor region, uses a typical flagellum for locomotion. The sperm are released into the lumen of the seminiferous tubule and leave the testes. They then enter the epididymis where they undergo their final maturation and become capable of fertilizing a female gamete.

Sperm production begins at puberty and continues throughout the life of a male. The entire process, beginning with a primary spermatocyte, takes about 74 days. After ejaculation, the sperm can live for about 48 hours in the female reproductive tract.

DUCT SYSTEM

Sperm cells pass through a series of ducts to reach the outside of the body. After they leave the testes, the sperm passes through the epididymis, ductus deferens, ejaculatory duct, and urethra.

Epididymis

Sperm leave the testes through a series of efferent ducts that enter the epididymis. Each epididymis is a long (about 6 meters) tube that is tightly coiled to form a comma-shaped organ located along the superior and posterior margins of the testes. When the sperm leave the testes, they are immature and incapable of fertilizing ova (female eggs). They complete their maturation process and become fertile as they move through the epididymis. Mature sperm are stored in the lower portion, or tail, of the epididymis.

Ductus Deferens

The ductus deferens, also called "vas deferens," is a fibromuscular tube that is continuous (or contiguous) with the epididymis. It begins at the bottom (tail) of the epididymis and then turns sharply upward along the posterior margin of the testes. The ductus deferens enters the abdominopelvic cavity through the inguinal canal and passes along the lateral pelvic wall. It crosses over the ureter and posterior portion of the urinary bladder and then descends along the posterior wall of the bladder toward the prostate gland. Just before it reaches the prostate gland, each ductus deferens enlarges to form an ampulla. Sperm are stored in the proximal portion of the ductus deferens, near the epididymis, and peristaltic movements propel the sperm through the tube.

The proximal portion of the ductus deferens is a component of the spermatic cord, which contains vascular and neural structures that supply the testes. The spermatic cord contains the ductus deferens, testicular artery and veins, lymph vessels, testicular nerve, the cremaster muscle that elevates the testes for warmth and at times of sexual stimulation, and a connective tissue covering.

Ejaculatory Duct

Each ductus deferens, at the ampulla, joins the duct from the adjacent seminal vesicle (one of the accessory glands) to form a short ejaculatory duct. Each ejaculatory duct passes through the prostate gland and empties into the urethra.

Urethra

The urethra extends from the urinary bladder to the external urethral orifice (terminal opening of the urethra) at the tip of the penis. It is a passageway for sperm and fluids from the reproductive system and urine from the urinary system. While reproductive fluids are passing through the urethra, sphincters contract tightly to keep urine from entering the urethra.

The male urethra is divided into three regions:

- **Prostatic urethra**. This region is the proximal portion that passes through the prostate gland. It receives the ejaculatory duct, which contains sperm and secretions from the seminal vesicles, and numerous ducts from the prostate glands.
- **Membranous urethra**. This next portion is a short region that passes through the pelvic floor.
- **Penile urethra**. Also called "spongy urethra" or "cavernous urethra," this is the longest portion which extends the length of the penis and opens to the outside at the external urethral orifice. The ducts from the bulbourethral glands open into the penile urethra.

ACCESSORY GLANDS

The accessory glands of the male reproductive system are the seminal vesicles, prostate gland, and bulbourethral glands. These glands secrete fluids that enter the urethra.

Seminal Vesicles

The paired seminal vesicles are saccular glands posterior to the urinary bladder. Each gland has a short duct that joins with the ductus deferens at the ampulla to form an ejaculatory duct, which then empties into the urethra. The fluid from the seminal vesicles is viscous and contains fructose, which provides an energy source for the sperm; prostaglandins, which contribute to the mobility and viability of the sperm; and proteins that cause slight coagulation reactions in the semen after ejaculation.

Prostate

The prostate gland is a firm, dense structure that is located just inferior to the urinary bladder. It is about the size of a walnut and encircles the urethra as it leaves the urinary bladder. Numerous short ducts from the substance of the prostate gland empty into the prostatic urethra. The secretions of the prostate are thin, milky, and alkaline. They function to enhance the motility of the sperm.

Bulbourethral Glands

The paired bulbourethral (Cowper) glands are small, about the size of a pea, and located near the base of the penis. A short duct from each gland enters the proximal end of the penile urethra. In response to sexual stimulation, the bulbourethral glands secrete an alkaline mucus-like fluid. This fluid neutralizes the acidity of the urine residue in the urethra, helps neutralize the acidity of the vagina, and provides some lubrication for the tip of the penis during intercourse.

Seminal Fluid

Seminal fluid, or semen, is a slightly alkaline mixture of sperm cells and secretions from the accessory glands. Secretions from the seminal vesicles make up about 60 percent of the volume of the semen, with most of the remainder coming from the prostate gland. The sperm and secretions from the bulbourethral gland contribute only a small volume.

The volume of semen in a single ejaculation may vary from 1.5 to 6.0 ml. There are usually between 50 and 150 million sperm per milliliter of semen. Sperm counts below 10–20 million per milliliter usually present fertility problems. Although only one sperm actually penetrates and fertilizes the ovum, it takes several million sperm in an ejaculation to ensure that fertilization will take place.

PENIS

The penis, the male copulatory organ, is a cylindrical pendant organ located anterior to the scrotum and functions to transfer sperm to the vagina. The penis consists of three columns of erectile tissue that are wrapped in connective tissue and covered with skin. The two dorsal columns are the corpora cavernosa. The single, midline ventral column surrounds the urethra and is called the "corpus spongiosum."

The penis has a root, body (shaft), and glans penis. The root of the penis attaches it to the pubic arch, and the body is the visible, pendant portion. The corpus spongiosum expands at the distal end to form the glans penis. The urethra, which extends throughout the length of the corpus spongiosum, opens through the external urethral orifice at the tip of the glans penis. A loose fold of the skin, called the "prepuce" or "foreskin," covers the glans penis.

MALE SEXUAL RESPONSE AND HORMONAL CONTROL

The male sexual response includes erection and orgasm accompanied by ejaculation of semen. Orgasm is followed by a variable time period during which it is not possible to achieve another erection.

Three hormones are the principal regulators of the male reproductive system: follicle-stimulating hormone (FSH) stimulates spermatogenesis; luteinizing hormone (LH) stimulates the production of testosterone; and testosterone stimulates the development of male secondary sex characteristics and spermatogenesis.[8]

---

[8] Surveillance, Epidemiology, and End Results (SEER) Program, "Male Reproductive System," National Cancer Institute (NCI), September 7, 2016. Available online. URL: https://training.seer.cancer.gov/anatomy/reproductive/male. Accessed May 19, 2023.

Chapter 2 | **Sexually Transmitted Diseases: An Overview**

Chapter Contents

Section 2.1 | Understanding Sexually Transmitted Diseases

Sexually transmitted diseases (STDs), also known as "sexually transmitted infections" (STIs), are typically caused by bacteria or viruses and are passed from person to person during sexual contact with the penis, vagina, anus, or mouth. The symptoms of STDs/STIs vary between individuals, depending on the cause, and many people may not experience symptoms at all.

Many STDs/STIs have significant health consequences. For instance, certain STIs can also increase the risk of getting and transmitting the human immunodeficiency virus (HIV)/acquired immune deficiency syndrome (AIDS) and alter the way the disease progresses. STIs can also cause long-term health problems, particularly in women and infants. Some of the health problems that arise from STIs include pelvic inflammatory disease (PID), infertility, tubal or ectopic pregnancy, cervical cancer, and perinatal or congenital infections in infants.

WHAT CAUSES SEXUALLY TRANSMITTED DISEASES OR SEXUALLY TRANSMITTED INFECTIONS?

The following are the three major causes of STDs/STIs:
- bacteria, including chlamydia, gonorrhea, and syphilis
- viruses, including HIV/AIDS, herpes simplex virus, human papillomavirus (HPV), hepatitis B virus, cytomegalovirus (CMV), and Zika
- parasites, such as *Trichomonas vaginalis*, or insects such as crab lice or scabies mites

Any STI can be spread through sexual activity, including sexual intercourse, and some STIs spread through oral sex and other sexual activity. Ejaculation does not have to occur for an STI to pass from person to person.

In addition, sharing contaminated needles, such as those used to inject drugs, or using contaminated body piercing or tattooing equipment can also transmit some infections, such as HIV, hepatitis B, and hepatitis C. A few infections can be sexually transmitted and are also spread through nonsexual, close contact. Some of these infections, such as CMV, are not considered STIs even though they can be transmitted through sexual contact.

Regardless of how a person is exposed, once a person is infected by an STI, he or she can spread the infection to other people through oral, vaginal, or anal sex, even if no symptoms.

WHAT ARE THE SYMPTOMS OF SEXUALLY TRANSMITTED DISEASES OR SEXUALLY TRANSMITTED INFECTIONS?

People with STDs/STIs may feel ill and notice some of the following signs and symptoms:

- unusual discharge from the penis or vagina
- sores or warts on the genital area
- painful or frequent urination
- itching and redness in the genital area
- blisters or sores in or around the mouth
- abnormal vaginal odor
- anal itching, soreness, or bleeding
- abdominal pain
- fever

In some cases, people with STIs have no symptoms. Over time, any symptoms that are present may improve on their own. It is also possible for a person to have an STI with no symptoms and then pass it on to others without knowing it.

If you are concerned that you or your sexual partner may have an STI, talk to your health-care provider. Even if you do not have symptoms, it is possible you may have an STI that needs treatment to ensure your and your partners' sexual health.[1]

---

[1] "Sexually Transmitted Diseases (STDs)," *Eunice Kennedy Shriver* National Institute of Child Health and Human Development (NICHD), January 31, 2017. Available online. URL: www.nichd.nih.gov/health/topics/stds. Accessed June 14, 2023.

Section 2.2 | **Factors Influencing the Spread of Sexually Transmitted Diseases**

Sexually transmitted diseases (STDs) refer to more than 35 infectious organisms that are transmitted primarily through sexual activities. STD prevention is an essential primary care strategy for improving reproductive health.

Despite their burdens, costs, and complications and the fact that they are largely preventable, STDs remain a significant public health problem in the United States. This problem is largely unrecognized by the public, policymakers, and health-care professionals. STDs cause many harmful, often irreversible, and costly clinical complications, such as:

- reproductive health problems
- fetal and perinatal health problems
- cancer
- facilitation of the sexual transmission of human immunodeficiency virus (HIV) infection

FACTORS THAT CONTRIBUTE TO THE SPREAD OF SEXUALLY TRANSMITTED DISEASES

Several factors contribute to the spread of STDs, and they are as follows:

- **Biological factors.** STDs are acquired during unprotected sex with an infected partner. Biological factors that affect the spread and complications of STDs include the following:
  - **Asymptomatic nature of STDs.** The majority of STDs either do not produce any symptoms or signs or produce symptoms so mild that they are unnoticed; consequently, many infected persons do not know that they need medical care.
  - **Gender disparities.** Women suffer more frequent and more serious STD complications than men. Among the most serious STD complications are pelvic inflammatory disease (PID), ectopic

25

pregnancy (pregnancy outside of the uterus), infertility, and chronic pelvic pain.
- **Age disparities**. Young people aged 15–24 account for half of all new STDs although they represent just 25 percent of the sexually experienced population. Adolescent females may have increased susceptibility to infection because of increased cervical ectopy.
- **Social, economic, and behavioral factors**. The spread of STDs is directly affected by social, economic, and behavioral factors. Such factors may cause serious obstacles to STD prevention due to their influence on social and sexual networks, access to and provision of care, willingness to seek care, and social norms regarding sex and sexuality. Among certain vulnerable populations, historical experience with segregation and discrimination exacerbates the influence of these factors. Social, economic, and behavioral factors that affect the spread of STDs include the following:
  - **Racial and ethnic disparities**. Certain racial and ethnic groups (mainly African American, Hispanic, and American Indian/Alaska Native populations) have high rates of STDs than Whites. Race and ethnicity in the United States are correlated with other determinants of health status, such as poverty, limited access to health care, fewer attempts to get medical treatment, and living in communities with high rates of STDs.
  - **Poverty and marginalization**. STDs disproportionately affect disadvantaged people and people in social networks where high-risk sexual behavior is common, and either access to care or health-seeking behavior is compromised.
  - **Access to health care**. Access to high-quality health care is essential for early detection, treatment, and behavior change counseling for STDs. Groups with the highest rates of STDs are often the same groups

for whom access to or use of health services is most limited.

- **Substance abuse.** Many studies document the association of substance abuse with STDs. The introduction of new illicit substances into communities often can alter sexual behavior drastically in high-risk sexual networks, leading to the epidemic spread of STDs.
- **Sexuality and secrecy.** Perhaps the most important social factors contributing to the spread of STDs in the United States are the stigma associated with STDs and the general discomfort of discussing intimate aspects of life, especially those related to sex. These social factors separate the United States from industrialized countries with low rates of STDs.
- **Sexual networks.** Sexual networks refer to groups of people who can be considered "linked" by sequential or concurrent sexual partners. A person may have only one sex partner, but if that partner is a member of a risky sexual network, then the person is at higher risk for STDs than a similar individual from a lower-risk network.[2]

---

[2] Office of Disease Prevention and Health Promotion (ODPHP), "Sexually Transmitted Diseases," U.S. Department of Health and Human Services (HHS), February 6, 2022. Available online. URL: www.healthypeople.gov/2020/topics-objectives/topic/sexually-transmitted-diseases. Accessed June 14, 2023.

Chapter 3 | Incidence Trends of Sexually Transmitted Diseases

Chapter Contents

Section 3.1 | Incidence, Prevalence, and Cost of Sexually Transmitted Infections in the United States

As noted in the 2021 National Academies of Sciences Engineering and Medicine (NASEM) report, Sexually Transmitted Infections (STIs): Adopting a Sexual Health Paradigm (www.nationalacademies.org/our-work/prevention-and-control-of-sexually-transmitted-infections-in-the-united-states), surveillance is key to understanding the magnitude of STIs in the United States and in subpopulations that are most affected.

Because STDs often do not show symptoms and screening is necessary for timely diagnosis and treatment, changes in access to sexual health care can affect the number of infections diagnosed and reported. Disruptions in STD-related prevention and care activities related to the U.S. response to the coronavirus disease 2019 (COVID-19) pandemic had a pronounced impact on trends in STD surveillance data collected during 2020. It is likely that some of the disruptions persisted in 2021; therefore, trends presented in STD Surveillance, 2021, should be interpreted cautiously.

CHLAMYDIA

In 2021, a total of 1,644,416 cases of *Chlamydia trachomatis* infection were reported to the Centers for Disease Control and Prevention (CDC), making it the most common notifiable STI in the United States for that year. This case count corresponds to a rate of 495.5 cases per 100,000 population, an increase of 3.9 percent compared with the rate in 2020. During 2020–2021, rates of reported chlamydia increased among both males and females, in all regions of the United States, among most age groups, and among all race/Hispanic ethnicity groups. Rates of reported chlamydia are highest among adolescents and young adults. In 2021, almost two-thirds (58%) of all reported chlamydia cases were among persons aged 15–24 (see Figures 3.1 and 3.2).

31

Weekly Percentage of Cases Reported
Compared to 2019

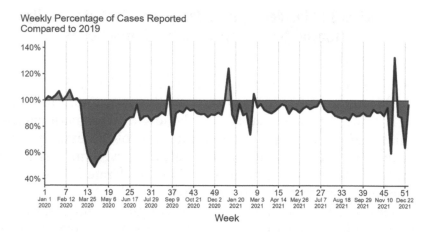

Figure 3.1. Chlamydia: Reported 2020 and 2021 Cases as a Percentage of 2019 by *MMWR* Week, United States

Note: The Morbidity and Mortality Weekly Report (MMWR) Week is the week of the epidemiologic year for which the case is assigned by the reporting local or state health department. For the weeks displayed, the midpoint of the date range (i.e., Wednesday of the week) is provided for reference. Adapted from Pagaoa et al., Sexually Transmitted Diseases, 2021. Centers for Disease Control and Prevention (CDC)

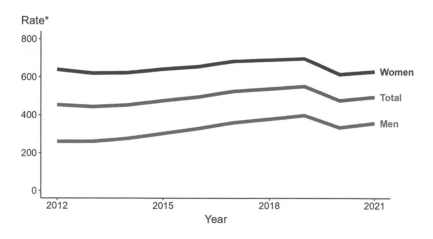

Figure 3.2. Chlamydia: Rates of Reported Cases by Sex, United States, 2012–2021

** Per 100,000
Centers for Disease Control and Prevention (CDC)*

The increases in rates of reported chlamydia during 2020–2021 follow a substantial decrease in rates during 2019–2020. The decrease in rates of reported chlamydia in 2020 was unlikely due to a reduction in new infections. As chlamydial infections are usually asymptomatic, case rates are heavily influenced by screening coverage. During the COVID-19 pandemic, many health-care clinics limited in-person visits to patients with symptoms or closed entirely, and it is likely that preventive health-care visits where STD screening usually happens, such as annual reproductive health visits for young women, decreased. During the initial shelter-in-place orders in March and April of 2020, the number of chlamydia cases decreased substantially when compared to the number of cases reported at the corresponding time in 2019 and the deficit persisted throughout the year. Although the rate of reported chlamydia increased during 2020–2021, the rate is still lower than the rate in 2019 suggesting that COVID-19-related challenges that are related to chlamydia screening may have persisted during 2021.

GONORRHEA

In 2021, a total of 710,151 cases of gonorrhea were reported to the CDC, making it the second most common notifiable sexually transmitted infection in the United States for that year. Rates of reported gonorrhea have increased 118 percent since their historic low in 2009. During 2020–2021, the overall rate of reported gonorrhea increased by 4.6 percent. During 2020–2021, rates increased among both males and females, in three regions of the United States (West, Northeast, and South), among most age groups, and among most racial/Hispanic ethnicity groups (see Figures 3.3 and 3.4).

During the initial shelter-in-place orders in March and April of 2020, the weekly number of cases of reported gonorrhea was lower compared to counts during the comparable time in 2019; however, later in 2020, the number of reported gonorrhea cases increased. The reasons for the increase are unclear but may have resulted from increased service utilization as health-care clinics reopened or increased transmission later in the year. During 2019–2020, the rate of reported gonorrhea increased in 35 states and

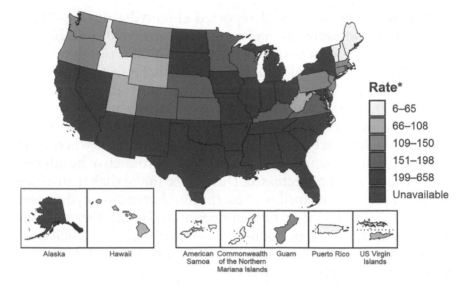

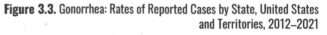

Figure 3.3. Gonorrhea: Rates of Reported Cases by State, United States and Territories, 2012–2021

* Per 100,000
Centers for Disease Control and Prevention (CDC)

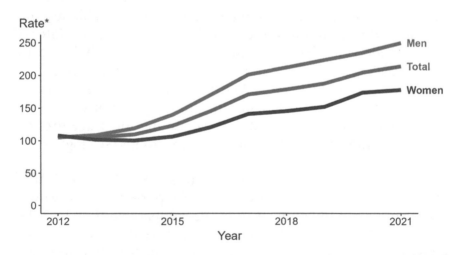

Figure 3.4. Gonorrhea: Rates of Reported Cases by Sex, United States, 2012–2021

* Per 100,000
Centers for Disease Control and Prevention (CDC)

two U.S. territories. This trend continued during 2020–2021, with increases in rates of reported gonorrhea in 27 states, the District of Columbia, and three U.S. territories.

During 2020–2021, rates of reported gonorrhea increased among both men (6.3%) and women (2.4%). Since 2013, rates of reported gonorrhea have been higher among men compared to women, likely reflecting cases identified in both gay, bisexual, and other men who have sex with men (MSM) and men who have sex with women only. Although there are limited data available on sexual behaviors of persons reported with gonorrhea at the national level, enhanced data from jurisdictions participating in a sentinel surveillance system, the STD Surveillance Network (SSuN), suggest that about a third of gonorrhea cases occurred among MSM in 2021.

SYPHILIS

In 2021, 176,713 cases of syphilis (all stages and congenital syphilis) were reported, including 53,767 cases of primary and secondary (P&S) syphilis, the most infectious stages of the disease. Since reaching a historic low in 2000 and 2001, the rate of P&S syphilis has increased almost every year, increasing 28.6 percent during 2020–2021. Rates increased among both males and females, in all regions of the United States, and in all age groups. Rates of P&S syphilis increased in all racial/Hispanic ethnicity groups, with the greatest increases among non-Hispanic American Indian or Alaska Native persons who also had the highest P&S syphilis rate in 2021 (see Figures 3.5 and 3.6).

MSM are disproportionately impacted by syphilis, accounting for almost half (46.5%) of all male P&S syphilis cases in 2021, and in areas with complete information on the sex of sex partners for male cases, rates of P&S syphilis among MSM increased in 27 states and the District of Columbia during 2020–2021. While rates of P&S syphilis are lower among women, they have substantially increased in recent years—rising by 55.3 percent during 2020–2021 and 217.4 percent during 2017–2021, highlighting the sustained increase in the heterosexual syphilis epidemic in the United States.

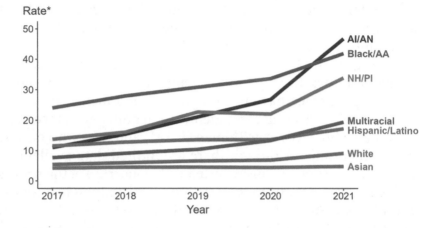

Figure 3.5. Primary and Secondary Syphilis: Rates of Reported Cases by Race/Hispanic Ethnicity, United States, 2017–2021

* Per 100,000
Abbreviations: AI/AN = American Indian or Alaska Native; Black/AA = Black or African American; NH/PI = Native Hawaiian or other Pacific Islander
Centers for Disease Control and Prevention (CDC)

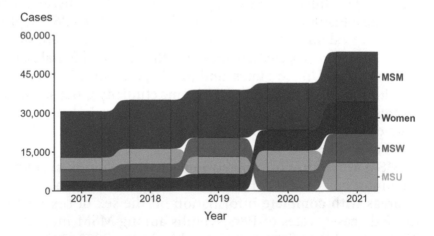

Figure 3.6. Primary and Secondary Syphilis: Reported Cases by Sex and Sex of Sex Partners, United States, 2017–2021

Abbreviations: MSM = gay, bisexual, and other men who have sex with men, MSU = men with unknown sex of sex partners, and MSW = men who have sex with women only
Note: Over the five-year period, 0.2 percent of cases were missing sex and were not included.
Centers for Disease Control and Prevention (CDC)

CONGENITAL SYPHILIS

The 2013 rate of congenital syphilis (9.2 cases per 100,000 live births) marked the first increase in congenital syphilis since 2008. Since 2013, the rate of congenital syphilis has increased each year. In 2021, 2,855 cases of congenital syphilis were reported, including 220 congenital syphilis-related stillbirths and infant deaths. Although the majority of congenital syphilis cases were reported from a few states, in 2021, almost all jurisdictions (46 states and the District of Columbia) reported at least one case of congenital syphilis; 37 states and the District of Columbia had increases in congenital syphilis during 2020–2021 (see Figures 3.7 and 3.8).

The national congenital syphilis rate of 77.9 cases per 100,000 live births in 2021 represents a 30.5 percent increase relative to 2020 and 219.3 percent increase relative to 2017. These increases mirror increases in syphilis among reproductive-aged women. During 2020–2021, the rate of P&S syphilis increased 52.3 percent among women aged 15–44, and rates increased in 45 states. Furthermore,

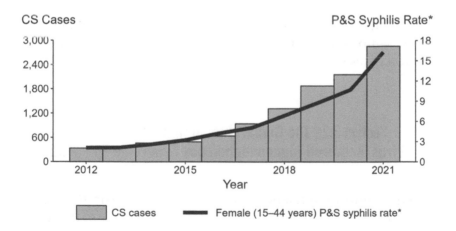

Figure 3.7. Congenital Syphilis: Reported Cases by Year of Birth and Rates of Reported Cases of Primary and Secondary Syphilis among Women Aged 15–44, United States, 2012–2021

Per 100,000
Abbreviations: CS = congenital syphilis and P&S syphilis = primary and secondary syphilis
Centers for Disease Control and Prevention (CDC)

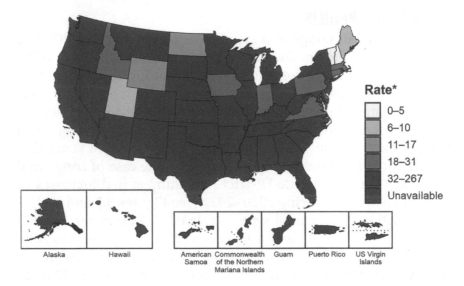

Figure 3.8. Primary and Secondary Syphilis: Rates of Reported Cases among Women Aged 15–44 by State, United States and Territories, 2012–2021

* Per 100,000
Centers for Disease Control and Prevention (CDC)

in 2012, there were only three states that had over 100 cases of P&S syphilis among women aged 15–44; in 2021, 29 states reported over 100 cases.[1]

Section 3.2 | The Global Human Immunodeficiency Virus/Acquired Immunodeficiency Syndrome Epidemic

Human immunodeficiency virus (HIV), the virus that causes acquired immunodeficiency syndrome (AIDS), is one of the world's most serious public health challenges. But there is a global commitment to stopping new HIV infections and ensuring that everyone with HIV has access to HIV treatment.

[1] "National Overview of STDs, 2021," Centers for Disease Control and Prevention (CDC), May 16, 2023. Available online. URL: www.cdc.gov/std/statistics/2021/overview.htm. Accessed May 29, 2023.

The latest statistics on HIV around the world from the Joint United Nations Programme on HIV/AIDS (UNAIDS) include the following:

- **Number of people with HIV**. There were approximately 38.4 million people across the globe with HIV in 2020. Of these, 36.7 million were adults, and 1.7 million were children (younger than 15 years old). In addition, 54 percent were women and girls.
- **New HIV infections**. An estimated 1.5 million individuals worldwide acquired HIV in 2021, marking a 32 percent decline in new HIV infections since 2010. New HIV infections, or "HIV incidence," refers to the estimated number of people who newly acquired HIV during a given period such as a year, which is different from the number of people diagnosed with HIV during a year. (Some people may have HIV but not know it.) Of these 1.5 million new HIV infections:
  - 1.3 million were among adults
  - 160,000 were among children (younger than 15 years old)
- **HIV testing**. Approximately 85 percent of people with HIV globally knew their HIV status in 2021. The remaining 15 percent (about 5.9 million people) did not know they had HIV and still needed access to HIV testing services. HIV testing is an essential gateway to HIV prevention, treatment, care, and support services.
- **HIV treatment access**. As of the end of 2021, 28.7 million people with HIV (75%) were accessing antiretroviral therapy (ART) globally. That means 9.7 million people are still waiting. HIV treatment access is key to the global effort to end AIDS as a public health threat. People with HIV who are aware of their status, take ART as prescribed, and get and keep an undetectable viral load can live long and healthy lives and will not transmit HIV to their HIV-negative partners through sex.
- **HIV care continuum**. The term HIV care continuum refers to the sequence of steps a person with HIV takes from diagnosis through receiving treatment until his or her

viral load is suppressed to undetectable levels. Each step in the continuum is marked by an assessment of the number of people who have reached that stage. The stages are being diagnosed with HIV, being linked to medical care, starting ART, adhering to the treatment regimen, and, finally, having HIV suppressed to undetectable levels in the blood. The UNAIDS reports that in 2021, of all people with HIV worldwide:

- 85 percent knew their HIV status
- 75 percent were accessing ART
- 68 percent were virally suppressed
- **Perinatal transmission**. In 2021, 81 percent of pregnant women with HIV had access to ART to prevent transmitting HIV to their babies during pregnancy and childbirth and to protect their own health.
- **AIDS-related deaths**. AIDS-related deaths have been reduced by 68 percent since the peak in 2004. In 2021, around 650,000 people died from AIDS-related illnesses worldwide, compared to 2 million people in 2004 and 1.4 million in 2010.
- **Regional impact**. The vast majority of people with HIV are in low- and middle-income countries. In 2021, there were 20.6 million people with HIV (53%) in Eastern and Southern Africa, 5 million (13%) in Western and Central Africa, 6 million (15%) in Asia and the Pacific, and 2.3 million (5%) in Western and Central Europe and North America.

CHALLENGES AND PROGRESS

Despite advances in our scientific understanding of HIV and its prevention and treatment as well as years of significant effort by the global health community and leading government and civil society organizations, too many people with HIV or at risk for HIV still do not have access to prevention, care, and treatment, and there is still no cure. Furthermore, the HIV epidemic not only affects the health of individuals but also impacts households, communities, and the development and economic growth of nations. Many of the countries hardest hit by HIV also suffer from other infectious diseases, food insecurity, and other serious problems.

Despite these challenges, there have been successes and promising signs. New global efforts have been mounted to address the epidemic, particularly in the last decade. The number of people who have newly acquired HIV has declined over the years. In addition, the number of people with HIV receiving treatment in resource-poor countries has dramatically increased in the past decade, and dramatic progress has been made in preventing perinatal transmission of HIV and keeping pregnant women alive.

However, despite the availability of a widening array of effective HIV prevention tools and methods and a massive scale-up of HIV treatment in recent years, the UNAIDS cautions there has been unequal progress in reducing new HIV infections, increasing access to treatment, and ending AIDS-related deaths, with too many vulnerable people and populations left behind. Stigma and discrimination, together with other social inequalities and exclusion, are proving to be key barriers, and our response to HIV/AIDS across the globe may be in danger.

U.S. RESPONSE TO THE GLOBAL EPIDEMIC

The U.S. President's Emergency Plan for AIDS Relief (PEPFAR) is the U.S. government's response to the global HIV/AIDS epidemic and represents the largest commitment by any nation to address a single disease in history. Through the PEPFAR, the United States has supported a world safer and more secure from infectious disease threats. It has demonstrably strengthened the global capacity to prevent, detect, and respond to new and existing risks—which ultimately enhances global health security and protects America's borders. Among other global results, the PEPFAR provided HIV testing services for more than 50 million people in fiscal year 2021 and, as of September 30, 2021, supported lifesaving ART for nearly 18.96 million men, women, and children. The PEPFAR also enabled 2.8 million babies to be born HIV-free to parents living with HIV.

In addition, the National Institutes of Health (NIH) represents the largest public investment in HIV/AIDS research in the world. The NIH is engaged in research around the globe to understand, diagnose, treat, and prevent HIV infection and its many associated conditions and to find a cure.[2]

Section 3.3 | U.S. Response to the Global Human Immunodeficiency Virus/Acquired Immunodeficiency Syndrome Epidemic

HOW ARE U.S. GOVERNMENT AGENCIES WORKING TO END HUMAN IMMUNODEFICIENCY VIRUS AND ACQUIRED IMMUNODEFICIENCY SYNDROME AROUND THE WORLD?

Agencies across the federal government are involved in implementing the President's Emergency Plan for AIDS Relief (PEPFAR), the largest commitment by any nation to address a single disease in history. These agencies support a range of global human immunodeficiency virus (HIV)/acquired immune deficiency syndrome (AIDS) activities from research to technical assistance and financial support to other countries to help prevent new HIV infections and assist people with HIV to access lifesaving treatment. These activities are coordinated through the PEPFAR.

U.S. Department of State

The Office of the U.S. Global AIDS Coordinator and Health Diplomacy (OGAC) of the U.S. Department of State (DOS) oversees implementation of the U.S. government's international HIV/AIDS efforts and ensures program and policy coordination among the relevant government agencies and departments. This includes managing the PEPFAR program. The PEPFAR partners closely with U.S. ambassadors globally, who oversee all aspects of the PEPFAR at their respective posts. The PEPFAR also works closely with the diplomatic corps in Washington, D.C., to advance U.S. global health diplomacy and connect health to other U.S. foreign

---

[2] HIV.gov, "Global HIV/AIDS Overview," U.S. Department of Health and Human Services (HHS), August 3, 2022. Available online. URL: www.hiv.gov/federal-response/pepfar-global-aids/global-hiv-aids-overview. Accessed May 29, 2023.

policy priorities, including economic growth, trade, education, and political stability.

U.S. Agency for International Development
The U.S. Agency for International Development (USAID) is an independent federal government agency that receives overall foreign policy guidance from the Secretary of State. As a key implementer of the PEPFAR, the USAID's Office of HIV/AIDS supports country-led efforts to combat the complex challenges of HIV in over 50 countries around the world. The agency's goal is to support and sustain the achievement of HIV epidemic control across these countries. It achieves this by providing global leadership in the development of programs that maximize impact and by supporting country-led strategies while applying the USAID's broad health and development expertise and specialized HIV technical competencies. In addition, the USAID leverages science, technology, and innovation to support cost-effective, sustainable, and appropriately integrated HIV interventions at scale.

U.S. Department of Health and Human Services
The U.S. Department of Health and Human Services (HHS) has a long history of HIV/AIDS work within the United States and internationally. Under the PEPFAR, the HHS supports the implementation of HIV prevention, treatment, and care programs in developing countries and conducts HIV research through the following agencies and offices.

CENTERS FOR DISEASE CONTROL AND PREVENTION
As a key implementing partner of the PEPFAR, the Centers for Disease Control and Prevention (CDC) works side by side with ministries of health, civil and faith-based organizations, private sector organizations, and other on-the-ground partners to improve methods for finding, treating, and preventing HIV. The CDC does so by supporting more than 10,000 labs or testing sites worldwide, getting lifesaving treatment to people with HIV around the world, and designing and enhancing surveillance systems and enabling

43

countries to understand which geographic areas require urgent HIV attention and services. Furthermore, the CDC's Division of Global HIV & TB (DGHT), through the PEPFAR, works to tackle HIV and tuberculosis (TB), the world's two most deadly diseases. These two epidemics are tragically interconnected, as TB is the leading cause of death for those with HIV. The CDC's experts are working on the front lines in more than 45 countries and regions around the globe, focused on a single mission: to fight these diseases and, ultimately, bring an end to the dual epidemics of HIV and TB.

FOOD AND DRUG ADMINISTRATION

The Food and Drug Administration (FDA) plays an integral role in the PEPFAR by ensuring safe and effective antiretroviral (ARV) drugs are available for procurement through the PEPFAR so that these drugs can get to countries with high rates of HIV infection in a timely manner. Since 2004, the FDA has encouraged sponsors worldwide to submit U.S. marketing applications for single-entity, fixed-combination, and co-packaged versions of previously approved ARV drugs. To speed up approval, the FDA uses its existing processes including expedited review for PEPFAR ARV drugs, while ensuring that these products meet the same standards as similar products for the U.S. market and its own citizens.

HEALTH RESOURCES AND SERVICES ADMINISTRATION

The Health Resources and Services Administration (HRSA) has been a significant contributor to the PEPFAR's achievements. The HRSA's Office of Special Health Initiatives in the Office of Global Health implements the agency's PEPFAR activities. The HRSA's work builds on the agency's domestic and international experience and expertise by improving outcomes along the treatment and prevention cascade for people living with HIV. The HRSA works with host countries and other key partners to assess the needs of each country and design a customized program of assistance that fits within the host country's strategic plan for HIV/AIDS and/or the health sector. This work is guided and reinforced by the HRSA's experience in building and strengthening the U.S. health system and leading the nation's response to the HIV epidemic by ensuring that each person living with HIV receives comprehensive care and treatment. Building on this experience, a major component of the HRSA's global efforts is related to ensuring the quality of services, building and strengthening local organizations, and ensuring the production and readiness of a strong health-care workforce across many cadres of facility and community service providers.

NATIONAL INSTITUTES OF HEALTH
The National Institutes of Health (NIH) provides the largest public investment in HIV/AIDS research globally. Coordinated by the Office of AIDS Research (OAR), the NIH's HIV research program encompasses basic, clinical, behavioral, and social sciences; translational and implementation science research on HIV infection, prevention, treatment, and cure; and research on HIV-associated coinfections, comorbidities, and complications. This research will lead to a better understanding of the basic biology of HIV/AIDS and the development of next-generation therapies to treat it. It will also foster the design of better countermeasures to prevent new infections, including vaccines and prophylaxis with ARV drugs and microbicides.

OFFICE OF GLOBAL AFFAIRS
The HHS's Office of Global Affairs (OGA), within the Office of the HHS Secretary, is the diplomatic voice of the HHS, fostering critical global relationships, coordinating international engagement across the HHS and the U.S. government, and providing leadership and expertise in global health diplomacy and policy to contribute to a safer, healthier world. The OGA works with the HHS and other agencies implementing the PEPFAR to ensure the federal government is leveraging the HHS's scientific and technical expertise to accelerate HIV epidemic control and achieve an AIDS-free generation.

SUBSTANCE ABUSE AND MENTAL HEALTH SERVICES ADMINISTRATION
The Substance Abuse and Mental Health Services Administration (SAMHSA) works through state and tribal governments and

faith- and community-based programs to support substance abuse and dependence and mental illness prevention, treatment, and recovery, including by supporting an educational and training center network that disseminates state-of-the-art information and best practices. This technical expertise and program experience is being applied to the PEPFAR to assist other countries in addressing serious substance use—including opioid-related—disorders and mental disorders that make the treatment and prevention of HIV more complicated.

U.S. Department of Commerce
The U.S. Department of Commerce (DOC) fosters public–private partnerships and makes presentations in industry/trade advisory committee meetings on how the private sector can contribute to global HIV/AIDS interventions. In addition, the U.S. Census Bureau, housed within the DOC, provides support for the PEPFAR by assisting with data management and analysis, survey support, and mapping of country-level activities. With funds from the PEPFAR, the U.S. Census Bureau maintains and annually updates the HIV/AIDS Surveillance Data Base to meet the needs of policy-makers and program planners around the world. This database is a compilation of information from widely scattered small-scale surveys on the HIV/AIDS pandemic in population groups in developing countries and hosts information from the medical and scientific literature, presentations at international conferences, and the press.

U.S. Department of Defense
The HIV/AIDS Prevention Program of the Department of Defense (DoD; DHAPP) is responsible for assisting foreign military partners with the development and implementation of culturally focused, military-specific HIV/AIDS prevention, care, and treatment programs in more than 55 countries around the globe. The DHAPP employs an integrated bilateral and regional strategy for HIV/AIDS cooperation and security assistance. The DHAPP is also the DoD implementing agency for the PEPFAR. As such, the DHAPP plans activities and sets targets based on the specific context of the

partner military and the clients seen at military health facilities and uses information from military HIV seroprevalence studies, programmatic data, and other sources to implement programs at military locations with a significant burden of HIV.

U.S. Department of Labor

The Department of Labor (DoL) implements PEPFAR work-place-targeted projects that focus on the prevention and reduction of HIV/AIDS-related stigma and discrimination. The DoL brings to these endeavors its unique experience in building strategic alliances with employers, unions, and Ministries of Labor, which are often overlooked and can be difficult to target.

Department of the Treasury

The Department of the Treasury (USDT) is working to promote financial effectiveness and fiscal sustainability of the HIV/AIDS response in partner countries, primarily in Africa. The goal of the USDT's work is to increase awareness and understanding of the economic and financial dimensions of HIV/AIDS, especially among finance ministries; include the disease response as part of national economic strategies; strengthen financial resource mobilization and efficient utilization; and build capacity to implement policy improvements. Its work entails both policy engagement and technical assistance to support the implementation of improved policies, generally in partnership with finance ministries. Illustrative examples include supporting HIV expenditure oversight committees, strengthening budget systems and execution in health and finance ministries, and developing capacity for health cost analysis.

Peace Corps

The Peace Corps contributes to the global response to HIV by partnering with people and communities to adopt healthy behaviors and mitigate the impact of the disease. The Peace Corps Volunteers around the world provide capacity development support to non-governmental, community-based, and faith-based organizations, with an emphasis on ensuring that community-initiated projects and programs provide holistic support to people with and affected by HIV/AIDS.[3]

[3] HIV.gov, "U.S. Government Global HIV/AIDS Activities," U.S. Department of Health and Human Services (HHS), November 30, 2021. Available online. URL: www.hiv.gov/federal-response/pepfar-global-aids/us-government-global-aids-activities. Accessed May 29, 2023.

Chapter 4 | Sexually Transmitted Diseases in General Population

Chapter Contents

Section 4.1 | Sexually Transmitted Diseases in Children

Identification of STIs in children past the neonatal period strongly indicates sexual abuse. The importance of identifying a sexually transmitted organism for such children as evidence of possible child sexual abuse varies by the pathogen. Postnatally acquired gonorrhea, syphilis, chlamydia, and *Trichomonas vaginalis* infection and nontransfusion, nonperinatally acquired human immunodeficiency virus (HIV) infection are indicative of sexual abuse. Sexual abuse should be suspected when anogenital herpes or anogenital warts are diagnosed. Investigation of sexual abuse among children who have an infection that might have been transmitted sexually should be conducted in compliance with recommendations by clinicians who have experience and training in all elements of the evaluation of child abuse, neglect, and assault. The social significance of an infection that might have been acquired sexually varies by the specific organism, as does the threshold for reporting suspected child sexual abuse. When any STI has been diagnosed in a child, efforts should be made in consultation with a specialist to evaluate the possibility of sexual abuse, including conducting a history and physical examination for evidence of abuse and diagnostic testing for other commonly occurring STIs.

The general rule that STIs beyond the neonatal period are evidence of sexual abuse has exceptions. For example, genital infection with *T. vaginalis* or rectal or genital infection with *Chlamydia trachomatis* among young children might be the result of perinatally acquired infection and has, in certain cases of chlamydial infection, persisted for as long as two to three years although perinatal chlamydial infection is now uncommon because of prenatal screening and treatment of pregnant women. Genital warts have been diagnosed among children who have been sexually abused but also among children who have no other evidence of sexual abuse; lesions appearing for the first time in a child older than five years of age are more likely to have been caused by sexual transmission. Bacterial vaginosis (BV) has been diagnosed among children who have been abused, but its presence alone does not prove sexual abuse. The majority of hepatitis B virus (HBV) infections among children result from household exposure to persons who have chronic HBV infection rather than sexual abuse.

REPORTING

All U.S. states and territories have laws that require reporting of child abuse. Although the exact requirements differ by state or territory, if a health-care provider has reasonable cause to suspect child abuse, a report must be made. Health-care providers should contact their state or local child protection service agency regarding child abuse reporting requirements.

EVALUATING CHILDREN FOR SEXUALLY TRANSMITTED INFECTIONS

Evaluating children for sexual assault or abuse should be conducted in a manner designed to minimize pain and trauma to the child. Examinations and collection of vaginal specimens in prepubertal girls can be extremely uncomfortable and should be performed by an experienced clinician to avoid psychological and physical trauma to the child. The decision to obtain genital or other specimens from a child to evaluate for STIs should be made on an individual basis. However, children who received a diagnosis of one STI should be screened for other STIs. History and reported type of sexual contact might not be a reliable indicator, and urogenital, pharyngeal, and rectal testing should be considered for preverbal children and children who cannot verbalize details of the assault. Factors that should lead the physician to consider testing for STIs include the following:

- The child has experienced penetration or has evidence of recent or healed penetrative injury to the genitals, anus, or oropharynx.
- The child has been abused by a stranger.
- The child has been abused by an assailant known to be infected with an STI or at high risk for STIs (e.g., injecting drug user, men who have sex with men (MSM), person with multiple sex partners, or person with a history of STIs).
- The child has a sibling, other relative, or another person in the household with an STI.

- The child lives in an area with a high rate of STIs in the community.
- The child has signs or symptoms of STIs (e.g., vaginal discharge or pain, genital itching or odor, urinary symptoms, or genital lesions or ulcers).
- The child or parent requests STI testing.
- The child is unable to verbalize details of the assault.

If a child has symptoms, signs, or evidence of an infection that might be sexually transmitted, the child should be tested for common STIs before initiation of any treatment that might interfere with diagnosing other STIs. Because of the legal and psychosocial consequences of a false-positive diagnosis, only tests with high specificities should be used. The potential benefit to the child of a reliable STI diagnosis justifies deferring presumptive treatment until specimens for highly specific tests are obtained by providers with experience in evaluating sexually abused and assaulted children.

Evaluations should be performed on a case-by-case basis, according to the history of assault or abuse and in a manner that minimizes the possibility for psychological trauma and social stigma. If the initial exposure was recent, the infectious organisms acquired through the exposure might not have produced sufficient concentrations to result in positive test results or examination findings. Alternatively, positive test results after a recent exposure might represent the assailant's secretions (but would nonetheless be an indication for treatment of the child). A second visit approximately two to six weeks after the most recent sexual exposure should be scheduled to include a repeat physical examination and collection of additional specimens to identify any infection that might not have been detected at the time of initial evaluation. A single evaluation might be sufficient if the child was abused for an extended period and if a substantial amount of time elapsed between the last suspected episode of abuse and the medical evaluation. Compliance with follow-up appointments might be improved when law enforcement personnel or child protective services are involved.

INITIAL EXAMINATION

Visual inspection of the genital, perianal, and oral areas for genital discharge, odor, bleeding, irritation, warts, and ulcerative lesions should be performed during the initial examination. The clinical manifestations of certain STIs are different for children than for adults. For example, typical vesicular lesions might be absent even in the presence of herpes simplex virus (HSV) infection. The following should be performed during the initial examination if STI testing is indicated:

- Testing for *Neisseria gonorrhoeae* and *C. trachomatis* can be performed from specimens collected from the pharynx and rectum, as well as the vagina for girls and urine for boys. Cervical specimens are not recommended for prepubertal girls. For boys with a urethral discharge, a meatal specimen discharge is an adequate substitute for an intraurethral swab specimen. Culture or nucleic acid amplification test (NAAT) can be used to test for *N. gonorrhoeae* and *C. trachomatis*. Only NAAT assays cleared by the U.S. Food and Drug Administration (FDA) should be used. Specimens (either NAAT or culture, including any isolates) obtained before treatment should be preserved for further validation if needed. When a specimen is positive, the result should be confirmed either by retesting the original specimen or obtaining another. Because of the overall low prevalence of *N. gonorrhoeae* and *C. trachomatis* among children, false-positive results can occur, and all specimens that are initially positive should be confirmed.

- Testing for *T. vaginalis* should not be limited to girls with vaginal discharge if other indications for vaginal testing exist because evidence indicates that asymptomatic sexually abused children might be infected with *T. vaginalis* and might benefit from treatment. NAAT can be used as an alternative or in addition to culture and wet mount, especially in settings where culture and wet mount of vaginal swab specimens are not obtainable. Consultation with an expert is necessary before using NAAT in this context to ensure correct interpretation of results. In the case of a positive specimen, the result should be confirmed either by retesting the original specimen or obtaining another. Because of the overall low prevalence of *T. vaginalis* among children, false-positive results can occur, and all specimens that are initially positive should be confirmed.

- HSV can be indicative of sexual abuse; therefore, specimens should be obtained from all vesicular or ulcerative genital or perianal lesions and sent for NAAT or viral culture.
- Wet mount can be used for a vaginal swab specimen for BV if discharge is present.
- Collection of serum samples should be evaluated, preserved for subsequent analysis, and used as a baseline for comparison with follow-up serologic tests. Sera can be tested for antibodies to *Treponema pallidum*, HIV, and HBV.

TREATMENT

The risk for a child acquiring an STI as a result of sexual abuse or assault has not been well studied. Presumptive treatment for children who have been sexually assaulted or abused is not recommended because the incidence of most STIs among children is low after abuse or assault, prepubertal girls appear to be at lower risk for ascending infection than adolescent or adult women, and regular follow-up of children usually can be ensured. However, certain children or their parent or guardian might be concerned about the possibility of infection with an STI, even if the health-care provider has perceived the risk to be low. Such concerns might be an indication for presumptive treatment in certain settings and might be considered after all relevant specimens for diagnostic tests have been collected.

OTHER MANAGEMENT CONSIDERATIONS

Children who are survivors of sexual assault or abuse are at increased risk for future unsafe sexual practices that have been linked to higher risk for human papillomavirus (HPV) acquisition and are more likely to engage in these behaviors at an earlier age; therefore, the Advisory Committee on Immunization Practices (ACIP) recommends vaccination of these children at nine years or older if they have not initiated or completed HPV vaccination (www.cdc.gov/vaccines/hcp/acip-recs/vacc-specific/hpv.html). Although the HPV vaccine will not protect against the progression of infection already acquired or promote clearance of the infection, the vaccine protects against HPV types not yet acquired.

FOLLOW-UP

If no infections were identified at the initial examination after the last suspected sexual exposure, and if this exposure was recent, a follow-up evaluation approximately two weeks after the last exposure can be considered. Likewise, if no physical examination or diagnostic testing was performed at the initial visit, a complete examination can be scheduled approximately two weeks after the last exposure to identify any evidence of STIs. In circumstances in which transmission of syphilis, HIV, HBV, or HPV is a concern but baseline tests for syphilis, HIV, and HBV are negative and examinations for genital warts are negative, follow-up serologic testing and examination approximately six weeks and less than three months after the last suspected sexual exposure is recommended to allow time for antibodies to develop and signs of infection to appear. In addition, results of hepatitis B surface antigen (HBsAg) testing should be interpreted carefully because HBV can be transmitted nonsexually.

RISK FOR ACQUIRING HUMAN IMMUNODEFICIENCY VIRUS INFECTION

Human immunodeficiency virus has been reported among children for whom sexual abuse was the only known risk factor. Serologic testing for HIV should be considered for sexually abused children. The decision to test for HIV should involve the family, if possible, and be made on a case-by-case basis depending on the likelihood of infection in the assailant. Although data are insufficient concerning the efficacy of postexposure prophylaxis (PEP) among children, treatment is well tolerated by infants and children with and without HIV, and children have a minimal risk for serious adverse reactions because of the short period recommended for prophylaxis.

RECOMMENDATIONS FOR POSTEXPOSURE HUMAN IMMUNODEFICIENCY VIRUS RISK ASSESSMENT OF CHILDREN LESS THAN 72 HOURS AFTER SEXUAL ASSAULT

Providers should do the following:
- Review local HIV epidemiology, assess risk for HIV in the assailant, and test for HIV.
- Evaluate the circumstances of the assault or abuse that might affect risk for HIV transmission.
- Perform HIV antigen or antibody testing (or antibody testing if antigen or antibody testing is unavailable) during the original assessment and again at follow-up visits, in accordance with Centers for Disease Control and Prevention (CDC) guidelines (https://stacks.cdc.gov/view/cdc/38856). In considering whether to offer PEP, health-care providers should consider whether the child can be treated soon after the sexual exposure (i.e., less than 72 hours), the likelihood that the assailant has HIV infection, and the likelihood of high compliance with the prophylactic regimen. The potential benefit of treating a sexually abused child should be weighed against the risk for adverse reactions.
- Consult with a provider specializing in evaluating or treating children with HIV infection to determine age-appropriate dosing and regimens and baseline laboratory testing, if PEP is being considered.
- Discuss PEP with the caregivers, including its toxicity, unknown efficacy, and possible benefits, for children determined to be at risk of HIV transmission from the assault or abuse.

- Provide adequate doses of medication, if PEP is begun, to last until the follow-up visit three to seven days after the initial assessment, at which time the child should be reevaluated and tolerance of medication assessed.[1]

Section 4.2 | Sexually Transmitted Diseases in Adolescents and Young Adults

In the United States, prevalence rates of certain sexually transmitted infections (STIs) are highest among adolescents and young adults. For example, reported rates of chlamydia and gonorrhea are highest among females during their adolescent and young adult years, and many persons acquire human papillomavirus (HPV) infection during that time.

Persons who initiate sex early in adolescence are at higher risk for STIs, as are adolescents living in detention facilities; those receiving services at sexually transmitted disease (STD) clinics; those who are involved in commercial sex exploitation or survival sex and are exchanging sex for drugs, money, food, or housing; young males who have sex with males (YMSM); transgender youths; and youths with disabilities, substance misuse, or mental health disorders. Factors contributing to increased vulnerability to STIs during adolescence include having multiple sex partners, having sequential sex partnerships of limited duration or concurrent partnerships, failing to use barrier protection consistently and correctly, having lower socioeconomic status, and facing multiple obstacles to accessing health care.

All 50 states and the District of Columbia explicitly allow minors to consent for their own STI services. No state requires parental consent for STI care although the age at which a minor can provide consent for specified health-care services (i.e., HPV vaccination and

---

[1] "Sexual Assault or Abuse of Children," Centers for Disease Control and Prevention (CDC), July 22, 2021. Available online. URL: www.cdc.gov/std/treatment-guidelines/sexual-assault-children.htm. Accessed May 29, 2023.

human immunodeficiency virus (HIV) testing and treatment) varies among states. In 2019, a total of 18 states allowed but did not require physicians to notify parents of a minor's receipt of STI services, including states where minors can legally provide their own consent to the service (www.cdc.gov/hiv/policies/law/states/minors.html).

Protecting confidentiality for STI care, particularly for adolescents enrolled in private health insurance plans, presents multiple problems. After a claim has been submitted, many states mandate that health plans provide a written statement to the beneficiary indicating the service performed, the charges covered, what the insurer allows, and the amount for which the patient is responsible (i.e., explanation of benefits (EOBs)). In addition, federal laws obligate notices to beneficiaries when claims are denied, including alerting beneficiaries who need to pay for care until the allowable deductible is reached. For STI testing and treatment-related care, an EOB or medical bill that is received by a parent might disclose services provided and list STI laboratory tests performed or treatment administered. Some states have instituted mechanisms for protecting adolescents' confidentiality and limiting EOBs. Additional risks to confidentiality breaches can inadvertently occur through electronic health records although technology continues to evolve to assist with ensuring confidential care. The American Academy of Pediatrics (AAP) and the Society for Adolescent Health and Medicine (SAHM) have published guidance on strategies to address emerging risks for confidentiality breaches associated with health information technology.

The AAP and the SAHM recommend that providers have time alone with their adolescent patients that includes assessment for sexual behavior. The AAP recommendations are available at https://services.aap.org/en/news-room/campaigns-and-toolkits/adolescent-health-care, and the SAHM recommendations are available at www.adolescenthealth.org/My-SAHM/Login-or-Create-an-Account.aspx?returnurl=%2fResources%2fClinical-Care-Resources%2fConfidentiality.aspx. Discussions concerning sexual behavior should be tailored to the patient's developmental level and be aimed at identifying risk behaviors (e.g., multiple partners; oral, anal, or vaginal sex; or drug misuse behaviors). Careful, nonjudgmental, and thorough counseling is particularly vital for adolescents who might not feel comfortable acknowledging their engagement in behaviors that make them more vulnerable to acquiring STIs.

SCREENING RECOMMENDATIONS

Recommendations for screening adolescents for STIs to detect asymptomatic infections are based on disease severity and sequelae, prevalence among the population, costs, medicolegal considerations (e.g., state laws), and other factors. Routine laboratory screening for common STIs is indicated for all sexually active adolescents. The following screening recommendations summarize published clinical prevention guidelines for sexually active adolescents from federal agencies and medical professional organizations.

Chlamydia

Routine screening for *Chlamydia trachomatis* infection on an annual basis is recommended for all sexually active females younger than 25 years of age. Rectal chlamydial testing can be considered for females on the basis of reported sexual behaviors and exposure through shared clinical decision-making between the patient and the provider. Evidence is insufficient to recommend routine screening for *C. trachomatis* among sexually active young males, on the basis of efficacy and cost-effectiveness. However, screening of sexually active young males should be considered in clinical settings serving populations of young men with a high prevalence of chlamydial infections (e.g., adolescent service clinics, correctional facilities, and STD clinics). Chlamydia screening, including pharyngeal or rectal testing, should be offered to all YMSM at least annually on the basis of sexual behavior and anatomic site of exposure.

Gonorrhea

Routine screening for *Neisseria gonorrhoeae* on an annual basis is recommended for all sexually active females younger than 25 years of age. Extragenital gonorrhea screening (pharyngeal or rectal) can be considered for females on the basis of reported sexual behaviors and exposure through shared clinical decisions between the patient and the provider. Gonococcal infection is more prevalent among certain geographic locations and communities. Clinicians should consider the communities they serve and consult local public health authorities for guidance regarding identifying groups that are more vulnerable to gonorrhea acquisition on the basis of local disease prevalence. Evidence is insufficient to recommend routine screening, on the basis of efficacy and cost-effectiveness, for *N. gonorrhoeae* among asymptomatic sexually active young males who have sex with females only. Screening for gonorrhea, including pharyngeal or rectal testing, should be offered to YMSM at least annually.

Providers might consider opt-out chlamydia and gonorrhea screening (i.e., the patient is notified that testing will be performed unless the patient declines, regardless of reported sexual activity) for adolescent and young adult females during clinical encounters. Cost-effectiveness analyses indicate that opt-out chlamydia screening among adolescent and young adult females might substantially increase screening, be cost-saving, and identify infections among patients who do not disclose sexual behavior.

Human Immunodeficiency Virus Infection
HIV screening should be discussed and offered to all adolescents. The frequency of repeat screenings should be based on the patient's sexual behaviors and the local disease prevalence. Persons with HIV infection should receive prevention counseling and linkage to care before leaving the testing site.

Cervical Cancer
Guidelines from the U.S. Preventive Services Task Force (USPSTF) and the American Congress of Obstetricians and Gynecologists (ACOG) recommend that cervical cancer screening begin at the age of 21. This recommendation is based on the low incidence of cervical cancer and the limited usefulness of screening for cervical cancer among adolescents. In contrast, the 2020 American Cancer Society (ACS) guidelines recommend that

cervical cancer screening begins at the age of 25 with HPV testing. This change is recommended because the incidence of invasive cervical cancer in women younger than 25 years of age is decreasing because of vaccination. Adolescents with HIV infection who have initiated sexual intercourse should have cervical screening cytology in accordance with HIV/acquired immunodeficiency syndrome (AIDS) guidelines (https://clinicalinfo.hiv. gov/en/guidelines/adult-and-adolescent-opportunistic-infection/ human-papillomavirus-disease?view=full).

Other Sexually Transmitted Infections

YMSM and pregnant females should be routinely screened for syphilis. Local disease prevalence can help guide decision-making regarding screening for *Trichomonas vaginalis*, especially among adolescent females in certain areas. Routine screening of adolescents and young adults who are asymptomatic for certain STIs (e.g., syphilis, trichomoniasis, bacterial vaginosis (BV), herpes simplex virus (HSV), hepatitis A virus (HAV), and hepatitis B virus (HBV)) is not typically recommended.

PRIMARY PREVENTION RECOMMENDATIONS

Primary prevention and anticipatory guidance for recognizing symptoms and behaviors associated with STIs are strategies that should be incorporated into all types of health-care visits for adolescents and young adults. The following recommendations for primary prevention of STIs (i.e., vaccination and counseling) are based on published clinical guidelines for sexually active adolescents and young adults from federal agencies and medical professional organizations:

- HPV vaccination is recommended through the age of 26 for those not vaccinated previously at the routine age of 11 or 12 (www.cdc.gov/vaccines/hcp/acip-recs/ vacc-specific/hpv.html).
- The HBV vaccination series is recommended for all adolescents and young adults who have not previously

received the universal HBV vaccine series during childhood.

- The HAV vaccination series should be offered to adolescents and young adults as well as those who have not previously received the universal HAV vaccine series during childhood (www.cdc.gov/vaccines/schedules/hcp/imz/child-indications.html#note-hepa).
- Information regarding HIV transmission, prevention, testing, and implications of infection should be regarded as an essential component of the anticipatory guidance provided to all adolescents and young adults as part of routine health care.
- The Centers for Disease Control and Prevention (CDC) and the USPSTF recommend offering HIV pre-exposure prophylaxis (PrEP) for adolescents weighing greater than or equal to 35 kg and adults who are HIV-negative and at substantial risk for HIV infection. YMSM should be offered PrEP in youth-friendly settings with tailored adherence support (e.g., text messaging and visits per existing guidelines). Indications for PrEP, initial and follow-up prescribing guidance, and laboratory testing recommendations are the same for adolescents and adults (www.cdc.gov/hiv/risk/prep).
- Medical providers who care for adolescents and young adults should integrate sexuality education into clinical practice. Health-care providers should counsel adolescents about the sexual behaviors that are associated with risk for acquiring STIs and should educate patients regarding evidence-based prevention strategies, which include a discussion about abstinence and other risk-reduction behaviors (e.g., consistent and correct condom use and reduction in the number of sex partners including concurrent partners). Interactive counseling approaches (e.g., patient-centered counseling and motivational interviewing) are effective STI and

HIV prevention strategies and are recommended by the USPSTF. Educational materials (e.g., handouts, pamphlets, and videos) can reinforce office-based educational efforts.[2]

Section 4.3 | Sexually Transmitted Diseases in Women

Sexually transmitted diseases (STDs) remain a major public health concern in the United States, especially among women, who disproportionately bear the long-term consequences of STDs. For example, each year untreated STDs cause infertility in at least 20,000 women in the United States, and a pregnant woman is highly likely to pass syphilis unto her unborn baby if left untested or untreated. Most STDs are preventable and curable. There is a vaccine to prevent human papillomavirus (HPV). Most STDs can be cured with antibiotics, averting serious health consequences and preventing transmission to others.[3]

WHO GETS SEXUALLY TRANSMITTED INFECTIONS?
Nearly 20 million people in the United States get an STI each year. These infections affect women and men of all backgrounds and economic levels. But half of all new infections are among young people aged 15–24.

HOW DO SEXUALLY TRANSMITTED INFECTIONS AFFECT WOMEN?
Women often have more serious health problems from STIs than men:
- Chlamydia and gonorrhea, left untreated, raise the risk of chronic pelvic pain and life-threatening ectopic

---

[2] "Adolescents," Centers for Disease Control and Prevention (CDC), July 22, 2021. Available online. URL: www.cdc.gov/std/treatment-guidelines/adolescents.htm. Accessed May 26, 2023.
[3] "How STDs Impact Women Differently from Men," Centers for Disease Control and Prevention (CDC), February 20, 2018. Available online. URL: www.cdc.gov/nchhstp/newsroom/docs/factsheets/stds-women.pdf. Accessed May 26, 2023.

pregnancy. Chlamydia and gonorrhea can also cause infertility.
- Untreated syphilis in pregnant women results in infant death up to 40 percent of the time.
- Women have higher risk than men of getting an STI during unprotected vaginal sex. Unprotected anal sex puts women at even more risk of getting an STI than unprotected vaginal sex.

HOW DO WOMEN GET SEXUALLY TRANSMITTED INFECTIONS?
Sexually transmitted infections are spread in the following ways:
- having unprotected (without a condom) vaginal, oral, or anal sex with someone who has an STI (It can be difficult to tell if someone has an STI. STIs can be spread even if there are no signs or symptoms.)
- during genital touching (It is possible to get some STIs, such as syphilis and herpes, without having sex.)
- through sexual contact between women who have sex only with other women (WSW)
- from a pregnant or breastfeeding woman to her baby

CAN SEXUALLY TRANSMITTED INFECTIONS CAUSE HEALTH PROBLEMS?
Yes. Each STI causes different health problems for women. Certain types of untreated STIs can cause or lead to:
- problems getting pregnant or permanent infertility
- problems during pregnancy and health problems for the unborn baby
- infection in other parts of the body
- organ damage
- certain types of cancer, such as cervical cancer
- death

Having certain types of STIs makes it easier for you to get human immunodeficiency virus (HIV; another STI) if you come into contact with it.

WHAT ARE THE SYMPTOMS OF SEXUALLY TRANSMITTED INFECTIONS?

Many STIs have only mild symptoms or no symptoms at all. When women have symptoms, they may be mistaken for something else, such as a urinary tract infection or yeast infection. Get tested so that you can be treated for the correct infection.

DO YOU NEED TO GET TESTED FOR SEXUALLY TRANSMITTED INFECTIONS?

If you are sexually active, talk to your doctor or nurse about STI testing. Which tests you will need and how often you need to get them will depend on your and your partner's sexual history.

You may feel embarrassed or that your sex life is too personal to share with your doctor or nurse. But being open and honest is the only way your doctor can help take care of you. Find out what screening tests you may need. Then talk to your doctor or nurse about what tests make sense for you.

HOW DO YOU GET TESTED FOR SEXUALLY TRANSMITTED INFECTIONS?

Ask your doctor or nurse about getting tested for STIs. Your doctor or nurse can tell you what test(s) you may need and how they are done. Testing for STIs is also called "STI screening."

STI testing can include the following:
- **Pelvic and physical exam**. Your doctor looks for signs of infection, such as warts, rashes, or discharge.
- **Blood test**. A nurse will draw some blood to test for an STI.
- **Urine test**. You urinate (pee) into a cup. The urine is then tested for an STI.
- **Fluid or tissue sample**. Your doctor or nurse uses a cotton swab to take fluid or discharge from an infected place on your body. The fluid is looked at under a microscope or sent to a lab for testing.

Find a clinic near you where you can get tested for STIs. Find a clinic near you where you can get vaccines for hepatitis B virus and HPV.

DOES A PAP TEST SCREEN FOR SEXUALLY TRANSMITTED INFECTIONS?

No. Papanicolaou (Pap) testing is mainly used to look for cell changes that could be cancer or precancer. However, your doctor may test you for HPV in addition to doing the Pap test if you are older than 30.

If you want to be tested for STIs, you must ask your doctor or nurse.

HOW CAN YOU GET FREE OR LOW-COST SEXUALLY TRANSMITTED INFECTION TESTING?

Under the Affordable Care Act (ACA), most health insurance plans must cover the cost of STI screening or counseling at no cost to you.

- If you have insurance, check with your insurance provider to find out what is included in your plan.
- If you do not have insurance, find free or reduced-cost testing and treatment for STIs.
- If you have Medicare, find out how and which STI tests are covered and how often.
- If you have Medicaid, the benefits covered are different in each state, but certain benefits must be covered by every Medicaid program. Check with your state's program to find out what is covered.

HOW ARE SEXUALLY TRANSMITTED INFECTIONS TREATED?

For some STIs, treatment may involve taking medicine by mouth or getting a shot. For other STIs that cannot be cured, such as herpes or HIV and acquired immunodeficiency syndrome (AIDS), medicines can help reduce the symptoms.

IF YOU HAVE A SEXUALLY TRANSMITTED INFECTION, DOES YOUR PARTNER HAVE IT TOO?

Maybe. If the tests show that you have an STI, your doctor might want your partner to come in for testing. Or the doctor may give you medicine to take home for your partner.

The STI may have spread to you or your partner from a former sex partner. This is why it is important to get tested after each new sex partner. Also, if you test positive for certain STIs (HIV, syphilis, or gonorrhea), some cities and states require you (or your doctor) to tell any past or current sex partners.

DO MEDICINES SOLD OVER THE INTERNET PREVENT OR TREAT SEXUALLY TRANSMITTED INFECTIONS?

No. Only use medicines prescribed or suggested by your doctor.

Some drugs sold over the Internet claim to prevent or treat STIs. And some of these sites claim their medicines work better than the medicines your doctor prescribes. But, in most cases, this is not true, and no one knows how safe these products are or even what is in them.

Buying prescription and over-the-counter (OTC) drugs on the Internet means you may not know exactly what you are getting. An illegal Internet pharmacy may try to sell you unapproved drugs, drugs with the wrong active ingredient, drugs with too much or too little of the active ingredient, or drugs with dangerous ingredients.

HOW CAN YOU PREVENT A SEXUALLY TRANSMITTED INFECTION?

The best way to prevent an STI is to not have vaginal, oral, or anal sex.

If you do have sex, lower your risk of getting an STI with the following steps:

- **Get vaccinated**. There are vaccines to protect against HPV and hepatitis B.
- **Use condoms**. Condoms are the best way to prevent STIs when you have sex. Because a man does not need to ejaculate (come) to give or get some STIs, make sure to put the condom on before the penis touches the vagina, mouth, or anus. Other methods of birth control, such as birth control pills, shots, implants, or diaphragms, will not protect you from STIs.
- **Get tested**. Be sure you and your partner are tested for STIs. Talk to each other about the test results before you have sex.

- **Be monogamous**. Having sex with just one partner can lower your risk for STIs. After being tested for STIs, be faithful to each other. That means that you have sex only with each other and no one else.
- **Limit your number of sex partners**. Your risk of getting STIs goes up with the number of partners you have.
- **Do not douche**. Douching removes some of the normal bacteria in the vagina that protect you from infection. This may increase your risk of getting STIs.
- **Do not abuse alcohol or drugs**. Drinking too much alcohol or using drugs increases risky behavior and may put you at risk for sexual assault and possible exposure to STIs.

The steps work best when used together. No single step can protect you from every single type of STI.[4]

SEXUALLY TRANSMITTED DISEASES AFFECT WOMEN DIFFERENTLY THAN MEN

- Women are less likely than men to have symptoms of common STDs such as chlamydia and gonorrhea.
  - If symptoms do occur, they can go away even though the infection may remain.
- Women are more likely than men to confuse symptoms of an STD for something else.
  - Women often have normal discharge or think that burning/itching is related to a yeast infection.
  - Men usually notice symptoms such as discharge because it is unusual.
- Women may not see symptoms as easily as men.
  - Genital ulcers (such as from herpes or syphilis) can occur in the vagina and may not be easily visible, while men may be more likely to notice sores on their penis.

---

[4] Office on Women's Health (OWH), "Sexually Transmitted Infections," U.S. Department of Health and Human Services (HHS), December 29, 2022. Available online. URL: www.womenshealth.gov/a-z-topics/sexually-transmitted-infections. Accessed May 26, 2023.

- Women typically see their doctor more often than men.
  - Women should use this time with their doctor as an opportunity to ask for STD testing and not assume STD testing is part of their annual exam. While the Pap test screens for cervical cancer, it is not a good test for other types of cancer or STDs.
- A woman's anatomy can place her at a unique risk for STD infection.
  - The lining of the vagina is thinner and more delicate than the skin on a penis, so it is easier for bacteria and viruses to penetrate.
  - The vagina is a good environment for bacteria to grow.
- STDs can lead to serious health complications and affect a woman's future reproductive plans.
  - Untreated STDs can lead to pelvic inflammatory disease (PID), which can result in infertility and ectopic pregnancy.
- Women who are pregnant can pass STDs to their babies.
  - Genital herpes, syphilis, and HIV can be passed to babies during pregnancy and at delivery.
  - The harmful effects of STDs in babies may include stillbirth, low birth weight (less than 5 pounds), brain damage, blindness, and deafness.
- HPV is the most common STI in women and is the main cause of cervical cancer.
  - While HPV is also very common in men, most do not develop any serious health problems.[5]

---

[5] See footnote [3].

Section 4.4 | **Sexually Transmitted Diseases in Men**

There are about 20 million estimated new sexually transmitted disease (STD) each year in the United States. There are 20 types of infections spread by sexual contact. These often show different signs of infection or no signs at all. You can have an STD and not know it.

CHLAMYDIA
How Is Chlamydia Spread?
Men get chlamydia through vaginal, oral, or anal sex (or sexual contact) with an infected partner.

What Are Signs of Chlamydia in Men?
There may be no signs or symptoms of infection.

Symptoms may not appear until several weeks after exposure and can include:
- pain/burning with urination
- watery/mucus discharge from the penis
- redness, swelling, or itching at the tip of the penis
- hard to start urination
- blood in semen or urine
- discomfort during sex
- rectal pain, bleeding, or discharge
- testicular pain, tenderness, and swelling (less common)

GENITAL HERPES
Genital herpes is a chronic, lifelong STD caused by two herpes simplex viruses (HSVs; HSV-1 and HSV-2).
- HSV-2 causes most genital herpes.
- HSV-1 can also cause genital herpes. More often, it causes blisters of the mouth and lips (e.g., cold sores or fever blisters).

The Centers for Disease Control and Prevention (CDC) estimates that over 50 million people or about one out of six people aged 14–49 in the United States has genital herpes. It occurs in about one in eight men. Many people with herpes have no signs of infection and do not know they have it. They can still pass it on to others.

How Does Genital Herpes Spread?

The herpes virus is spread by skin-to-skin contact with a person who has it:

- most often from herpes sores or blisters
- less often from normal-looking skin where the virus first entered the body
- during vaginal, anal, or oral sexual contact or skin-to-skin contact (This may happen even without visible sores.)
- the herpes virus getting into the body from:
  - the lining of the mouth
  - regular skin that has small cracks or cuts

Those with a weak immune system can get herpes infection more easily. A weak immune system is caused by some diseases (e.g., cancer and human immunodeficiency virus/acquired immunodeficiency syndrome (HIV/AIDS)) and by some medicines used to treat serious diseases.

What Are the Signs of Genital Herpes in Men?

Men who have the herpes virus may have no outbreaks or signs of infection. Many do not know they have the virus. Once you are infected, the virus stays in your nerve cells for life. When the virus is not active, there is no sign of infection. When the virus becomes active, a herpes outbreak occurs. Some men may:

- not have any outbreaks
- have only one outbreak
- have multiple outbreaks

FIRST OUTBREAK

The first herpes outbreak often occurs within two weeks after sexual contact with an infected person. Sometimes, the first outbreak will not occur until months or years after the first infection. The first signs may include:

- itching, tingling, or burning feeling in the genital area
- flu-like symptoms, including fever
- swollen glands
- pain or tingling in the legs, buttocks, or anal area
- headache
- a feeling of pressure in the area below the stomach

After a few days, painful sores, blisters, or ulcers may appear where the virus entered the body. These areas include:

- the genital or anal area
- the mouth
- the urinary tract
- the buttocks or thighs
- other parts of your body where the virus has entered

OTHER OUTBREAKS

After the first outbreak, you may have more outbreaks. For most, these occur less often over time. The signs of herpes infection are mostly milder than during the first outbreak, and they go away faster.

For those with a weak immune system, outbreaks can be severe and long-lasting.

GENITAL WARTS
How Are Genital Warts Spread?

Men can get genital warts from sexual contact with someone who has human papillomavirus (HPV). Genital warts are spread by skin-to-skin contact, usually from contact with the warts. It can be spread by vaginal, anal, oral, or hand-genital sexual contact. Genital warts will spread HPV while visible and after recent treatment. Long-term sexual partners usually have the same type of wart-causing HPV.

What Are Signs of Genital Warts in Men?

Genital warts can grow anywhere in the genital area:

- on the groin
- under the foreskin of the uncircumcised penis
- on the shaft of the circumcised penis
- in or around the anus
- in the mouth or throat (rare)

Genital warts:

- can be of any size from so small they cannot be seen to big clusters and lumps
- can be smooth with a "mosaic" pattern or bumpy like a cauliflower
- are soft, moist, and flesh-colored
- can cause itching, burning, or pain

Not all HPV infections cause genital warts. HPV infections often do not have any signs that you can see or feel. Some HPV infections can be more serious.

GONORRHEA
How Is Gonorrhea Spread?

Men get gonorrhea from sexual contact with someone who is infected. Anyone who has gonorrhea can spread it to others. Gonorrhea can be spread through oral, vaginal, and anal contact between:

- men and women
- men and men

What Are the Signs of Gonorrhea in Men?

Some women and men can have gonorrhea without any signs. For men, signs include:

- painful or burning urination
- white, yellow, or green discharge from the penis
- testicular/scrotal pain
- anal discharge, pain/itching, bleeding, or painful bowel movements

- fever, abdominal pain, rashes, and swelling or pain in joints over time
- sore throat
- red or itchy eyes
- eye discharge

HUMAN IMMUNODEFICIENCY VIRUS

If you are infected with HIV, you are said to be "HIV-positive." Over time as HIV weakens your immune system, you are more likely to get other infections. The late stage of HIV infection is known as AIDS. With medicines, the virus can be controlled, so AIDS may not occur.

How Is Human Immunodeficiency Virus Spread?

Each year in the United States, about 50,000 people get infected with HIV. More than 1.2 million people in the United States are living with HIV infection, and approximately 13 percent are not aware they are infected. Men account for 76 percent of all adults and adolescents living with HIV. HIV is found only in certain body fluids:

- blood
- vaginal fluid
- semen
- breast milk

Contact with infected body fluids can spread HIV by:
- sexual contact
  - vaginal and anal sex
  - sharing unclean sex toys
  - oral sex, very rarely
  - body fluids with HIV (It can enter tiny breaks or rips in the linings of the rectum or mouth. Rips and tears may not be seen or felt.)
- needle sharing
  - used or unclean needles
  - during illegal drug use

- breastfeeding
  - HIV can be spread to babies and others who drink breast milk from a woman who is HIV-positive.
- pregnancy and birth
  - HIV-positive women can spread the virus to their babies during pregnancy and birth.

HIV is rarely spread from a blood transfusion because:
- all donated blood is tested for HIV
- there is no risk of getting HIV when donating blood

HIV is not spread by:
- tears
- sweat
- feces
- urine
- saliva

What Are Signs of Human Immunodeficiency Virus?

Most people with HIV will not show signs of HIV until years after getting the virus. Those who have been infected with HIV may have:
- fever
- chills
- night sweats
- headache
- sore throat
- swollen lymph nodes, mainly on the neck
- tiredness
- rash
- sores or infections in the mouth
- body aches

What Can Happen If You Have a Human Immunodeficiency Virus for a Long Time?

If HIV is not diagnosed and treated, it can progress into AIDS. AIDS is the late stage of HIV infection. When you have AIDS, the virus has greatly weakened your immune system. If HIV is not treated, other infections can occur that can be life-threatening. The only way to know if you have AIDS is through a medical exam and testing by your health-care provider. Signs of AIDS are:

- rapid weight loss
- fevers
- night sweats
- extreme tiredness
- swelling of the lymph nodes in the armpits, groin, or neck that does not go away
- diarrhea that lasts for more than a week
- sores of the mouth, anus, or genitals
- infections such as pneumonia, tuberculosis, and certain cancers
- red, brown, pink, or purplish blotches on or under the skin or inside the mouth, nose, or eyelids
- depression
- memory loss and other brain or nerve problems

If you have HIV, do the following:
- See a health-care provider regularly.
- Take medicines as prescribed.
- Tell current and recent sex partners that you have HIV.
- Avoid spreading HIV to others by:
  - using condoms during all sexual contact
  - not sharing used or unclean needles and sex toys

HUMAN PAPILLOMAVIRUS

There are over 100 known types of HPV. About 40 types can infect female and male genital areas.

Genital HPV is grouped into the following two types:
- Low-risk types can cause genital warts or may be harmless.
- High-risk types can raise the chances for cancer of the penis and anus.

How Is Human Papillomavirus Spread?

HPV is spread by skin-to-skin contact. Men get HPV from sexual contact with someone who has it. HPV can be spread by vaginal, anal, oral, or hand-genital sexual contact. Some may have no signs of HPV but can still spread it to others. People can have more than one type of HPV. Long-term sex partners with HPV often have the same HPV types.

Risk of having HPV rises if you:
- have been sexually active at an earlier age
- have multiple sex partners
- smoke
- have a weak immune system due to:
  - a medical condition (cancer or HIV)
  - medicines

What Are the Signs of Human Papillomavirus in Men?

If you have HPV, you may not be able to see or feel it. You can have HPV even if years passed since your last sexual contact with an infected person. You may never know which sex partner gave you HPV. HPV infection may cause:
- genital warts (low-risk HPV)
- cancer (high-risk HPV)
  - cancer of the penis (more common)
  - cancers of the anus, throat, tongue, or tonsils (less common)

What Can Happen If You Have Human Papillomavirus for a Long Time?

Some types of low-risk HPV can cause genital warts. If not treated, genital warts may:
- go away
- remain unchanged
- increase in size or number

High-risk HPV can cause cancer. See your provider if you have strange growths, lumps, or sores on your penis, scrotum, anus, mouth, or throat.

If you have HPV, do the following:
- Talk to your health-care provider.
- Know that longtime sex partners often share the same HPV types, even if both have no signs.

SYPHILIS
How Is Syphilis Spread?

Men get syphilis from sexual contact with someone who has it. Anyone with syphilis can spread it to others. Those who have it may not show signs or know they have it. Syphilis can be spread by contact with a syphilis sore that occurs on external genitals, on the vagina, on the anus, or in the rectum. Syphilis can be spread between:
- men and women
- men and men

What Are Signs of Syphilis in Men?

There are four stages of syphilis. Each is defined by how long the person has had it. Signs vary in each stage.
- **Primary stage**. The first sign of syphilis is often a small, round, firm sore. These sores appear at the place where they entered the body such as the penis, tongue, or lips. Most do not cause pain. There can also be more than one sore. Signs often go away in about three to six weeks even without treatment. If not treated in this stage, it will progress into the other stages.
- **Secondary stage**. This stage can start with a rash over one or more areas of the body. These appear mostly on the palms of the hands and the bottoms of the feet. Other signs may be:
  - sores in the mouth or anus
  - sore throat
  - swollen glands
  - large, raised gray/white lesions in the mouth, underarm, or groin area
  - fever

- hair loss in patches
- head and muscle aches
- weight loss
- tiredness

If not treated in this stage, signs will still go away. However, the syphilis bacteria are still in the body. The infection will progress into the latent stage.

- **Latent stage**. This stage is also called the "hidden stage." It can last many years. Syphilis remains in the body with no signs of infection. Without treatment, syphilis can pass to the late stage. This can take 10–20 years.
- **Late stage**. Syphilis in this stage can cause:
  - numbness
  - problems with blood vessels
  - damage to bones and joints
  - difficulty walking
  - blindness
  - paralysis
  - brain damage
  - dementia
  - heart disease
  - death

TRICHOMONIASIS
How Is Trichomoniasis Spread?

Men get trichomoniasis from sexual contact. Anyone who has it can spread it to others. It can be spread between:

- men and women
- men and men

What Are the Signs of Trichomoniasis in Men?

Most men show no signs of trichomoniasis. Others have signs that include:

- itching and irritation inside the penis
- burning after urination or ejaculation

- discharge from the penis
- painful intercourse

THE ROLE OF CIRCUMCISION
What Is Circumcision?

Male circumcision is the surgical removal of some or the entire foreskin covering the tip of the penis. Germs can grow under the foreskin and create hygiene problems.

Why Do Men Get Circumcised?

- decision made by the parents when they were an infant
- religious, social, or cultural reasons
- medical reasons (to prevent infections or fix tight foreskin)

Benefits of Circumcision

Research studies have shown that male circumcision lowers the risk of:

- acquiring HIV, genital herpes, HPV, and syphilis
- penile cancer over a lifetime
- cervical cancer in sex partners
- urinary tract infections (UTIs) in the first year of life

Uncircumcised men can speak with their health-care provider about the following:

- How circumcision may impact disease and infections?
- How circumcision may impact sexual sensitivity?
- What are the benefits and risks of the procedure?
- Who will perform the procedure?[6]

---

[6] "Men's Health: A Guide to Preventing Infections," U.S. Department of Veterans Affairs (VA), September 15, 2014. Available online. URL: www.prevention.va.gov/docs/mens-health-guide/STIs.pdf. Accessed July 7, 2023.

Chapter 5 | Sexually Transmitted Diseases in Special Populations

Chapter Contents

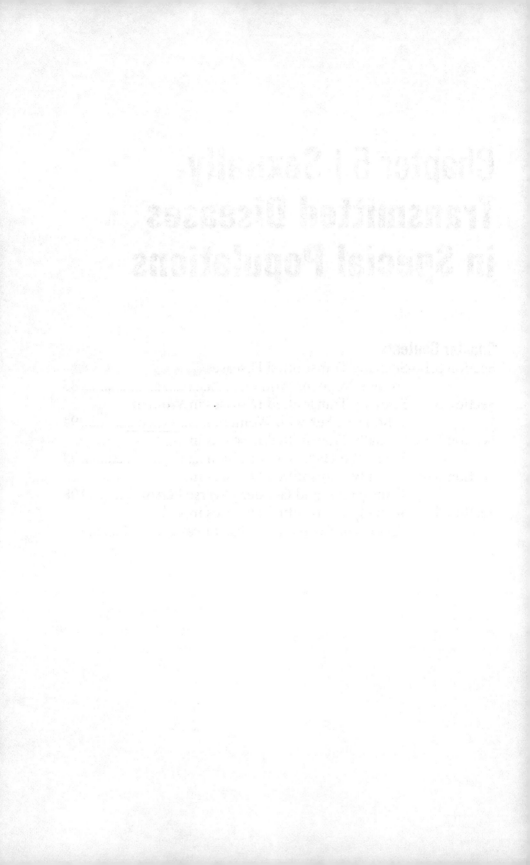

Section 5.1 | Sexually Transmitted Diseases among Pregnant Women

HOW DO DIFFERENT TYPES OF SEXUALLY TRANSMITTED DISEASES IMPACT PREGNANCY?
Bacterial Vaginosis

Bacterial vaginosis (BV), a common cause of vaginal discharge in women of childbearing age, is a polymicrobial clinical syndrome resulting from a change in the vaginal community of bacteria. Although BV is often not considered a sexually transmitted disease (STD), it has been linked to sexual activity. Women may have no symptoms or may complain of a foul-smelling, fishy, vaginal discharge. BV during pregnancy has been associated with serious pregnancy complications, including premature rupture of the membranes surrounding the baby in the uterus, preterm labor, premature birth, chorioamnionitis, as well as endometritis. While there is no evidence to support screening for BV in pregnant women at high risk for preterm delivery, symptomatic women should be evaluated and treated. There are no known direct effects of BV on the newborn.

Chlamydia

Chlamydia is the most common STD caused by bacteria in the United States. Although the majority of chlamydial infections (including those in pregnant women) do not have symptoms, infected women may have abnormal vaginal discharge, bleeding after sex, or itching/burning with urination. Untreated chlamydial infection has been linked to problems during pregnancy, including preterm labor, premature rupture of membranes, and low birth weight. The newborn may also become infected during delivery as the baby passes through the birth canal. Exposed newborns can develop eye and lung infections.

Gonorrhea

Gonorrhea is a common STD in the United States. Untreated gono-coccal infection in pregnancy has been linked to miscarriages, premature birth and low birth weight, premature rupture of mem-branes, and chorioamnionitis. Gonorrhea can also infect an infant during delivery as the infant passes through the birth canal. If untreated, infants can develop eye infections. Because gonorrhea can cause problems in both the mother and her baby, it is import-ant for providers to accurately identify the infection, treat it with effective antibiotics, and closely follow up to make sure that the infection has been cured.

Hepatitis B

Hepatitis B is a liver infection caused by hepatitis B virus (HBV). A mother can transmit the infection to her baby during pregnancy. While the risk of an infected mother passing HBV to her baby varies, depending on when she becomes infected, the greatest risk happens when mothers become infected close to the time of deliv-ery. Infected newborns also have a high risk (up to 90%) of becom-ing chronic HBV carriers themselves. Infants who have a lifelong infection with HBV are at increased risk for developing chronic liver disease (CLD) or liver cancer later in life. Approximately 25 percent of infants who develop chronic HBV infection will even-tually die from CLD. By screening your pregnant patients for the infection and providing treatment to at-risk infants shortly after birth, you can help prevent mother-to-child transmission of HBV.

Hepatitis C

Hepatitis C is a liver infection caused by hepatitis C virus (HCV) and can be passed from an infected mother to her child during pregnancy. In general, an infected mother will transmit the infec-tion to her baby 10 percent of the time, but the chances are higher in certain subgroups, such as women who are also infected with HIV. In some studies, infants born to HCV-infected women have been shown to have increased risk for being small for gestational age, premature, and having a low birth weight. Newborn infants with HCV infection usually do not have symptoms, and a majority will clear the infection without any medical help.

Herpes Simplex Virus

Herpes simplex virus (HSV) has two distinct virus types that can infect the human genital tract: HSV-1 and HSV-2. Infections of the newborn can be of either type, but most are caused by HSV-2. Generally, the symptoms of genital herpes are similar in pregnant and nonpregnant women; however, the major concern regarding HSV infection relates to complications linked to infection of the newborn. Although transmission may occur during pregnancy and after delivery, the risk of transmission to the neonate from an infected mother is high among women who acquire genital herpes near the time of delivery and low among women with recurrent herpes or who acquire the infection during the first half of pregnancy. HSV infection can have very serious effects on newborns, especially if the mother's first outbreak occurred during the third trimester. Cesarean section is recommended for all women in labor with active genital herpes lesions or early symptoms, such as vulvar pain and itching.

Human Immunodeficiency Virus

Human immunodeficiency virus (HIV) is the virus that causes acquired immunodeficiency syndrome (AIDS). HIV destroys specific blood cells that are crucial to helping the body fight diseases. According to Centers for Disease Control and Prevention (CDC) HIV surveillance data, women make up 19 percent of all new HIV diagnoses in the United States and dependent areas. The most common ways that HIV passes from the mother to the child are during pregnancy, childbirth, or breastfeeding. However, when HIV is diagnosed before or early during pregnancy and appropriate steps are taken, the risk of mother-to-child transmission can be less than 1 percent. A mother who knows early in her pregnancy that she has HIV has more time to consult with her health-care provider and decide on effective ways to protect her health and that of her unborn baby.

Human Papillomavirus

Human papillomaviruses (HPVs) are viruses that most commonly involve the lower genital tract, including the cervix, vagina, and external genitalia. Genital warts frequently increase in number and size during pregnancy. Genital warts often appear as small cauliflower-like clusters, which may burn or itch. If a woman has genital warts during pregnancy, you may elect to delay treatment until after delivery. When large or spread out, genital warts can complicate a vaginal delivery. In cases where there are large genital warts that are blocking the birth canal, a cesarean section may be recommended. Infection of the mother may be linked to the development of laryngeal papillomatosis in the newborn—a rare, noncancerous growth in the larynx.

Syphilis

Syphilis is primarily a sexually transmitted disease, but it may be transmitted to a baby by an infected mother during pregnancy. Transmission of syphilis to a developing baby can lead to a serious multisystem infection, known as "congenital syphilis." Recently, there has been a sharp increase in the number of congenital syphilis cases in the United States. Syphilis has been linked to premature births, stillbirths, and, in some cases, death shortly after birth. Untreated infants that survive tend to develop problems in multiple organs, including the brain, eyes, ears, heart, skin, teeth, and bones.

Trichomoniasis

Vaginal infection due to the sexually transmitted parasite *Trichomonas vaginalis* is very common. Although most people report no symptoms, others complain of itching, irritation, unusual odor, discharge, and pain during urination or sex. If a pregnant patient has symptoms of trichomoniasis, she should be evaluated for *T. vaginalis* and treated appropriately. Infection in pregnancy has been linked to premature rupture of membranes, preterm birth, and low-birth-weight infants. Rarely, the female newborn can acquire the infection when passing through the birth canal during delivery and have vaginal discharge after birth.

Screening and prompt treatment are recommended at least annually for all HIV-infected women, based on the high prevalence of *T. vaginalis* infection, the increased risk for pelvic inflammatory disease (PID) associated with this infection, and the ability of treatment to reduce genital tract viral load and vaginal HIV shedding. This includes HIV-infected women who are pregnant, as *T. vaginalis* infection is a risk factor for vertical transmission of HIV. For other pregnant women, screening may be considered at the discretion of the treating clinician, as the benefit of routine screening for pregnant women has not been established. Screening might be considered for persons receiving care in high-prevalence settings (e.g., STD clinics or correctional facilities) and for asymptomatic persons at high risk for infection. Decisions about screening might be informed by local epidemiology of *T. vaginalis* infection. However, data are lacking on whether screening and treatment for asymptomatic trichomoniasis in high-prevalence settings or persons at high risk can reduce any adverse health events and health disparities or reduce the community burden of infection.[1]

SCREENING RECOMMENDATIONS
Human Immunodeficiency Virus Infection

All pregnant women in the United States should be tested for human immunodeficiency virus (HIV) at the first prenatal visit, even if they have been previously tested. Testing pregnant women for HIV and prompt linkage to care of women with HIV infection are vital for women's health and reducing perinatal transmission of HIV through antiretroviral therapy (ART) and obstetrical interventions. HIV testing should be offered as part of the routine panel of prenatal tests (i.e., opt-out testing). For women who decline HIV testing, providers should address their concerns and, when appropriate, continue to encourage testing. Partners of pregnant patients should be offered HIV testing if their status is unknown.

Retesting in the third trimester (preferably before 36-week gestation) is recommended for women at high risk for acquiring HIV

---

[1] "STDs during Pregnancy," Centers for Disease Control and Prevention (CDC), April 11, 2023. Available online. URL: www.cdc.gov/std/pregnancy/stdfact-pregnancy-detailed.htm. Accessed July 7, 2023.

infection. Examples of women at high risk include those who inject drugs, have STIs during pregnancy, have multiple sex partners during pregnancy, have a new sex partner during pregnancy, or have partners with HIV infection; those who are receiving care in health-care facilities in settings with HIV incidence greater than or equal to 1 per 1,000 women per year; those who are incarcerated; those who live in areas with high rates of HIV infection; or those who have signs or symptoms of acute HIV infection (e.g., fever, lymphadenopathy, skin rash, myalgia, arthralgia, headache, oral ulcers, leukopenia, thrombocytopenia, or transaminase elevation).

Rapid HIV testing should be performed for any woman in labor who has not been tested for HIV during pregnancy or whose HIV status is unknown, unless she declines. If a rapid HIV test result is positive, ART should be administered without waiting for the results of confirmatory testing (https://clinicalinfo.hiv.gov/sites/default/files/inline-files/PerinatalGL.pdf).

Syphilis

During 2012–2019, congenital syphilis rates in the United States increased from 8.4 to 48.5 cases per 100,000 births, a 477.4 percent increase. At least 45 states have a prenatal syphilis testing requirement, with high variability among those requirements. In the United States, all pregnant women should be screened for syphilis at the first prenatal visit, even if they have been tested previously. Prenatal screening for syphilis has been reported to be suboptimal in the United States. Testing in the third trimester and at delivery can prevent congenital syphilis cases. Partners of pregnant women with syphilis should be evaluated, tested, and treated.

When access to prenatal care is not optimal, a stat rapid plasma reagin (RPR) card test and treatment, if that test is reactive, should be administered at the time that a pregnancy is confirmed or when the pregnancy test is performed if follow-up is uncertain. Pregnant women should be retested for syphilis at 28-week gestation and at delivery if the mother lives in a community with high syphilis rates or is at risk for syphilis acquisition during pregnancy (e.g., misusing drugs or having an STI during pregnancy, having multiple sex partners, having a new sex partner, or having a sex partner with an STI). Neonates should not be discharged from the hospital unless the syphilis serologic status of the mother has been determined at least once during pregnancy. Any woman who delivers a stillborn infant should be tested for syphilis.

Hepatitis B

All pregnant women should be routinely tested for hepatitis B surface antigen (HBsAg) at the first prenatal visit even if they have been previously vaccinated or tested. Women who are HBsAg-positive should be provided with, or referred for, counseling and medical management. Women who are HBsAg-negative but at risk for hepatitis B virus (HBV) infection should be vaccinated. Women who were not screened prenatally, those who engage in behaviors that put them at high risk for infection (e.g., having had more than one sex partner during the previous six months, having been evaluated or treated for an STI, having had recent or current injection drug use, or having an HBsAg-positive sex partner), and those with clinical hepatitis should be tested at the time of admission to the hospital for delivery. To avoid misinterpreting a transient positive HBsAg result during the 21 days after vaccination, HBsAg testing should be performed before the vaccine administration. All laboratories that conduct HBsAg tests should test initially reactive specimens with a licensed neutralizing confirmatory test. When pregnant women are tested for HBsAg at the time of admission for delivery, shortened testing protocols can be used, and initially, reactive results should prompt expedited administration of immunoprophylaxis to neonates. Pregnant women who are HBsAg-positive should be reported to the local or state health department to ensure that they are entered into a case management system and that timely and age-appropriate prophylaxis is provided to their infants. Information concerning the pregnant woman's HBsAg status should be provided to the hospital where delivery is planned and to the health-care provider who will care for the newborn. In addition, household and sexual contacts of women who are HBsAg-positive should be vaccinated.

Chlamydia

All pregnant women younger than 25 years of age as well as older women at increased risk for chlamydia (e.g., those aged 25 or over who have a new sex partner, more than one sex partner, a sex partner with concurrent partners, or a sex partner who has an STI) should be routinely screened for *Chlamydia trachomatis* at the first prenatal visit. Pregnant women who remain at increased risk for chlamydial infection should also be retested during the third trimester to prevent maternal postnatal complications and chlamydial infection in the neonate. Pregnant women identified as having chlamydia should be treated immediately and have a test of cure to document chlamydial eradication by a nucleic acid amplification test (NAAT) four weeks after treatment. All persons diagnosed with a chlamydial infection should be rescreened three months after the treatment.

Gonorrhea

All pregnant women younger than 25 years of age as well as women aged 25 or over at increased risk for gonorrhea (e.g., those with other STIs during pregnancy or those with a new sex partner, more than one sex partner, a sex partner with concurrent partners, or a sex partner who has an STI or is exchanging sex for money or drugs) should be screened for *Neisseria gonorrhoeae* at the first prenatal visit. Pregnant women who remain at high risk for gonococcal infection should also be retested during the third trimester to prevent maternal postnatal complications and gonococcal infection in the neonate. Clinicians should consider the communities they serve and might choose to consult local public health authorities for guidance on identifying groups that are more vulnerable to gonorrhea acquisition on the basis of local disease prevalence. Gonococcal infection, in particular, is concentrated among specific geographic locations and communities (www.cdc.gov/std/statistics/2019/default.htm). Pregnant women identified as having gonorrhea should be treated immediately. All persons diagnosed with gonorrhea should be rescreened three months after the treatment.

Hepatitis C Virus

The rate of HCV infection has increased among pregnant women in these years. HCV screening should be performed for all pregnant women during each pregnancy, except in settings where the HCV infection (HCV positivity) rate is less than 0.1 percent. The most important risk factor for HCV infection is past or current injecting drug use. Additional risk factors include having had a blood transfusion or organ transplantation before July 1992, having received clotting factor concentrates produced before 1987, having received an unregulated tattoo, having been on long-term hemodialysis, having other percutaneous exposures, or having HIV infection. All women with HCV infection should receive counseling, supportive care, and linkage to care (www. hcvguidelines.org). No vaccine is available for preventing HCV transmission.

Cervical Cancer

Pregnant women should undergo cervical cancer screening at the same frequency as nonpregnant women; however, management differs slightly during pregnancy. Colposcopy is recommended for the same indications during pregnancy as for nonpregnant women. However, biopsies may be deferred, and endocervical sampling should not be performed. Treatment should not be performed during pregnancy unless cancer is detected.

Bacterial Vaginosis, Trichomoniasis, and Genital Herpes

Evidence does not support routine screening for BV among asymptomatic pregnant women at high risk for preterm delivery. Symptomatic women should be evaluated and treated. Evidence does not support routine screening for *T. vaginalis* among asymptomatic pregnant women. Women who report symptoms should be evaluated and treated. In addition, the evidence does not support routine HSV-2 serologic screening among asymptomatic pregnant women. However, type-specific serologic tests might be useful for identifying pregnant women at risk for HSV-2 infection and for guiding counseling regarding the risk for acquiring genital herpes during pregnancy. Routine serial cultures for herpes simplex virus (HSV) are not indicated for women in the third trimester who have a history of recurrent genital herpes.[2]

Section 5.2 | Sexually Transmitted Diseases in Women Who Have Sex with Women

Women who have sex with women (WSW) and women who have sex with women and men (WSWM) comprise diverse groups with variations in sexual identity, practices, and risk behaviors. Studies indicate that certain WSW, particularly adolescents, young women, and WSWM, might be at increased risk for sexually transmitted infections (STIs) and human immunodeficiency virus (HIV) on the basis of reported risk behaviors. Studies have highlighted the diversity of sexual practices and examined the use of protective or risk-reduction strategies among WSW populations. The use of barrier protection with female partners (e.g., gloves during digital-genital sex, external condoms with sex toys, and latex or plastic barriers (also known as "dental dams" for oral-genital sex)) was infrequent in all studies. Although health organizations have online materials directed to patients, few comprehensive and reliable resources of sexual health information for WSW are available.

The studies regarding STI rates among WSW and WSWM indicate that WSWM experience higher rates of STIs than WSW, with rates comparable with women who have sex with men (WSM) in all studies reviewed. These studies indicate that WSW might experience STIs at lower rates than WSWM and WSM although still at significant rates. One study reported higher sexual risk behaviors among adolescent WSWM and WSW than among adolescent WSM. WSW report reduced knowledge of STI risks, and both

---

[2] "Pregnant Women," Centers for Disease Control and Prevention (CDC), July 22, 2021. Available online. URL: www.cdc.gov/std/treatment-guidelines/pregnant.htm. Accessed July 7, 2023.

WSW and WSWM experience barriers to care, especially Black WSW and WSWM. In addition, a continuum of sexual behaviors reported by WSW and WSWM indicates the need for providers to not assume lower risk for WSW, highlighting the importance of an open discussion about sexual health.

Few data are available regarding the risk for STIs conferred by sex between women; however, transmission risk probably varies by the specific STI and sexual practice (e.g., oral-genital sex; vaginal or anal sex using hands, fingers, or penetrative sex items; and oral-anal sex). Practices involving digital-vaginal or digital-anal contact, particularly with shared penetrative sex items, present a possible means for transmission of infected cervicovaginal or anal secretions. This possibility is most directly supported by reports of shared trichomonas infections and by concordant drug-resistance genotype testing and phylogenetic linkage analysis identifying HIV transmitted sexually between women. The majority of WSW (53–97%) have had sex with men in the past and continue to do so, with 5–28 percent of WSW reporting male partners during the previous year.

HUMAN PAPILLOMAVIRUS

Human papillomavirus (HPV) can be transmitted through skin-to-skin contact, and sexual transmission of HPV likely occurs between WSW. HPV deoxyribonucleic acid (DNA) has been detected through methods based on polymerase chain reaction (PCR) from the cervix, vagina, and vulva among 13–30 percent of WSW and can persist on fomites, including sex toys. Among WSW who report no lifetime history of sex with men, 26 percent had antibodies to HPV type 16 (HPV-16), and 42 percent had antibodies to HPV type 6 (HPV-6). High-grade squamous intraepithelial lesions (HSIL) and low-grade squamous intraepithelial lesions (LSIL) have been detected on Papanicolaou smears (Pap tests) among WSW who reported no previous sex with men. WSWM are at risk for acquiring HPV from both their female partners and male partners and, thus, are at risk for cervical cancer. Therefore, routine cervical cancer screening should be offered to all women, regardless of sexual orientation or practices, and young adult WSW and WSWM should be offered HPV vaccination in accordance with recommendations (www.cdc.gov/vaccines/hcp/acip-recs/vacc-specific/hpv.html).

HERPES SIMPLEX VIRUS

Genital transmission of herpes simplex virus type 2 (HSV-2) between female sex partners is inefficient but can occur. A U.S. population-based survey among women aged 18–59 demonstrated an HSV-2 seroprevalence of 30 percent among women reporting same-sex partners during the previous year, 36 percent among women reporting same-sex partners in their lifetime, and 24 percent among women reporting no lifetime same-sex behavior. HSV-2 seroprevalence among women self-identifying as homosexual or lesbian was 8 percent, similar to a previous clinic-based study of WSW, but was 26 percent among Black WSW in one study. The relatively frequent practice of orogenital sex among WSW and WSWM might place them at higher risk for genital infection with herpes simplex virus type 1 (HSV-1), a hypothesis supported by the recognized association between HSV-1 seropositivity and previous number of female partners. Thus, the sexual transmission of HSV-1 and HSV-2 can occur between female sex partners. This information should be communicated to women as part of sexual health counseling.

PROTOZOAL AND BACTERIAL SEXUALLY TRANSMITTED INFECTIONS

Trichomonas is a relatively common infection among WSW and WSWM, with prevalence rates higher than for chlamydia or gonorrhea, and direct transmission of trichomonas between female partners has been demonstrated.

Limited information is available regarding the transmission of bacterial STIs between female partners. Transmission of syphilis between female sex partners, probably through oral sex, has been reported. Although the rate of transmission of *Chlamydia trachomatis* or *Neisseria gonorrhoeae* between women is unknown, infection may also be acquired from past or current male partners. Data indicate that *C. trachomatis* infection among WSW can occur. Data are limited regarding gonorrhea rates among WSW and WSWM. Reports of same-sex behavior among women should not deter providers from offering and providing screening for STIs, including chlamydia, according to guidelines.

Bacterial vaginosis (BV) is common among women and even more so among women with female partners. Epidemiologic data strongly demonstrate that BV is sexually transmitted among women with female partners. Evidence continues to support the association of such sexual behaviors as having a new partner, having a partner with BV, having receptive oral sex, and having digital-vaginal and digital-anal sex with incident BV. A study including monogamous couples demonstrated that female sex partners frequently share identical genital *Lactobacillus* strains. Within a community-based cohort of WSW, extravaginal (i.e., oral and rectal) reservoirs of BV-associated bacteria were a risk factor for incident BV. Studies have examined the impact of specific sexual practices on the vaginal microflora and on recurrent or incident BV among WSW. A BV pathogenesis study in WSW reported that *Prevotella bivia*, *Gardnerella vaginalis*, and *Atopobium vaginae* might have substantial roles in the development of incident BV. These studies have continued to support, although not proven, the hypothesis that sexual behaviors, specific BV-associated bacteria, and possibly exchange of vaginal or extravaginal microbiota (e.g., oral bacterial communities) between partners might be involved in the pathogenesis of BV among WSW.

Although BV is common among WSW, routine screening for asymptomatic BV is not recommended. Results of one randomized trial used a behavioral intervention to reduce persistent BV among WSW through reduced sharing of vaginal fluid on hands or sex toys. Women randomly assigned to the intervention were 50 percent less likely to report receptive digital-vaginal contact without gloves than control subjects, and they reported sharing sex toys infrequently. However, these women had no reduction in persistent BV at one month after treatment and no reduction in incident episodes of recurrent BV. Trials have not been reported examining the benefits of treating female partners of women with BV. Recurrent BV among WSW is associated with having a same-sex partner and a lack of condom use. Increasing awareness of signs and symptoms of BV among women and encouraging healthy sexual practices (e.g., avoiding shared sex toys, cleaning shared sex toys, and using barriers) may benefit women and their partners.

Sexually active women are at risk for acquiring bacterial, viral, and protozoal STIs from current and previous partners, both male and female. WSW should not be presumed to be at low or no risk for STIs on the basis of their sexual orientation. The report of same-sex behavior among women should not deter providers from considering and performing screening for STIs and cervical cancer according to guidelines. Effective screening requires that care providers and their female patients engage in a comprehensive and open discussion of sexual and behavioral risks that extends beyond sexual identity.[3]

Section 5.3 | Sexually Transmitted Diseases in Men Who Have Sex with Men

Men who have sex with men (MSM) comprise a diverse group in terms of behaviors, identities, and health-care needs. The term "MSM" is often used clinically to refer to "sexual behavior alone," regardless of sexual orientation (e.g., a person might identify as heterosexual but still be classified as MSM). Sexual orientation is independent of gender identity. Classification of MSM can vary in the inclusion of transgender men and women on the basis of whether men are defined by sex at birth (i.e., transgender women included) or current gender identity (i.e., transgender men included). Therefore, sexual orientation, as well as gender identity of individual persons and their sex partners, should be obtained during health-care visits. MSM might be at increased risk for human immunodeficiency virus (HIV) and other sexually transmitted infections (STIs) because

---

[3] "Women Who Have Sex with Women (WSW) and Women Who Have Sex with Women and Men (WSWM)," Centers for Disease Control and Prevention (CDC), July 22, 2021. Available online. URL: www.cdc.gov/std/treatment-guidelines/wsw.htm. Accessed May 26, 2023.

of their sexual network or behavioral or biologic factors, including a number of concurrent partners, condomless sex, anal sex, or substance use. These factors, along with sexual network or higher community disease prevalence, can increase the risk for STIs among MSM compared with other groups.

Performing a detailed and comprehensive sexual history is the first step in identifying vulnerability and providing tailored counseling and care. Factors associated with increased vulnerability to STI acquisition among MSM include having multiple partners, anonymous partners, and concurrent partners. Repeat syphilis infections are common and might be associated with HIV infection, substance use (e.g., methamphetamines), Black race, and multiple sex partners. Similarly, gonorrhea incidence has increased among MSM and might be more likely to display antimicrobial resistance compared with other groups. Gonococcal infection among MSM has been associated with similar risk factors to syphilis, including having multiple anonymous partners and substance use, especially methamphetamines. Disparities in gonococcal infection are also more pronounced among certain racial and ethnic groups of MSM.

HUMAN IMMUNODEFICIENCY VIRUS RISK AMONG MEN WHO HAVE SEX WITH MEN

Men who have sex with men are disproportionately at risk for HIV infection. In the United States, the estimated lifetime risk for HIV infection among MSM is one in six, compared with heterosexual men at 1 in 524 and heterosexual women at 1 in 253. These disparities are further exacerbated by race and ethnicity, with African American/Black and Hispanic/Latino MSM having a one in two and a one in four lifetime risk for HIV infection, respectively. For HIV, transmission occurs much more readily through receptive anal sex, compared with penile-vaginal sex. Similar to other STIs, multiple partners, anonymous partners, condomless sex, and substance use are all associated with HIV infection. Importantly, other STIs might also significantly increase the risk for HIV infection. An estimated 10 percent of new HIV infections were attributable to chlamydial or gonococcal infection. A substantial number of MSM remain unaware of their HIV diagnosis. Clinical care involving MSM, including those who have HIV infection, should involve asking about STI-related risk factors and routine STI testing. Clinicians should routinely ask MSM about their sexual behaviors and symptoms consistent with common STIs, including urethral discharge, dysuria, ulcers, rash, lymphadenopathy, and anorectal symptoms that might be consistent with proctitis (e.g., discharge, rectal bleeding, pain on defecation, or pain during anal sex). However, certain STIs are asymptomatic, especially at rectal and pharyngeal sites, and routine testing is recommended. In addition, clinicians should provide education and counseling regarding evidence-based safer sex approaches that have demonstrated effectiveness in reducing STI incidence.

PRE-EXPOSURE PROPHYLAXIS FOR HUMAN IMMUNODEFICIENCY VIRUS PREVENTION

Pre-exposure prophylaxis (PrEP) is the use of medications for preventing an infection before exposure. Studies have demonstrated that a daily oral medication tenofovir (TDF)/emtricitabine (FTC) is effective in preventing HIV acquisition, specifically among MSM. PrEP guidelines provide information regarding sexually active persons who are at substantial risk for acquiring HIV infection (having had anal or vaginal sex during the previous six months with either a partner with HIV infection, a bacterial STI in the past six months, or inconsistent or no condom use with a sex partner) or persons who inject drugs (injecting a partner with HIV infection or sharing injection equipment). Those guidelines provide information regarding daily PrEP use for either TDF/FTC (men or women) or tenofovir alafenamide and emtricitabine for MSM. Screening for bacterial STIs should occur at least every six months for all sexually active patients and every three months among MSM or among patients with ongoing risk behaviors. MSM taking PrEP might compensate for decreased HIV acquisition risk by using condoms less frequently or modifying their behavior in other ways although data regarding this behavior are inconsistent. Studies have reported that MSM taking PrEP have high rates of STIs, and frequent screening is warranted.

IMPORTANCE OF RECTAL AND PHARYNGEAL TESTING

Rectal and pharyngeal testing by nucleic acid amplification testing (NAAT) for gonorrhea and chlamydia is recognized as an important sexual health consideration for MSM. Rectal gonorrhea and chlamydia are associated with HIV infection, and men with repeat rectal infections can be at substantially higher risk for HIV acquisition. Pharyngeal infections with gonorrhea or chlamydia might be a principal source of urethral infections. Studies have demonstrated that among MSM, the prevalence of rectal gonorrhea and chlamydia ranges from 0.2 to 24 percent and from 2.1 to 23 percent, respectively, and the prevalence of pharyngeal gonorrhea and chlamydia ranges from 0.5 to 16.5 percent and from 0 to 3.6 percent, respectively. Approximately 70 percent of gonococcal and chlamydial infections might be missed if urogenital-only testing is performed among MSM because most pharyngeal and rectal infections are asymptomatic. Self-collected swabs have been reported to be an acceptable means of collection for pharyngeal and rectal specimens, which can enhance patient comfort and reduce clinical workloads.

A detailed sexual history should be taken for all MSM to identify anatomic locations exposed to infection for screening. Clinics that provide services for MSM at high risk should consider implementing routine extragenital screening for *Neisseria gonorrhoeae* and *Chlamydia trachomatis* infections, and screening is likely to be cost-effective.

SCREENING RECOMMENDATIONS

Sexually transmitted infection screening among MSM has been reported to be suboptimal. In a cross-sectional sample of MSM in the United States, approximately one-third reported not having had an STI test during the previous three years, and MSM with multiple sex partners reported less frequent screening. MSM living with HIV infection and engaged in care also experience suboptimal rates of STI testing. Limited data exist regarding the optimal frequency of screening for gonorrhea, chlamydia, and syphilis among MSM, with the majority of evidence derived from mathematical modeling. Models from Australia have demonstrated that increasing syphilis screening frequency from two times a year to four times a year resulted in a relative decrease of 84 percent from peak prevalence. In a compartmental model applied to different populations in Canada, quarterly syphilis screening averted more than twice the number of syphilis cases, compared with semiannual screening. Furthermore, MSM screening coverage needed for eliminating syphilis among a population is substantially reduced from 62 percent with annual screening to 23 percent with quarterly screening. In an MSM transmission model that explored the impact of HIV PrEP use on STI prevalence, quarterly chlamydia and gonorrhea screening was associated with an 83 percent reduction in incidence. The only empiric data available that examined the impact of screening frequency come from an observational cohort of MSM using HIV PrEP, in which quarterly screening identified more bacterial STIs, and semiannual screening would have resulted in delayed treatment of 35 percent of total identified STI infections. In addition, quarterly screening was reported to have prevented STI exposure in a median of three sex partners per STI infection. On the basis of the available evidence, quarterly screening for gonorrhea, chlamydia, and syphilis for certain sexually active MSM can improve case finding, which can reduce the duration of infection at the population level, ongoing transmission, and, ultimately, prevalence among this population.

Preventive screening for common STIs is indicated for all MSM. The following screening recommendations summarize published federal agency and U.S. Preventive Services Task Force (USPSTF) clinical prevention guidelines for MSM and should be performed at least annually.

Human Immunodeficiency Virus Infection
HIV serologic testing is indicated if HIV status is unknown or if HIV-negative and the patient or their sex partner has had more than one sex partner since the most recent HIV test.

Syphilis
Syphilis serologic testing is indicated to establish whether persons with reactive tests have untreated syphilis, have partially treated

syphilis, or are manifesting a slow or inadequate serologic response to recommended previous therapy.

Gonorrhea and Chlamydia

The following testing is recommended for MSM:

- a test for urethral infection* with *N. gonorrhoeae* and *C. trachomatis* among men who have had insertive intercourse during the preceding year (Urine NAAT is preferred.)
- a test for rectal infection* with *N. gonorrhoeae* and *C. trachomatis* among men who have had receptive anal intercourse during the preceding year (Rectal NAAT is preferred.)
- a test for pharyngeal infection* with *N. gonorrhoeae* among men who have had receptive oral intercourse during the preceding year (Pharyngeal NAAT is preferred.)
- no recommended testing for *C. trachomatis* pharyngeal infection

* *Regardless of condom use during exposure.*

Basing screening practices solely on history might be suboptimal because providers might feel uncomfortable taking a detailed sexual history, men might also feel uncomfortable sharing personal sexual information with their provider, and rectal and pharyngeal infections can be identified even in the absence of reported risk behaviors. Furthermore, the role of saliva, kissing, and rimming (i.e., oral-rectal contact) in the transmission of *N. gonorrhoeae* and *C. trachomatis* has not been well studied.

Rectal and pharyngeal testing (provider-collected or self-collected specimens) should be performed for all MSM who report exposure at these sites. Testing can be offered to MSM who do not report exposure at these sites after a detailed explanation, due to known underreporting of risk behaviors. All MSM with HIV infection entering care should be screened for gonorrhea and chlamydia at appropriate anatomic sites of exposure as well as for syphilis.

More frequent STI screening (i.e., for syphilis, gonorrhea, and chlamydia) at three- to six-month intervals is indicated for MSM, including those taking PrEP and those with HIV infection, if risk behaviors persist or if they or their sex partners have multiple partners. In addition, providers can consider the benefits of offering more frequent HIV screening (e.g., every three to six months) to MSM at increased risk for acquiring HIV infection.

Hepatitis B Virus

All MSM should be screened with hepatitis B surface antigen (HBsAg), hepatitis B virus (HBV) core antibody, and HBV surface antibody testing to detect HBV infection. Vaccination against both hepatitis A virus (HAV) and HBV is recommended for all MSM for whom previous infection or vaccination cannot be documented. Serologic testing can be considered before vaccinating if the patient's vaccination history is unknown; however, vaccination should not be delayed. Vaccinating persons who have had previous infection or vaccination does not increase the risk for vaccine-related adverse events.

Hepatitis C Virus

The Centers for Disease Control and Prevention (CDC) recommends hepatitis C virus (HCV) screening at least once for all adults aged 18 or over, except in settings where the prevalence of HCV infection (HCV ribonucleic acid (RNA) positivity) is less than 0.1 percent. The American Association for the Study of Liver Diseases (AASLD)/Infectious Diseases Society of America (IDSA) guidelines recommend all MSM with HIV infection be screened for HCV during the initial HIV evaluation and at least annually thereafter (www.hcvguidelines.org). More frequent screening depends on ongoing risk behaviors, high-risk sexual behavior, and concomitant ulcerative STIs or STI-related proctitis. Sexual transmission of HCV can occur and is most common among MSM with HIV infection. Screening for HCV in this setting is cost-effective. Screening should be performed by using HCV antibody assays followed by HCV RNA testing for those with a positive antibody test. Suspicion for acute HCV infection (e.g., clinical evidence of hepatitis and risk behaviors) should prompt consideration for HCV RNA testing, despite a negative antibody test.

Human Papillomavirus

Human papillomavirus (HPV) infection and associated conditions (e.g., anogenital warts and anal squamous intraepithelial lesions) are highly prevalent among MSM. The HPV vaccination is recommended for all men, including MSM and transgender persons or immunocompromised males, including those with HIV infection, through the age of 26.

A digital anorectal examination (DARE) should be performed to detect early anal cancer among persons with HIV and MSM without HIV but who have a history of receptive anal intercourse. Data are insufficient to recommend routine anal cancer screening with anal cytology in populations at risk for anal cancer. Health centers that initiate a cytology-based screening program should only do so if referrals to high-resolution anoscopy (HRA) and biopsy are available.

Herpes Simplex Virus-2

Evaluation for herpes simplex virus-2 (HSV-2) infection with type-specific serologic tests can also be considered if the infection status is unknown among persons with previously undiagnosed genital tract infection.

POST- AND PRE-EXPOSURE PROPHYLAXIS FOR SEXUALLY TRANSMITTED INFECTION PREVENTION

Studies have reported that a benefit might be derived from STI postexposure prophylaxis (PEP) and PrEP for STI prevention. One study demonstrated that monthly oral administration of a 1-g dose of azithromycin reduced infection with *N. gonorrhoeae* and *C. trachomatis* but did not decrease the incidence of HIV transmission. Among MSM, doxycycline taken as PEP in a single oral dose less than or equal to 24 hours after sex decreased infection with

Treponema pallidum and *C. trachomatis*; however, no substantial effect was observed for infection with *N. gonorrhoeae*. Doxycycline taken as STI PrEP as 100 mg orally once daily also demonstrated a substantial reduction in gonorrhea, chlamydia, and syphilis among MSM. However, these studies had limitations because of the small sample size, short duration of therapy, and concerns about antibiotic resistance, specifically regarding *N. gonorrhoeae*. Further study is needed to determine the effectiveness of using antimicrobials for STI PrEP or PEP.

ENTERIC INFECTIONS AMONG MEN WHO HAVE SEX WITH MEN
The importance of sexual transmission of enteric pathogens among MSM has been recognized since the 1970s, after the first report of MSM-associated shigellosis was reported in San Francisco. Global increases in the incidence of shigellosis among adult MSM have been more recently observed. Sporadic outbreaks of *Shigella sonnei* and *Shigella flexneri* have been reported among MSM. Transmission occurs through oral-anal contact or sexual contact, and transmission efficiency is enhanced by both biologic or host and behavioral factors. HIV without viral suppression can be an independent risk factor that can contribute to transmission by increasing the shedding of the enteric pathogen, increasing susceptibility of the host, or both. Surveillance data in England during 2004–2015 demonstrated that 21 percent of nontravel-associated *Shigella* diagnoses among MSM were among persons with HIV infection.

Other enteric organisms might also cause disease among MSM through sexual activities leading to oral-anal contact, including bacteria such as *Escherichia coli* and *Campylobacter jejuni* or *Campylobacter coli*; viruses such as HAV; and parasites such as *Giardia lamblia* or *Entamoeba histolytica*. Behavioral characteristics associated with the sexual transmission of enteric infections are broadly similar to those associated with other STIs (e.g., gonorrhea, syphilis, and lymphogranuloma venereum (LGV)). This includes multiple sex partners and online hookup sites that increase opportunities for sexual mixing, which might create dense sexual networks that facilitate STI transmission among MSM.

Specific behaviors associated with sexually transmitted enteric infections among MSM involve attendance at sex parties and recreational drug use including chem sex (i.e., using crystal methamphetamine, gamma-butyrolactone, or mephedrone before or during sex), which might facilitate condomless sex, group sex, fisting, use of sex toys, and scat play. The growing number of sexually transmitted enteric infections might be attributable in part to the emergence of antimicrobial resistance. This is well reported regarding *Shigella* species, for which rapid intercontinental dissemination of an *S. flexneri* 3a lineage with high-level resistance to azithromycin through sexual transmission among MSM and clusters of multidrug-resistant *Shigella* cases among MSM have recently been reported. Multidrug-resistant *Campylobacter* species have also been documented. For MSM patients with diarrhea, clinicians should request laboratory examinations, including stool culture; provide counseling about the risk for infection with enteric pathogens during sexual activity (oral-anal, oral-genital, anal-genital, and digital-anal contact) that could expose them to enteric pathogens; and choose treatment, when needed, according to antimicrobial drug susceptibility.

COUNSELING AND EDUCATION APPROACHES

Different counseling and STI prevention strategies are needed to effectively engage different groups of MSM. Outreach efforts should be guided by local surveillance efforts and community input. Engaging MSM at risk through social media, specifically online hookup sites, is an important outreach effort to consider. Hookup sites are Internet sites and mobile telephone applications that men might use for meeting other men for sex. Internet use might facilitate sexual encounters and STI transmission among MSM, and many men report using hookup sites to meet partners. The ease and accessibility of meeting partners online might reduce stigma and barriers of meeting partners through other settings. Moreover, these sites offer an opportunity for effective STI prevention messaging although the cost might be limiting. Different groups of MSM might use different hookup sites, and efforts should be guided by local community input. Studies have demonstrated the acceptability and feasibility of reaching MSM through these hookup sites to promote STI prevention efforts.[4]

Section 5.4 | Sexually Transmitted Diseases in Transgender and Gender Diverse Persons

Transgender persons often experience high rates of stigma and socio-economic and structural barriers to care that negatively affect health-care usage and increase susceptibility to human immunodeficiency virus (HIV) and sexually transmitted infections (STIs). Persons who are transgender have a gender identity that differs from the sex that they were assigned at birth. Transgender women (also known as "trans women," "transfeminine persons," or "women of transgender experience") are women who were assigned male sex at birth (born with male anatomy). Transgender men (also known as "trans men," "transmasculine persons," or "men of transgender experience") are men who were assigned female sex at birth (i.e., born with female anatomy). In addition, certain persons might identify outside the gender binary of male or female or move back and forth between different gender identities and use such terms as "gender nonbinary," "genderqueer," or "gender fluid" to describe themselves. Persons who use terms such as "agender" or "null gender" do not identify with having any gender. The term "cisgender" is used to describe persons who identify with their assigned sex at birth. Prevalence studies of transgender persons among the overall population have been limited and often are based on small convenience samples.

Gender identity is independent of sexual orientation. Sexual orientation identities among transgender persons are diverse. Persons who are transgender or gender-diverse might have sex with cisgender men, cisgender women, or other transgender or gender nonbinary persons.

---

[4] "Men Who Have Sex with Men (MSM)," Centers for Disease Control and Prevention (CDC), July 22, 2021. Available online. URL: www.cdc.gov/std/treatment-guidelines/msm.htm. Accessed May 29, 2023.

IMPROVING TRANSGENDER HEALTH BY BUILDING SAFE CLINICAL ENVIRONMENTS

Providers should create welcoming environments that facilitate disclosure of gender identity and sexual orientation. Clinics should document gender identity and sex assigned at birth for all patients to improve sexual health care for transgender and gender nonbinary persons.

Lack of medical provider knowledge and other barriers to care (e.g., discrimination in health-care settings or denial of services) often result in transgender and gender nonbinary persons avoiding or delaying preventive care services and incurring missed opportunities for HIV and STI prevention services. Gender-inclusive and trauma-guided health care might increase the number of transgender patients who seek sexual health services, including STI testing, because transgender persons are at high risk for sexual violence.

TRANSGENDER WOMEN

A systematic review and meta-analysis of HIV infection among transgender women estimated that HIV prevalence in the United States is 14 percent among transgender women, with the highest prevalence among Black (44%) and Hispanic (26%) transgender women. Data also demonstrate high rates of HIV infection among transgender women worldwide. Bacterial STI prevalence varies among transgender women and is based largely on convenience samples. Despite limited data, international and U.S. studies have indicated elevated incidence and prevalence of gonorrhea and chlamydia among transgender women similar to rates among cisgender MSM. A study using data from the STD Surveillance Network revealed that the proportions of transgender women with extragenital chlamydial or gonococcal infections were similar to those of cisgender MSM.

Providers caring for transgender women should have knowledge of their patients' current anatomy and patterns of sexual behavior before counseling them about STI and HIV prevention. The majority of transgender women have not undergone genital affirmation surgery and therefore might retain a functional penis; in these instances, they might engage in insertive oral, vaginal, or anal sex as well as receptive oral or anal sex. In the U.S. Transgender Survey, 12 percent of transgender women had undergone vaginoplasty surgery, and approximately 50 percent more were considering surgical intervention (see Figure 5.1). Providers should have knowledge about the type of tissue used to construct the neovagina, which can affect future STI and HIV preventive care and screening recommendations. The majority of vaginoplasty surgeries conducted in the United States use penile and scrotal tissue to create the neovagina. Other surgical techniques use intestinal tissue (e.g., sigmoid colon graft) or split-skin grafts. Although these surgeries involve penectomy and orchiectomy, the prostate remains intact. Transgender women who have had a vaginoplasty might engage in receptive vaginal, oral, or anal sex.

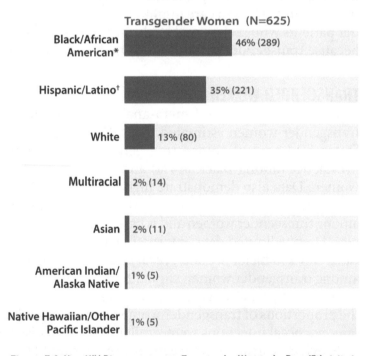

Figure 5.1. New HIV Diagnoses among Transgender Women by Race/Ethnicity in the United States and Dependent Areas, 2019

Centers for Disease Control and Prevention (CDC)
*Black refers to people having origins in any of the Black racial groups of Africa. African American is a term often used for people of African descent with ancestry in North America.
†Hispanic/Latino people can be of any race.

TRANSGENDER MEN

The few studies of HIV prevalence among transgender men indicated that they have a lower prevalence of HIV infection than transgender women. A recent estimate of HIV prevalence among transgender men was 2 percent (see Figure 5.2). However, transgender men who have sex with cisgender men might be at elevated risk for HIV infection. Data are limited regarding STI prevalence among transgender men, and the majority of studies have used clinic-based data or convenience sampling. Recent data from the STD Surveillance Network demonstrated a higher prevalence of gonorrhea and chlamydia among transgender men, similar to rates reported among cisgender MSM.

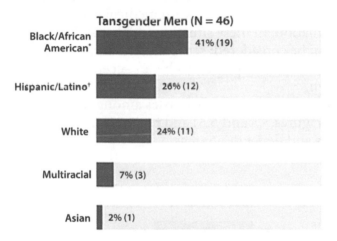

Figure 5.2. New HIV Diagnoses among Transgender Men by Race/Ethnicity in the United States and Dependent Areas, 2019

Centers for Disease Control and Prevention (CDC)
*Black refers to people having origins in any of the Black racial groups of Africa. African American is a term often used for people of African descent with ancestry in North America.
† Hispanic/Latino people can be of any race.

The U.S. Transgender Survey indicated that the proportion of transgender men and gender-diverse persons assigned female sex at birth who have undergone gender affirmation genital surgery is low. Providers should consider the anatomic diversity among transgender men because a person can undergo a metoidioplasty (a procedure to increase the length of the clitoris), with or without urethral lengthening, and might not have a hysterectomy and oophorectomy and therefore be at risk for bacterial STIs, human papillomavirus (HPV), herpes simplex virus (HSV), HIV, and cervical cancer. For transgender men using gender-affirming hormone therapy, the decrease in estradiol levels caused by exogenous testosterone can lead to vaginal atrophy and is associated with a high prevalence of unsatisfactory sample acquisition. The impact of these hormonal changes on mucosal susceptibility to HIV and STIs is unknown.

Transgender men who have not chosen to undergo hysterectomy with the removal of the cervix remain at risk for cervical cancer. These persons often avoid cervical cancer screening because of multiple factors, including discomfort with medical examinations and fear of discrimination. In these situations, high-risk HPV testing using a swab can be considered; self-collected swabs for high-risk HPV testing have been reported to be an acceptable option for transgender men.

The following figures show HIV diagnoses among transgender people by age (see Figures 5.3 and 5.5) and region (see Figure 5.4) in the United States and dependent areas.

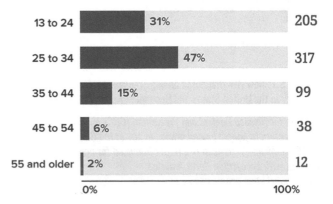

Figure 5.3. New HIV Diagnoses among Transgender People by Age in the United States and Dependent Areas, 2019

Centers for Disease Control and Prevention (CDC)
The total may exceed 100 percent due to rounding.

Sexually Transmitted Diseases in Special Populations

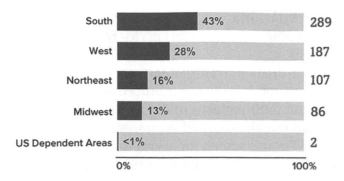

Figure 5.4. New HIV Diagnoses among Transgender People by Region in the United States and Dependent Areas, 2019

Centers for Disease Control and Prevention (CDC)

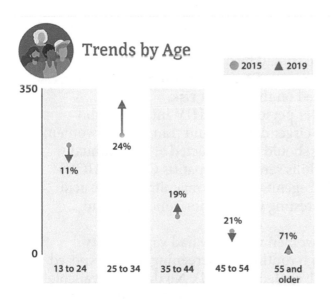

Figure 5.5. HIV Diagnoses among Transgender People in the United States and Dependent Areas, 2015–2019

Centers for Disease Control and Prevention (CDC)

SCREENING RECOMMENDATIONS

The following are screening recommendations for transgender and gender-diverse persons:

- Because of the diversity of transgender persons regarding surgical gender-affirming procedures, hormone use, and their patterns of sexual behavior, providers should remain aware of symptoms consistent with common STIs and screen for asymptomatic infections on the basis of the patient's sexual practices and anatomy.
- Gender-based screening recommendations should be adapted on the basis of anatomy (e.g., routine screening for trachomatis and *Neisseria gonorrhoeae*) as recommended for all sexually active females younger than 25 years of age on an annual basis and should be extended to transgender men and nonbinary persons with a cervix among this age group.
- HIV screening should be discussed and offered to all transgender persons. Frequency of repeat screenings should be based on the level of risk.
- For transgender persons with HIV infection who have sex with cisgender men and transgender women, STI screening should be conducted at least annually, including syphilis serology, hepatitis C virus (HCV) testing, and urogenital and extragenital nucleic acid amplification testing (NAAT) for gonorrhea and chlamydia.
- Transgender women who have had vaginoplasty should undergo routine STI screening for all exposed sites (e.g., oral, anal, or vaginal). No data are available regarding the optimal screening method (urine or vaginal swab) for bacterial STIs of the neovagina. The usual techniques for creating a neovagina do not result in a cervix; therefore, no rationale exists for cervical cancer screening.
- If transgender men have undergone metoidioplasty with urethral lengthening and have not had a

vaginectomy, assessment of genital bacterial STIs should include a cervical swab because a urine specimen will be inadequate for detecting cervical infections.

- Cervical cancer screening for transgender men and nonbinary persons with a cervix should follow current screening guidelines.[5]

Section 5.5 | Sexually Transmitted Diseases in Persons in Correctional Facilities

Multiple studies have demonstrated that persons entering correctional facilities have a high prevalence of sexually transmitted infections (STIs), human immunodeficiency virus (HIV), and viral hepatitis, especially those aged 35 or younger. Risk behaviors for acquiring STIs (e.g., having condomless sex, having multiple sex partners, substance misuse, and engaging in commercial, survival, or coerced sex) are common among incarcerated populations. Before their incarceration, many persons have had limited access to medical care. Other social determinants of health (e.g., insufficient social and economic support or living in communities with high local STI prevalence) are common. Addressing STIs in correctional settings is vital for addressing the overall STI impact among affected populations.

Growing evidence demonstrates the usefulness of expanded STI screening and treatment services in correctional settings, including short-term facilities (jails), long-term institutions (prisons), and juvenile detention centers. For example, in jurisdictions with comprehensive, targeted jail screening, more chlamydial infections among females (and males if screened) are detected and subsequently treated in the correctional setting than in any other single

---

[5] "Transgender and Gender Diverse Persons," Centers for Disease Control and Prevention (CDC), July 22, 2021. Available online. URL: www.cdc.gov/std/treatment-guidelines/trans.htm. Accessed July 7, 2023.

reporting source and might represent the majority of reported cases in certain jurisdictions. Screening in the jail setting has the potential to reach substantially more persons at risk than screening among the prison population alone.

Both males and females aged 35 and younger in juvenile and adult detention facilities have been reported to have higher rates of chlamydia and gonorrhea than nonincarcerated persons in the community. Syphilis seroprevalence rates, which can indicate previously treated or current infection, are considerably higher among incarcerated adult men and women than among adolescents, which are consistent with the overall national syphilis trends. Detection and treatment of early syphilis in correctional facilities might affect rates of transmission among adults and the prevention of congenital syphilis.

In jails, approximately half of the entrants are released back into the community within 48 hours. As a result, treatment completion rates for those screened for STIs and who receive STI diagnoses in short-term facilities might not be optimal. However, because of the mobility of incarcerated populations in and out of the community, the impact of screening in correctional facilities on the prevalence of infections among detainees and subsequent transmission in the community after release might be considerable. Moreover, treatment completion rates of greater than or equal to 95 percent in short-term facilities can be achieved by offering screening at or shortly after intake, thus facilitating earlier receipt of test results, and if needed, follow-up of untreated persons can be conducted through public health outreach.

Universal, opt-out screening for chlamydia and gonorrhea among females aged 35 and younger entering juvenile and adult correctional facilities is recommended. Males younger than 30 years of age entering juvenile and adult correctional facilities should also be screened for chlamydia and gonorrhea. Opt-out screening has the potential to substantially increase the number tested and the number of chlamydia and gonorrhea infections detected. Point-of-care (POC) nucleic acid amplification testing (NAAT) might also be considered if the tests have demonstrated sufficient sensitivity and specificity. Studies have demonstrated a high prevalence of trichomoniasis among incarcerated females.

SCREENING RECOMMENDATIONS
Chlamydia and Gonorrhea
Females aged 35 and younger and males younger than 30 years of age housed in correctional facilities should be screened for chlamydia and gonorrhea. This screening should be conducted at intake and offered as opt-out screening.

Trichomonas
Females aged 35 and younger housed in correctional facilities should be screened for trichomonas. This screening should be conducted at intake and offered as opt-out screening.

Syphilis
Opt-out screening for incarcerated persons should be conducted on the basis of the local area and institutional prevalence of early (primary, secondary, or early latent) infectious syphilis. Correctional facilities should stay apprised of local syphilis prevalence. In short-term facilities, screening at entry might be indicated.

Viral Hepatitis
All persons housed in juvenile and adult correctional facilities should be screened at the entry for hepatitis B and hepatitis C. All persons who are susceptible to hepatitis B virus (HBV) infection should be offered the hepatitis B vaccine, per Advisory Committee on Immunization Practices (ACIP) recommendations (www.cdc.gov/vaccines/hcp/acip-recs/vacc-specific/hepb.html). During outbreaks in the facility or the surrounding community, all unvaccinated persons should be offered the hepatitis A vaccine; regardless of outbreak conditions, all persons who are at risk for hepatitis A virus (HAV) infection or severe disease should be offered the hepatitis A vaccine, per ACIP recommendations (www.cdc.gov/vaccines/hcp/acip-recs/vacc-specific/hepa.html).

Cervical Cancer

Women and transgender men who are housed in correctional facilities should be screened for cervical cancer as for women who are not incarcerated.

Human Immunodeficiency Virus Infection

All persons being housed in juvenile and adult correctional facilities should be screened at entry for HIV infection; screening should be offered as opt-out screening. For those identified as being at risk for HIV infection (e.g., with diagnosed gonorrhea or syphilis or persons who inject drugs) and being released into the community, starting HIV pre-exposure prophylaxis (PrEP; or providing linkage to a community clinic for HIV PrEP) for HIV prevention should be considered. Persons are likely to engage in high-risk activities immediately after release from incarceration. For those identified with HIV infection, treatment should be initiated. Those persons receiving PrEP or HIV treatment should have a linkage to care established before release. Correctional settings should consider implementing other STI prevention approaches, both during incarceration and upon release, which might include educational and behavioral counseling interventions, vaccination (e.g., for human papillomavirus (HPV)), condom distribution, expedited partner therapy (EPT), and PrEP to prevent HIV infection.[6]

---

[6] "Persons in Correctional Facilities," Centers for Disease Control and Prevention (CDC), September 21, 2022. Available online. URL: www.cdc.gov/std/treatment-guidelines/correctional.htm. Accessed May 29, 2023.

Chapter 6 | **Sexually Transmitted Diseases in Racial and Ethnic Minorities**

Health equity is achieved when everyone has an equal chance to be healthy regardless of their background. This includes a person's race, ethnicity, income, gender, religion, sexual identity, and disability.

Research shows that there are higher rates of sexually transmitted diseases (STDs) among some racial or ethnic minority groups than among Whites. It is important to understand that these higher rates are not caused by ethnicity or heritage but by social conditions that are more likely to affect minority groups. Factors such as poverty, large gaps between the rich and the poor, fewer jobs, and low education levels can make it more difficult for people to stay sexually healthy.

- People who cannot afford basic needs may have trouble accessing quality sexual health services.
- Many racial/ethnic minorities may distrust the health-care system, fearing discrimination from doctors and other health-care providers. This could create negative feelings around getting tested and treated for STDs.
- In communities with higher STD rates, sexually active people may be more likely to get an STD because they have greater odds of selecting a partner who is infected.[1]

---

[1] "STD Health Equity," Centers for Disease Control and Prevention (CDC), March 2, 2020. Available online. URL: www.cdc.gov/std/health-disparities/default.htm. Accessed July 10, 2023.

DISPARITIES IN SEXUALLY TRANSMITTED DISEASES

Disparities continue to persist in rates of reported STDs among some racial minority or Hispanic ethnicity groups when compared with rates among non-Hispanic White persons. In 2021, 31 percent of all cases of chlamydia (Figure 6.1), gonorrhea (Figure 6.2), primary and secondary (P&S) syphilis (Figure 6.3), and congenital syphilis (Figure 6.4) were among non-Hispanic Black persons, even though they made up only approximately 12 percent of the U.S. population. Although American Indian or Alaska Native persons contributed only 0.7 percent of all live births in the United States, they made up 3.6 percent of all congenital syphilis cases.

It is important to note that these disparities are unlikely explained by differences in sexual behavior and rather reflect differential access to quality sexual health care, as well as differences in sexual network characteristics. For example, in communities with higher prevalence of STDs, with each sexual encounter, people face a greater chance of encountering an infected partner than those in lower-prevalence settings, regardless of similar sexual behavior patterns. Acknowledging inequities in STD rates is a critical first step toward empowering affected groups and the public health community to collaborate in addressing systemic inequities in the burden of disease—with the ultimate goal of minimizing the health impacts of STDs on individuals and populations.[2]

---

[2] "National Overview of STDs, 2021," Centers for Disease Control and Prevention (CDC), May 16, 2023. Available online. URL: www.cdc.gov/std/statistics/2021/overview.htm. Accessed July 10, 2023.

Sexually Transmitted Diseases in Racial and Ethnic Minorities

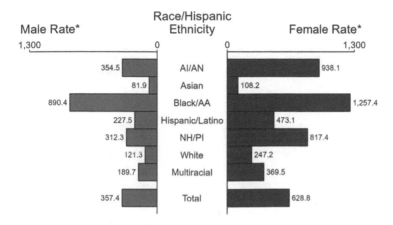

Figure 6.1. Chlamydia: Rates of Reported Cases by Race/Hispanic Ethnicity and Sex, United States, 2021

Centers for Disease Control and Prevention (CDC)
*Per 100,000
Abbreviations: *AI/AN = American Indian or Alaska Native, Black/AA = Black or African American, and NH/PI = Native Hawaiian or other Pacific Islander*
Note: *Total includes all cases including those with unknown race/Hispanic ethnicity.*

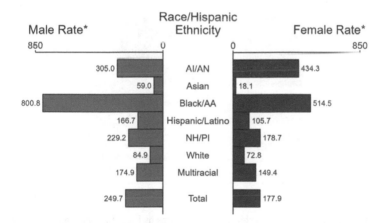

Figure 6.2. Gonorrhea: Rate of Reported Cases by Race/Hispanic Ethnicity and Sex, United States, 2021

Centers for Disease Control and Prevention (CDC)
*Per 100,000
Abbreviations: *AI/AN = American Indian or Alaska Native, Black/AA = Black or African American, and NH/PI = Native Hawaiian or other Pacific Islander*
Note: *Total includes all cases including those with unknown race/Hispanic ethnicity.*

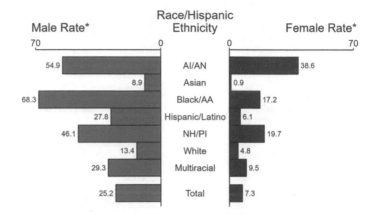

Figure 6.3. Primary and Secondary Syphilis: Rates of Reported Cases by Race/ Hispanic Ethnicity and Sex, United States, 2021

Centers for Disease Control and Prevention (CDC)
*Per 100,000
***Abbreviations**: AI/AN = American Indian or Alaska Native, Black/AA = Black or African American, and NH/PI = Native Hawaiian or other Pacific Islander*
***Note**: Total includes all cases including those with unknown race/Hispanic ethnicity.*

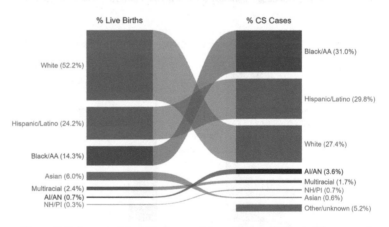

Figure 6.4. Congenital Syphilis: Reported Cases by Race/Hispanic Ethnicity of the Mother, United States, 2021

Centers for Disease Control and Prevention (CDC)
***Note**: In 2021, a total of 149 congenital syphilis cases (5.2%) had missing, unknown, or other race and were not reported to be of Hispanic ethnicity. These cases are included in the "other/unknown" category.*
***Abbreviations**: AI/AN = American Indian or Alaska Native, Black/AA = Black or African American, and NH/PI = Native Hawaiian or other Pacific Islander*

WHAT IS THE IMPACT OF HUMAN IMMUNODEFICIENCY VIRUS ON RACIAL AND ETHNIC MINORITIES IN THE UNITED STATES?

Human immunodeficiency virus can affect anyone regardless of sexual orientation, race, ethnicity, gender, age, or where they live. However, in the United States, some racial/ethnic groups are more affected than others, compared to their percentage of the population. This is because some population groups have higher rates of HIV in their communities, thus raising the risk of new infections with each sexual or injection drug use encounter. Additionally, a range of social, economic, and demographic factors, such as stigma, discrimination, income, education, and geographic region, can affect people's risk for HIV as well as their HIV-related outcomes.

Black/African American and Hispanic/Latinx communities are disproportionately affected by HIV compared to other racial/ethnic groups. For example, in 2019, Blacks/African Americans represented 13 percent of the U.S. population but 40 percent of people with HIV. Hispanics/Latinx represented 18.5 percent of the population but 25 percent of people with HIV.

The disproportionate impact of HIV on Black/African American and Hispanic/Latinx communities is also evident in incidence (new HIV infections), showing that effective prevention and treatment are not adequately reaching people who could benefit most.

Certain subpopulations within racial and ethnic minority groups are disproportionately affected as well. For example, gay, bisexual, and other men who have sex with men (MSM) are by far the most affected group in the United States. They account for about 66 percent of new infections each year, even though they make up only 2 percent of the population, with the highest burden among Black and Latinx gay and bisexual men. According to the Centers for Disease Control and Prevention (CDC), in 2019, 26 percent of new HIV infections were among Black gay and bisexual men; 23 percent were among Latinx gay and bisexual men; and 45 percent among gay and bisexual men under the age of 35.

Among women, disparities also exist. Black women are disproportionately affected by HIV as compared to women of other races/ethnicities. Although annual HIV infections remained stable overall among Black women from 2015 to 2019, the rate of new HIV infections among Black women is 11 times that of White women and four times that of Latina women.

Furthermore, over 1 million people identify as transgender in the United States. In 2019, adult and adolescent transgender people composed 2 percent (669) of new HIV diagnoses in the United States and dependent areas. Most of those new HIV diagnoses were among Black/African American transgender women.[3]

[3] HIV.gov, "Impact on Racial and Ethnic Minorities," U.S. Department of Health and Human Services (HHS), January 20, 2023. Available online. URL: www.hiv.gov/hiv-basics/overview/data-and-trends/impact-on-racial-and-ethnic-minorities. Accessed July 10, 2023.

Part 2 | **Types of Sexually Transmitted Diseases**

Chapter 7 | **Chancroid**

Chancroid is a bacterial infection that is spread through sexual contact. It is caused by a type of bacteria called "*Haemophilus ducreyi.*" Chancroid is characterized by a small bump on the genital that becomes a painful ulcer. Men may have just one ulcer, but women often develop four or more. About half of the people who are infected with chancroid will develop enlarged inguinal lymph nodes, the nodes located in the fold between the leg and the lower abdomen. In some cases, the nodes will break through the skin and cause draining abscesses. The swollen lymph nodes and abscesses are often called "buboes."[1]

CLINICAL PRESENTATION

Chancroid is caused by the bacterium *H. ducreyi* and results in painful, superficial ulcers, often with regional lymphadenopathy. Chancroid occurs in Asia, Africa, and the Caribbean and is an important cofactor of human immunodeficiency virus (HIV) transmission. The genital ulcer from chancroid is painful, tender, and nonindurated. Symptoms usually occur 4–10 days after exposure. The lesion at the site of infection is, initially, a pustule that breaks down to form a painful, soft ulcer with a necrotic base and irregular borders. Multiple lesions and inguinal adenopathy often develop. With lymph node involvement, fever, chills, and malaise may also develop. Other symptoms of chancroid include painful urination, vaginal discharge, rectal bleeding, pain with bowel movements, and dyspareunia.

---

[1] Genetic and Rare Diseases Information Center (GARD), "Chancroid," National Center for Advancing Translational Sciences (NCATS), February 2023. Available online. URL: https://rarediseases.info.nih.gov/diseases/9522/chancroid. Accessed May 29, 2023.

DIAGNOSTIC TESTING

The combination of a painful genital ulcer and tender suppurative inguinal adenopathy suggests the diagnosis of chancroid. A probable diagnosis of chancroid can be made if:

- one or more painful genital ulcers are present (Regional lymphadenopathy is also typical.)
- no evidence of *Treponema pallidum* infection is found by darkfield examination of ulcer exudate or by syphilis serologic testing performed at least seven days after onset of ulcers
- test for herpes simplex virus (HSV) performed on the ulcer exudate is negative

A definitive diagnosis of chancroid requires the identification of *H. ducreyi* on special culture media. However, culture media for chancroid are not widely available. Nucleic acid amplification tests (NAATs) can be performed in clinical laboratories that have developed their own tests.[2]

DIAGNOSTIC CONSIDERATIONS

A definitive diagnosis of chancroid requires identifying *H. ducreyi* on special culture media that is not widely available from commercial sources; even when these media are used, sensitivity is less than 80 percent. There is no NAAT approved by the U.S. Food and Drug Administration (FDA) for *H. ducreyi* available in the United States; however, such testing can be performed by clinical laboratories that have developed their own NAAT and have conducted Clinical Laboratory Improvement Amendments (CLIA) verification studies on genital specimens.

The combination of one or more deep and painful genital ulcers and tender suppurative inguinal adenopathy indicates the chancroid diagnosis; inguinal lymphadenitis typically occurs in less than 50 percent of cases. For both clinical and surveillance purposes, a

[2] "Chancroid," Centers for Disease Control and Prevention (CDC), April 6, 2017. Available online. URL: www.cdc.gov/immigrantrefugeehealth/guidelines/domestic/sexually-transmitted-diseases/chancroid.html. Accessed May 29, 2023.

probable diagnosis of chancroid can be made if all of the following four criteria are met:
- The patient has one or more painful genital ulcers.
- The clinical presentation, the appearance of genital ulcers, and, if present, regional lymphadenopathy are typical for chancroid.
- The patient has no evidence of *T. pallidum* infection by darkfield examination or NAAT (i.e., ulcer exudate or serous fluid) or by serologic tests for syphilis performed at least 7–14 days after the onset of ulcers.
- Herpes simplex virus type 1 (HSV-1) or herpes simplex virus type 2 (HSV-2) NAAT or HSV culture performed on the ulcer exudate or fluid is negative.

TREATMENT

Successful antimicrobial treatment for chancroid cures the infection, resolves the clinical symptoms, and prevents transmission to others. In advanced cases, genital scarring and rectal or urogenital fistulas from suppurative buboes can result despite successful therapy.

Recommended Regimens

One of the following regimens can be used:
- azithromycin: 1 g orally in a single dose
- ceftriaxone: 250 mg intramuscular (IM) in a single dose
- ciprofloxacin: 500 mg orally two times a day for three days
- erythromycin base: 500 mg orally three times a day for seven days

Azithromycin and ceftriaxone offer the advantage of single-dose therapy. Worldwide, several isolates with intermediate resistance to either ciprofloxacin or erythromycin have been reported. However, because cultures are not routinely performed and chancroid is uncommon, data are limited regarding the prevalence of *H. ducreyi* antimicrobial resistance.

OTHER MANAGEMENT CONSIDERATIONS

Men who are uncircumcised and persons with HIV infection do not respond as well to treatment as persons who are circumcised or are HIV-negative. Patients should be tested for HIV at the time chancroid is diagnosed. If the initial HIV test results are negative, the provider can consider the benefits of offering more frequent testing and HIV pre-exposure prophylaxis (PrEP) to persons at increased risk for HIV infection.

FOLLOW-UP

Patients should be reexamined three to seven days after therapy initiation. If treatment is successful, ulcers usually improve symptomatically within three days and objectively within seven days after therapy. If no clinical improvement is evident, the clinician should consider whether the diagnosis is correct, another sexually transmitted infection (STI) is present, the patient has HIV infection, the treatment was not used as instructed, or the *H. ducreyi* strain causing the infection is resistant to the prescribed antimicrobial. The time required for complete healing depends on the size of the ulcer; large ulcers might require more than two weeks. In addition, healing can be slower for uncircumcised men who have ulcers under the foreskin. Clinical resolution of fluctuant lymphadenopathy is slower than that of ulcers and might require needle aspiration or incision and drainage despite otherwise successful therapy. Although needle aspiration of buboes is a simpler procedure, incision and drainage might be preferred because of the reduced need for subsequent drainage procedures.

MANAGEMENT OF SEX PARTNERS

Regardless of whether disease symptoms are present, sex partners of patients with chancroid should be examined and treated if they had sexual contact with the patient during the 10 days preceding the patient's symptom onset.

SPECIAL CONSIDERATIONS
Pregnancy
Data indicate ciprofloxacin presents a low risk to the fetus during pregnancy but has the potential for toxicity during breastfeeding. Alternative drugs should be used if the patient is pregnant or lactating. No adverse effects of chancroid on pregnancy outcomes have been reported.

Human Immunodeficiency Virus Infection
Persons with HIV infection who have chancroid infection should be monitored closely because they are more likely to experience chancroid treatment failure and to have ulcers that heal slowly. Persons with HIV might require repeated or longer courses of therapy, and treatment failures can occur with any regimen. Data are limited concerning the therapeutic efficacy of the recommended single-dose azithromycin and ceftriaxone regimens among persons with HIV infection.

Children
Because sexual contact is the major primary transmission route among U.S. patients, diagnosis of chancroid ulcers among infants and children, especially in the genital or perineal region, is highly suspicious of sexual abuse. However, *H. ducreyi* is recognized as a major cause of nonsexually transmitted cutaneous ulcers among children in tropical regions and, specifically, countries where yaws (a chronic skin infection caused by the bacterium *T. pallidum* subspecies *pertenue*, which belongs to the same group of bacteria that causes venereal syphilis) is endemic. Acquisition of a lower-extremity ulcer attributable to *H. ducreyi* in a child without genital ulcers and reported travel to a region where yaws is endemic should not be considered evidence of sexual abuse.[3]

---

[3] "Chancroid," Centers for Disease Control and Prevention (CDC), July 22, 2021. Available online. URL: www.cdc.gov/std/treatment-guidelines/chancroid.htm. Accessed May 29, 2023.

Chapter 8 | **Chlamydia**

WHAT IS CHLAMYDIA?

Chlamydia is a common sexually transmitted disease (STD) that can cause infection among both men and women. It can cause permanent damage to a woman's reproductive system. This can make it difficult or impossible to get pregnant later. Chlamydia can also cause a potentially fatal ectopic pregnancy (pregnancy that occurs outside the womb).

HOW IS CHLAMYDIA SPREAD?

You can get chlamydia by having vaginal, anal, or oral sex with someone who has chlamydia. Also, you can still get chlamydia even if your sex partner does not ejaculate (cum). A pregnant person with chlamydia can give the infection to their baby during childbirth.

HOW CAN YOU REDUCE YOUR RISK OF GETTING CHLAMYDIA?

The only way to completely avoid STDs is to avoid vaginal, anal, or oral sex.

If you are sexually active, the following things can lower your chances of getting chlamydia:
- being in a long-term, mutually monogamous relationship with a partner who has been tested and does not have chlamydia
- using condoms the right way every time you have sex

ARE YOU AT RISK FOR CHLAMYDIA?

Sexually active people can get chlamydia through vaginal, anal, or oral sex without a condom with a partner who has chlamydia.

Sexually active young people are at a higher risk of getting chlamydia. This is due to behaviors and biological factors common among young people. Gay and bisexual men are also at risk since chlamydia can spread through oral and anal sex.

If you are sexually active, have an honest and open talk with your health-care provider. Ask them if you should get tested for chlamydia or other STDs. Gay or bisexual men and pregnant women should also get tested for chlamydia. If you are a sexually active woman, you should get tested for chlamydia every year if you are:

- younger than 25 years old
- twenty-five years and older with risk factors, such as new or multiple sex partners or a sex partner who has a sexually transmitted infection (STI)

IF YOU ARE PREGNANT, HOW DOES CHLAMYDIA AFFECT YOUR BABY?

If you are pregnant and have chlamydia, you can give the infection to your baby during delivery. This can cause an eye infection or pneumonia in your baby. Having chlamydia may also make it more likely to deliver your baby early.

If you are pregnant, you should receive testing for chlamydia at your first prenatal visit. Talk to your health-care provider about getting the correct examination, testing, and treatment. Testing and treatment are the best ways to prevent health problems.

HOW DO YOU KNOW IF YOU HAVE CHLAMYDIA?

Chlamydia often has no symptoms, but it can cause serious health problems, even without symptoms. If symptoms occur, they may not appear until several weeks after having sex with a partner who has chlamydia.

Even when chlamydia has no symptoms, it can damage a woman's reproductive system. Women with symptoms may notice:

- an abnormal vaginal discharge
- a burning sensation when peeing

Symptoms in men can include:
- a discharge from their penis
- a burning sensation when peeing
- pain and swelling in one or both testicles (although this is less common)

Men and women can also get chlamydia in their rectum. This happens either by having receptive anal sex or by spreading from another infected site (such as the vagina). While these infections often cause no symptoms, they can cause:
- rectal pain
- discharge
- bleeding

See a health-care provider if you notice any of the following symptoms. You should also see a provider if your partner has an STD or symptoms of one. Symptoms can include:
- an unusual sore
- a smelly discharge
- burning when peeing
- bleeding between periods

HOW WILL YOUR HEALTH-CARE PROVIDER KNOW IF YOU HAVE CHLAMYDIA?

Laboratory tests can diagnose chlamydia. Your health-care provider may ask you to provide a urine sample for testing, or they might use (or ask you to use) a cotton swab to get a vaginal sample.

IS THERE A CURE FOR CHLAMYDIA?

Yes, the right treatment can cure chlamydia. It is important that you take all of the medicine your health-care provider gives you to cure your infection. Do not share medicine for chlamydia with anyone. When taken properly, it will stop the infection and could decrease your chances of having problems later. Although medicine will stop the infection, it will not undo any permanent damage caused by the disease.

Repeat infection with chlamydia is common. You should receive testing again about three months after your treatment, even if your sex partner receives treatment.

WHEN CAN YOU HAVE SEX AGAIN AFTER YOUR CHLAMYDIA TREATMENT?

You should not have sex again until you and your sex partner(s) complete treatment. If given a single dose of medicine, you should wait seven days after taking the medicine before having sex. If given medicine to take for seven days, wait until you finish all the doses before having sex.

If you have had chlamydia and took medicine in the past, you can still get it again. This can happen if you have sex without a condom with a person who has chlamydia.

WHAT HAPPENS IF YOU DO NOT GET TREATED?

The initial damage that chlamydia causes often goes unnoticed. However, chlamydia can lead to serious health problems.

In women, untreated chlamydia can cause pelvic inflammatory disease (PID). Some of the complications of PID are as follows:

- formation of scar tissue that blocks fallopian tubes
- ectopic pregnancy (pregnancy outside the womb)
- infertility (not being able to get pregnant)
- long-term pelvic/abdominal pain

Men rarely have health problems from chlamydia. The infection can cause a fever and pain in the tubes attached to the testicles. This can, in rare cases, lead to infertility.

Untreated chlamydia may also increase your chances of getting or giving human immunodeficiency virus (HIV).[1]

HOW COMMON IS CHLAMYDIA?

The Centers for Disease Control and Prevention (CDC) estimates that there were 4 million chlamydial infections in 2018. Chlamydia

---

[1] "Chlamydia," Centers for Disease Control and Prevention (CDC), April 12, 2022. Available online. URL: www.cdc.gov/std/chlamydia/stdfact-chlamydia.htm. Accessed May 29, 2023.

is also the most frequently reported bacterial STI in the United States. It is difficult to account for many cases of chlamydia. Most people with the infection have no symptoms and do not seek testing. Chlamydia is most common among young people. Two-thirds of new chlamydial infections occur among youth aged 15–24 years. Estimates show that 1 in 20 sexually active young women aged 14–24 years has chlamydia.

Disparities persist among racial and ethnic minority groups. In 2021, chlamydia rates for African Americans/Blacks were six times that of Whites. Chlamydia is also common among men who have sex with men (MSM). Among MSM screened for rectal chlamydial infection, positivity ranges from 3.0 to 10.5 percent. Among MSM screened for pharyngeal chlamydial infection, positivity ranges from 0.5 to 2.3 percent.

CHLAMYDIA AND HUMAN IMMUNODEFICIENCY VIRUS
Untreated chlamydia may increase a person's chances of getting or transmitting HIV.

WHO SHOULD TEST FOR CHLAMYDIA?
Anyone with the following genital symptoms should not have sex until they see a health-care provider:
- a discharge
- a burning sensation when peeing
- unusual sores or a rash

Anyone having oral, anal, or vaginal sex with a partner recently diagnosed with an STD should see a health-care provider.

Because chlamydia usually has no symptoms, screening is necessary to identify most infections. Screening programs can reduce rates of adverse sequelae in women. The CDC recommends yearly chlamydia screening of all sexually active women younger than 25. The CDC also recommends screening for older women with risk factors, such as new or multiple partners or a sex partner who has an STI. Women who are sexually active should discuss their risk factors with a health-care provider to determine if more frequent screening is necessary.

Routine screening is not necessary for men. However, consider screening sexually active young men in clinical settings with a high prevalence of chlamydia. This can include adolescent clinics, correctional facilities, and STD clinics. Consider this when resources permit and do not hinder screening efforts in women.

Screen sexually active MSM who have insertive intercourse for urethral chlamydial infection. Also, screen MSM who have receptive anal intercourse for rectal infection at least yearly. Screening for pharyngeal infection is not recommended. MSM, including those with HIV, should receive more frequent chlamydia screening at three- to six-month intervals if risk behaviors persist or if they or their sexual partners have multiple partners.

At the initial HIV care visit, providers should test all sexually active people for chlamydia. Test at least each year during HIV care. A patient's health-care provider might determine more frequent screening is necessary based on the patient's risk factors.

HOW IS CHLAMYDIA DIAGNOSED?

Diagnose chlamydia with nucleic acid amplification tests (NAATs), cell culture, and other types of tests. NAATs are the most sensitive tests to use on easy-to-obtain specimens. These include vaginal swabs (either clinician- or patient-collected) or urine.

To diagnose genital chlamydia in women using an NAAT, vaginal swabs are the optimal specimen. Urine is the specimen of choice for men. Urine is an effective alternative specimen type for women. Self-collected vaginal swab specimens perform as well as other approved specimens using NAATs. Patients may prefer self-collected vaginal swabs or urine-based screening to more invasive specimen collection. Adolescent girls may be good candidates for self-collected vaginal swab- or urine-based screening.

Diagnose rectal or pharyngeal infection by testing at the anatomic exposure site. While useful for these specimens, culture is not widely available. Additionally, NAATs have better sensitivity and specificity compared with culture for detecting *Chlamydia trachomatis* at nongenital sites. Most tests, including NAATs, are not approved by the U.S. Food and Drug Administration (FDA) for use with rectal or pharyngeal swab specimens. NAATs have better sensitivity and specificity compared with culture for the detection of *C. trachomatis* at rectal sites. However, some laboratories have met set requirements and have validated NAATs on rectal and pharyngeal swab specimens.

NOTIFYING PARTNERS

People treated for chlamydia should tell their recent sex partners, so the partner can see a health-care provider. Recent partners include anyone the patient had anal, vaginal, or oral sex within the 60 days before symptom onset or diagnosis. This will help protect the partner from health problems and prevent reinfection.

Patients treated with single-dose antibiotics should not have sex for seven days. Patients treated with a seven-day course of antibiotics should not have sex until they complete treatment and their symptoms go away.

In some states, health-care providers may give people with chlamydia extra medicine or prescriptions to give to their sex partner(s). This is called "expedited partner therapy" (EPT). Clinical trials comparing EPT to asking the patient to refer their partners in for treatment find that EPT leads to fewer reinfections in the index patient and more partner treatment. EPT is another strategy providers use to manage the partners of people with chlamydial infection. Partners should still seek medical care, regardless of whether they receive EPT.

HOW CAN CHLAMYDIA BE PREVENTED?

Condoms, when used correctly every time someone has sex, can reduce the risk of getting or giving chlamydia. The only way to completely avoid chlamydia is to not have vaginal, anal, and oral sex. Another option is being in a long-term, mutually monogamous relationship with a partner who has been tested and does not have chlamydia.[2]

---

[2] "Chlamydia," Centers for Disease Control and Prevention (CDC), April 11, 2023. Available online. URL: www.cdc.gov/std/chlamydia/stdfact-chlamydia-detailed.htm. Accessed May 29, 2023.

Chapter 9 | **Donovanosis**

Granuloma inguinale (donovanosis) is a genital ulcerative disease caused by the intracellular Gram-negative bacterium *Klebsiella granulomatis* (formerly known as "*Calymmatobacterium granulomatis*"). The disease rarely occurs in the United States; however, sporadic cases have been described in India, South Africa, and South America. Although granuloma inguinale was previously endemic in Australia, it is now extremely rare. Clinically, the disease is characterized as painless, slowly progressive ulcerative lesions on the genitals or perineum without regional lymphadenopathy; subcutaneous granulomas (pseudobuboes) might also occur. The lesions are highly vascular (i.e., beefy red appearance) and can bleed. Extragenital infection can occur with infection extension to the pelvis, or it can disseminate to intra-abdominal organs, bones, or the mouth. The lesions can also develop secondary bacterial infection and can coexist with other sexually transmitted pathogens.

DIAGNOSTIC CONSIDERATIONS

The causative organism of granuloma inguinale is difficult to culture, and diagnosis requires visualization of dark-staining Donovan bodies on tissue crush preparation or biopsy. Although there is no molecular test for the detection of *K. granulomatis* deoxyribonucleic acid (DNA) approved by the U.S. Food and Drug Administration (FDA), molecular assays might be useful for identifying the causative agent.

TREATMENT FOR DONOVANOSIS

Multiple antimicrobial regimens have been effective; however, only a limited number of controlled trials have been published. Treatment has been reported to halt the progression of lesions, and healing typically proceeds inward from the ulcer margins. Prolonged therapy is usually required to permit granulation and reepithelialization of the ulcers. Relapse can occur 6–18 months after apparently effective therapy.

Recommended Regimen

The following regimen can be used:
- azithromycin: 1 g orally once weekly or 500 mg daily for more than three weeks and until all lesions have completely healed

Alternative Regimens

One of the following regimens can be used:
- doxycycline: 100 mg orally two times a day for at least three weeks and until all lesions have completely healed
- erythromycin base: 500 mg orally four times a day for more than three weeks and until all lesions have completely healed
- trimethoprim-sulfamethoxazole: one double-strength (160 mg/800 mg) tablet orally two times a day for more than three weeks and until all lesions have completely healed

The addition of another antibiotic to these regimens can be considered if improvement is not evident within the first few days of therapy.

OTHER MANAGEMENT CONSIDERATIONS

Patients should be followed clinically until signs and symptoms have resolved. All persons who receive a diagnosis of granuloma inguinale should be tested for human immunodeficiency virus (HIV).

FOLLOW-UP
Patients should be followed clinically until signs and symptoms resolve.

MANAGEMENT OF SEX PARTNERS
Persons who have had sexual contact with a patient who has granuloma inguinale within the 60 days before the onset of the patient's symptoms should be examined and offered therapy. However, the value of empiric therapy in the absence of clinical signs and symptoms has not been established.

SPECIAL CONSIDERATIONS
Pregnancy
The use of doxycycline in pregnancy might be associated with discoloration of teeth; however, the risk is not well-defined. Doxycycline is compatible with breastfeeding. Sulfonamides can be associated with neonatal kernicterus among those with glucose-6-phosphate dehydrogenase deficiency and should be avoided during the third trimester and while breastfeeding. For these reasons, pregnant and lactating women with granuloma inguinale should be treated with a macrolide regimen (erythromycin or azithromycin).

Human Immunodeficiency Virus Infection
Persons with granuloma inguinale and HIV infection should receive the same regimens as those who do not have HIV.[1]

---

[1] "Granuloma Inguinale (Donovanosis)," Centers for Disease Control and Prevention (CDC), July 22, 2021. Available online. URL: www.cdc.gov/std/treatment-guidelines/donovanosis.htm. Accessed May 30, 2023

Chapter 10 | Gonorrhea

WHAT IS GONORRHEA?

Gonorrhea is a sexually transmitted disease (STD) caused by infection with the *Neisseria gonorrhoeae* bacterium. *N. gonorrhoeae* infects the mucous membranes of the reproductive tract, including the cervix, uterus, and fallopian tubes in women and the urethra in women and men. *N. gonorrhoeae* can also infect the mucous membranes of the mouth, throat, eyes, and rectum.

HOW COMMON IS GONORRHEA?

Gonorrhea is a very common infectious disease. As per Sexually Transmitted Disease Surveillance 2021, a total of 710,151 cases of gonorrhea were reported to the Centers for Disease Control and Prevention (CDC), making it the second most common notifiable sexually transmitted infection (STI) in the United States. Rates of reported gonorrhea have increased 118 percent since their historic low in 2009. During 2020–2021, the overall rate of reported gonorrhea increased by 4.6 percent. During 2020–2021, rates increased among both males and females, in three regions of the United States (West, Northeast, and South), among most age groups, and among most racial/Hispanic ethnicity groups. However, many infections are asymptomatic, so reported cases only capture a fraction of the true burden.

HOW DO PEOPLE GET GONORRHEA?

Gonorrhea is transmitted through sexual contact with the penis, vagina, mouth, or anus of an infected partner. Ejaculation does not have to occur for gonorrhea to be transmitted or acquired.

Gonorrhea can also be spread perinatally from the mother to the baby during childbirth.

People who have had gonorrhea and received treatment may be reinfected if they have sexual contact with a person infected with gonorrhea.

ARE YOU AT RISK FOR GONORRHEA?
Any sexually active person can be infected with gonorrhea. In the United States, the highest reported rates of infection are among sexually active teenagers, young adults, and African Americans.

WHAT ARE THE SIGNS AND SYMPTOMS OF GONORRHEA?
Many men with gonorrhea are asymptomatic. When present, signs and symptoms of urethral infection in men include dysuria or a white, yellow, or green urethral discharge that usually appears 1–14 days after infection. In cases where urethral infection is complicated by epididymitis, men with gonorrhea may also complain of testicular or scrotal pain.

Most women with gonorrhea are asymptomatic. Even when a woman has symptoms, they are often so mild and nonspecific that they are mistaken for a bladder or vaginal infection. The initial symptoms and signs in women include dysuria, increased vaginal discharge, or vaginal bleeding between periods. Women with gonorrhea are at risk of developing serious complications from the infection, regardless of the presence or severity of symptoms.

Symptoms of rectal infection in both men and women may include discharge, anal itching, soreness, bleeding, or painful bowel movements. Rectal infection may also be asymptomatic. Pharyngeal infection may cause a sore throat but usually is asymptomatic.

WHAT ARE THE COMPLICATIONS OF GONORRHEA?
Untreated gonorrhea can cause serious and permanent health problems in both women and men.

In women, gonorrhea can spread into the uterus or fallopian tubes and cause pelvic inflammatory disease (PID). The symptoms may be quite mild or can be very severe and can include abdominal pain and fever. PID can lead to internal abscesses and chronic pelvic pain. PID can also damage the fallopian tubes enough to cause infertility or increase the risk of ectopic pregnancy.

In men, gonorrhea may be complicated by epididymitis. In rare cases, this may lead to infertility.

If left untreated, gonorrhea can also spread to the blood and cause disseminated gonococcal infection (DGI). DGI is usually characterized by arthritis, tenosynovitis, and/or dermatitis. This condition can be life-threatening.

GONORRHEA AND HUMAN IMMUNODEFICIENCY VIRUS

Untreated gonorrhea can increase a person's risk of acquiring or transmitting human immunodeficiency virus (HIV), the virus that causes acquired immunodeficiency syndrome (AIDS).[1]

HOW DOES GONORRHEA AFFECT PREGNANCY?

For pregnant women, untreated gonorrhea raises the risk of:
- miscarriage
- premature birth—babies born before 37 weeks of pregnancy (Premature birth is the most common cause of infant death and can lead to long-term health and developmental problems in children.)
- low birth weight
- water breaking too early (This can lead to premature birth.)

Babies born to infected mothers are at risk of:
- blindness (Treating the newborn's eyes with medicine right after birth can prevent eye infection. The U.S. Preventive Services Task Force (USPSTF) strongly recommends—and most states require by law—that all babies be treated with medicated eye ointments soon after birth.)

---

[1] "Gonorrhea," Centers for Disease Control and Prevention (CDC), April 11, 2023. Available online. URL: www.cdc.gov/std/gonorrhea/stdfact-gonorrhea-detailed.htm. Accessed June 2, 2023.

- joint infection
- life-threatening blood infection

Treatment of gonorrhea as soon as it is found in pregnant women will lower the risk of these problems for both the mother and the baby. Your baby will get antibiotics if you have gonorrhea or if your baby has a gonorrheal eye infection.[2]

WHO SHOULD BE TESTED FOR GONORRHEA?

Any sexually active person can be infected with gonorrhea. Anyone with genital symptoms such as discharge, burning during urination, unusual sores, or rash should stop having sex and see a health-care provider immediately.

Also, anyone with an oral, anal, or vaginal sex partner who has been recently diagnosed with an STD should see a health-care provider for evaluation.

Some people should be tested (screened) for gonorrhea even if they do not have symptoms or know of a sex partner who has gonorrhea. Anyone who is sexually active should discuss his or her risk factors with a health-care provider and ask whether he or she should be tested for gonorrhea or other STDs.

The CDC recommends yearly gonorrhea screening for all sexually active women younger than 25 years, as well as older women with risk factors such as new or multiple sex partners or a sex partner who has an STI.

People who have gonorrhea should also be tested for other STDs.[3]

- If you are 24 or younger and have sex, you need to get tested for gonorrhea. Gonorrhea is most common in women between the ages of 15 and 24. You need to get tested if you have had any symptoms of gonorrhea since your last negative test result or if your sex partner has gonorrhea.

---

[2] Office on Women's Health (OWH), "Gonorrhea," U.S. Department of Health and Human Services (HHS), February 22, 2021. Available online. URL: www.womenshealth.gov/a-z-topics/gonorrhea. Accessed June 2, 2023.
[3] See footnote [1].

- If you are older than 24, you need to get tested if, in the past year or since your last test, you:
  - had a new sex partner
  - had your sex partner tell you they have gonorrhea
  - have had gonorrhea or another STI in the past
  - traded sex for money or drugs in the past
  - do not use condoms during sex and are in a relationship that is not monogamous, meaning you or your partner has sex with other people

You also need to get tested if you have any symptoms of gonorrhea.

Testing is very important because women with untreated gonorrhea can develop serious health problems. If you are tested for gonorrhea, you also need to get tested for other STIs, including chlamydia, syphilis, and HIV.

HOW IS GONORRHEA DIAGNOSED?

The following are the two ways that a doctor or nurse tests for gonorrhea:

- **A urine test**. This is the most common. You urinate (pee) into a cup. Your urine is then tested for gonorrhea.
- **A swab test**. Your doctor or nurse uses a cotton swab to take a fluid sample from an infected place (cervix, rectum, or throat). The fluid is then tested for gonorrhea.

A Pap test is not used to detect gonorrhea.[4]

Urogenital gonorrhea can be diagnosed by testing urine, urethral (for men), or endocervical or vaginal (for women) specimens using a nucleic acid amplification test (NAAT). It can also be diagnosed using gonorrhea culture, which requires endocervical or urethral swab specimens.

Rectal and oral diagnostic tests for gonorrhea cleared by the U.S. Food and Drug Administration (FDA; as well as chlamydia) have been validated for clinical use.

---

[4] See footnote [2].

WHAT IS THE TREATMENT FOR GONORRHEA?

Gonorrhea can be cured with the right treatment. The CDC now recommends a single 500 mg intramuscular dose of ceftriaxone for the treatment of gonorrhea. Alternative regimens are available when ceftriaxone cannot be used to treat urogenital or rectal gonorrhea. Although medication will stop the infection, it will not repair any permanent damage done by the disease. Antimicrobial resistance in gonorrhea is of increasing concern, and successful treatment of gonorrhea is becoming more difficult. A test of cure—follow-up testing to be sure the infection was treated successfully—is not needed for genital and rectal infections; however, if a person's symptoms continue for more than a few days after receiving treatment, he or she should return to a health-care provider to be reevaluated. A test of cure is needed 7–14 days after treatment for people who are treated for pharyngeal (infection of the throat) gonorrhea.

Because reinfection is common, men and women with gonorrhea should be retested three months after treatment of the initial infection, regardless of whether they believe that their sex partners were successfully treated.

Health-care providers and health departments can report suspected gonorrhea cephalosporin treatment failure or any *N. gonorrhoeae* specimen with decreased cephalosporin susceptibility through the Suspected Gonorrhea Treatment Failure Consultation Form (https://airc.cdc.gov/surveys/?s=JACPEYPPAJ3T779W).

NOTIFYING PARTNERS

If a person has been diagnosed and treated for gonorrhea, he or she should tell all recent anal, vaginal, or oral sex partners, so they can see a health-care provider and be treated. This will reduce the risk that the sex partners will develop serious complications from gonorrhea and will also reduce the person's risk of becoming reinfected. A person with gonorrhea and all of his or her sex partners must avoid having sex until they have completed their treatment for gonorrhea and until they no longer have symptoms. For tips on talking to partners about sex and STD testing, visit www.gytnow. org/talking-to-your-partner.[5]

CAN WOMEN WHO HAVE SEX WITH WOMEN GET GONORRHEA?

Yes. It is possible to get gonorrhea, or any other STIs, if you are a woman who has sex only with women.

Talk to your partner about her sexual history before having sex and ask your doctor about getting tested if you have signs or symptoms of gonorrhea.

HOW CAN YOU PREVENT GONORRHEA?

The best way to prevent gonorrhea or any STI is to not have vaginal, oral, or anal sex.

If you do have sex, lower your risk of getting an STI with the following steps:

- **Use condoms.** Condoms are the best way to prevent STIs when you have sex. Because a man does not need to ejaculate to give or get gonorrhea, make sure to put the condom on before the penis touches the vagina, mouth, or anus. Other methods of birth control, such as birth control pills, shots, implants, or diaphragms, will not protect you from STIs.
- **Get tested.** Be sure you and your partner are tested for STIs. Talk to each other about your test results before you have sex.
- **Be monogamous.** Having sex with just one partner can lower your risk for STIs. After being tested for STIs, be faithful to each other. That means that you have sex only with each other and no one else.
- **Limit your number of sex partners.** Your risk of getting STIs goes up with the number of partners you have.
- **Do not douche.** Douching removes some of the normal bacteria in the vagina and may increase your risk of getting STIs.

---

[5] See footnote [1].

- **Do not abuse alcohol or drugs**. Drinking too much alcohol or using drugs increases risky behavior and may put you at risk of sexual assault and possible exposure to STIs.

The steps work best when used together. No single step can protect you from every single type of STI.[6]

---

[6] See footnote [2].

Chapter 11 | **Genital Herpes**

Genital herpes is a sexually transmitted infection (STI). Genital herpes is usually spread by having vaginal, oral, or anal sex. One in five women aged 14–49 has genital herpes. There is no cure for herpes. But you can take medicine to prevent outbreaks and to lower your risk of passing genital herpes to your partner.

WHAT IS GENITAL HERPES?

Genital herpes is an STI caused by herpes simplex virus type 1 (HSV-1) and herpes simplex virus type 2 (HSV-2). HSV-1 and HSV-2 cause the same symptoms, are both contagious, and are treated with the same medicine. But they are different in some ways:

- HSV-1 most often causes infections of the mouth and lips, called "cold sores" or "fever blisters." Symptoms are often milder than genital herpes, and you may get fewer outbreaks. It can spread to the genital area during oral sex and cause genital herpes. If HSV-1 spreads to the genital area, it is still HSV-1.
- HSV-2 is the most common cause of genital herpes. It is spread through vaginal, oral, or anal sex. HSV-2 can spread to the mouth during oral sex. If HSV-2 spreads to the mouth or lips during oral sex, it is still HSV-2.

WHO GETS GENITAL HERPES?

Genital herpes is more common in women than in men. One in five women aged 14–49 has genital herpes, compared with one in ten men aged 14–49.

A woman's anatomy (body) puts her more at risk for genital herpes than men. Small tears in vaginal tissue can make it easier to get genital herpes.

Genital herpes is also much more common in African American women. One in two African American women between the ages of 14 and 49 is infected with HSV-2 that causes genital herpes.

HOW DO YOU GET GENITAL HERPES?

Genital herpes is spread through:
- vaginal, oral, or anal sex (The herpes virus is usually spread through contact with open sores. But you can also get herpes from someone without any symptoms or sores.)
- genital touching
- childbirth from a mother to her baby
- breastfeeding if a baby touches an open sore

DOES A COLD SORE ON YOUR MOUTH MEAN YOU HAVE GENITAL HERPES?

No, a cold sore on your mouth usually means you have HSV-1. You can get HSV-1 by kissing someone or sharing utensils, towels, razors, or lipstick with someone who has HSV-1.

HSV-1 cannot turn into HSV-2 (the type of genital herpes spread by sexual contact), but you can get a cold sore on your mouth from HSV-2 if you give oral sex to someone with HSV-2. Cold sores caused by HSV-1 or HSV-2 are contagious. You can spread it to other people or other parts of your body if you touch an open sore and then touch another part of your body. That means if you have a cold sore and give oral sex to someone, that person will get the herpes virus on his or her genitals.

Avoid touching your cold sore as much as possible. If you touch your cold sore, wash your hands right away to avoid spreading the infection to other parts of your body or other people.

WHAT IS THE DIFFERENCE BETWEEN GENITAL HERPES AND GENITAL WARTS?

Both genital herpes and genital warts are STIs, are spread through skin-to-skin contact, and are caused by a virus. But the viruses that cause genital herpes and genital warts are different:
- Herpes simplex virus (HSV) is the virus that causes genital herpes.

- Human papillomavirus (HPV) is the virus that causes genital warts.

There is no cure for either genital herpes or genital warts. But different medicines can help manage the symptoms of herpes and treat the complications of HPV infections that can cause genital warts.

WHAT ARE THE SYMPTOMS OF GENITAL HERPES?

Most women with genital herpes do not know they have it. But, if you get symptoms with the first outbreak of genital herpes, they can be severe. Genital herpes can also be severe and long-lasting in people whose immune systems do not work properly, such as women with human immunodeficiency virus (HIV).

Within a few days of sexual contact with someone who has the herpes virus, sores (small red bumps that may turn into blisters) may show up where the virus entered your body, such as on your mouth or vagina. Some women might confuse mild sores for insect bites or something else. After a few days, sores become crusted and then heal without scarring. Sometimes, a second set of sores appear soon after the first outbreak, and symptoms can happen again.

The first signs of genital herpes usually show up two to twelve days after having sexual contact with someone who has herpes. Symptoms can last from two to four weeks. The following are the other early symptoms of genital herpes:
- feeling of pressure in the abdomen
- flu-like symptoms, including fever
- itching or burning feeling in the genital or anal area
- pain in the legs, buttocks, or genital area
- swollen glands
- unusual vaginal discharge

If you have any symptoms of genital herpes, see a doctor or nurse.

HOW IS GENITAL HERPES DIAGNOSED?

Often, your doctor can diagnose genital herpes by looking at visible sores. Your doctor or nurse may also use a cotton swab to take a fluid sample from a sore to test in a lab.

Genital herpes can be hard to diagnose, especially between outbreaks. Blood tests that look for antibodies to the herpes virus can help diagnose herpes in women without symptoms or between outbreaks.

A Pap test is not used to detect genital herpes.

HOW IS GENITAL HERPES TREATED?

Herpes has no cure. But antiviral medicines can prevent or shorten outbreaks during the time you take the medicine. Also, daily suppressive therapy (e.g., daily use of antiviral medicine) for herpes can lower your chance of spreading the infection to your partner.

Your doctor will give you antiviral medicine either to take right after getting outbreak symptoms or to take regularly to try to stop outbreaks from happening. Talk to your doctor about treatment options.

During outbreaks, you can take the following steps to speed healing and prevent spreading herpes to other parts of your body or to other people:

- Keep sores clean and dry.
- Try not to touch the sores.
- Wash your hands after any contact with the sores.
- Avoid all sexual contact from the time you first notice symptoms until the sores have healed.

CAN GENITAL HERPES COME BACK?

Yes. Genital herpes symptoms can come and go, but the virus stays inside your body even after all signs of the infection have gone away. The virus becomes "active" from time to time, leading to an outbreak. Some people have outbreaks only once or twice. Other people may have four or five outbreaks within a year. Over time, the outbreaks usually happen less often and are less severe.

Experts do not know what causes the virus to become active. Some women say the virus comes back when they are sick, under stress, out in the sun or during their period.

WHAT SHOULD YOU DO IF YOU HAVE GENITAL HERPES?
If you have genital herpes, do the following:
- See a doctor or nurse as soon as possible for testing and treatment.
- Take all of the medicine. Even if symptoms go away, you need to finish all of the antiviral medicine.
- Tell your sex partner(s), so they can be tested and treated if necessary.
- Avoid any sexual contact while you are being treated for genital herpes or while you have an outbreak.
- Remember that genital herpes is a lifelong disease. Even though you may not have a genital herpes outbreak for long periods of time, you can still pass the virus to another person at any time. Talk with your doctor or nurse about how to prevent passing the virus to another person.

HOW DOES GENITAL HERPES AFFECT PREGNANCY?
- If you get genital herpes during pregnancy, you can spread genital herpes to your baby during delivery.
- If you had genital herpes before pregnancy, your baby is still at risk of getting herpes, but the risk is lower.

Most women with genital herpes have healthy babies. But babies who get herpes from their mothers have neonatal herpes. Neonatal herpes is a serious condition that can cause problems in a newborn baby, such as brain damage, eye problems, or even death.

CAN PREGNANT WOMEN TAKE GENITAL HERPES MEDICINE?
Researchers do not know if all antiviral medicines for genital herpes are safe for pregnant women. If you are pregnant, make sure you tell your doctor or nurse that you have genital herpes, even if you are not having an outbreak.

CAN YOU BREASTFEED IF YOU HAVE GENITAL HERPES?

Yes, you can breastfeed if you have genital herpes, but not if you have a herpes sore on one of your breasts. If you have genital herpes, it is possible to spread the infection to any part of your breast, including your nipple and areola.

If you have any genital herpes sores on one or both of your breasts, you may have to do the following:

- You can keep breastfeeding as long as your baby or pumping equipment does not touch a herpes sore.
- Do not breastfeed from the breast with sores. Herpes is spread through contact with sores and can be dangerous to a newborn baby.
- Pump or hand-express your milk from the breast with sores until the sores heal. Pumping will help keep up your milk supply and prevent your breast from getting overly full and painful. You can store your milk to give to your baby in a bottle for another feeding. But, if parts of your pump also touch the sore(s) while pumping, throw the milk away.

CAN GENITAL HERPES CAUSE OTHER PROBLEMS?

For most women, genital herpes does not usually cause serious health problems.

Women with HIV can have severe herpes outbreaks that are long-lasting. Herpes may also play a role in the spread of HIV. Herpes sores can make it easier for HIV to get into your body. Also, herpes can make people who are HIV-positive more likely to spread the infection to someone else.

HOW CAN YOU PREVENT GENITAL HERPES?

The best way to prevent genital herpes or any STI is to avoid vaginal, oral, or anal sex.

If you do have sex, lower your risk of getting an STI with the following steps:

- **Use condoms**. Condoms are the best way to prevent STIs when you have sex. Because a man does not need to ejaculate (come) to give or get some STIs, make sure to put the condom on before the penis touches the vagina, mouth, or anus. Other methods of birth control, such as birth control pills, shots, implants, or diaphragms, will not protect you from STIs.

- **Get tested.** Be sure you and your partner are tested for STIs. Talk to each other about the test results before you have sex.
- **Be monogamous.** Having sex with just one partner can lower your risk for STIs. After being tested for STIs, be faithful to each other. That means that you have sex only with each other and no one else.
- **Limit your number of sex partners.** Your risk of getting STIs goes up with the number of partners you have.
- **Do not douche.** Douching removes some of the normal bacteria in the vagina that protect you from infection. This may increase your risk of getting STIs.
- **Do not abuse alcohol or drugs.** Drinking too much alcohol or using drugs increases risky behavior and may put you at risk of sexual assault and possible exposure to STIs.

The steps work best when used together. No single step can protect you from every single type of STI.

CAN WOMEN WHO HAVE SEX WITH WOMEN GET GENITAL HERPES?

Yes. It is possible to get genital herpes, or any other STI, if you are a woman who has sex only with women.

Talk to your partner about her sexual history before having sex and ask your doctor or nurse about getting tested if you have signs or symptoms of genital herpes. Use a dental dam during oral sex and avoid sexual activity during an outbreak.[1]

---

[1] Office on Women's Health (OWH), "Genital Herpes," U.S. Department of Health and Human Services (HHS), January 6, 2023. Available online. URL: www.womenshealth.gov/a-z-topics/genital-herpes. Accessed May 31, 2023.

Chapter 12 | Human Immunodeficiency Virus and Acquired Immunodeficiency Syndrome

Chapter Contents

Section 12.1 | Human Immunodeficiency Virus/Acquired Immunodeficiency Syndrome: The Basics

WHAT ARE HUMAN IMMUNODEFICIENCY VIRUS AND ACQUIRED IMMUNODEFICIENCY SYNDROME?

Human immunodeficiency virus (HIV) is the virus that causes HIV infection. The abbreviation "HIV" can refer to the virus or to HIV infection. The structure of HIV is shown in Figure 12.1.

Acquired immunodeficiency syndrome (AIDS) is the most advanced stage of HIV infection.

HIV attacks and destroys the infection-fighting CD4 cells (CD4 T lymphocyte) of the immune system. The loss of CD4 cells makes it difficult for the body to fight off infections and certain cancers. Without treatment, HIV can gradually destroy the immune system, and HIV infection advances to AIDS.[1]

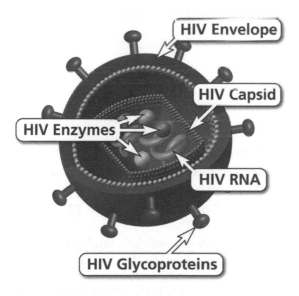

Figure 12.1. Human Immunodeficiency Virus

HIVinfo, U.S. Department of Health and Human Services (HHS)

---

[1] HIVinfo, "HIV and AIDS: The Basics," U.S. Department of Health and Human Services (HHS), January 31, 2023. Available online. URL: https://hivinfo.nih.gov/understanding-hiv/fact-sheets/hiv-and-aids-basics. Accessed May 30, 2023.

WHERE DID HUMAN IMMUNODEFICIENCY VIRUS COME FROM?

- Human immunodeficiency virus in humans came from a type of chimpanzee in Central Africa. Studies show that HIV may have jumped from chimpanzees to humans as far back as the late 1800s.
- The chimpanzee version of the virus is called "simian immunodeficiency virus" (SIV). It was probably passed to humans when humans hunted these chimpanzees for meat and came in contact with their infected blood.
- Over decades, HIV slowly spread across Africa and later into other parts of the world. The virus has existed in the United States since at least the mid-1970s to late 1970s.[2]

HOW IS HUMAN IMMUNODEFICIENCY VIRUS SPREAD?

The spread of HIV from person to person is called "HIV transmission." HIV is spread only through certain body fluids from a person who has HIV. These body fluids include:

- blood
- semen
- pre-seminal fluid
- vaginal fluids
- rectal fluids
- breast milk

HIV transmission is only possible through contact with HIV-infected body fluids. In the United States, HIV is spread mainly by:

- having anal or vaginal sex with someone who has HIV without using a condom or taking medicines to prevent or treat HIV
- sharing injection drug equipment (works), such as needles or syringes, with someone who has HIV

The spread of HIV from a woman with HIV to her child during pregnancy, childbirth, or breastfeeding is called "perinatal transmission of HIV."

---

[2] "About HIV," Centers for Disease Control and Prevention (CDC), June 30, 2022. Available online. URL: www.cdc.gov/hiv/basics/whatishiv.html. Accessed May 30, 2023.

You cannot get HIV by shaking hands or hugging a person who has HIV. You cannot also get HIV from contact with objects, such as dishes, toilet seats, or doorknobs, used by a person with HIV. HIV is not spread through the air or water or by mosquitoes, ticks, or other blood-sucking insects.

WHAT ARE THE SYMPTOMS OF HUMAN IMMUNODEFICIENCY VIRUS AND ACQUIRED IMMUNODEFICIENCY SYNDROME?

Within two to four weeks after infection with HIV, some people may have flu-like symptoms, such as fever, chills, or rash (Figure 12.2). The symptoms may last for a few days to several weeks. Other possible symptoms of HIV include night sweats, muscle aches, sore throat, fatigue, swollen lymph nodes, and mouth ulcers. Having these symptoms does not mean you have HIV. Other illnesses can cause the same symptoms. Some people may not feel sick during early HIV infection (called "acute HIV infection"). During this earliest stage of HIV infection, the virus multiplies rapidly. After the initial stage of infection, HIV continues to multiply but at very low levels.

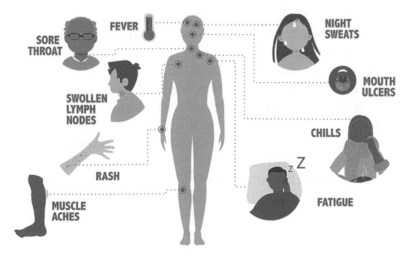

Figure 12.2. Human Immunodeficiency Virus Symptoms

Centers for Disease Control and Prevention (CDC)

More severe symptoms of HIV infection, such as a badly damaged immune system and signs of opportunistic infections, generally do not appear for many years until HIV has advanced to AIDS. People with AIDS have badly damaged immune systems that make them prone to opportunistic infections. (Opportunistic infections are infections and infection-related cancers that occur more frequently or are more severe in people with weakened immune systems than in people with healthy immune systems.)

Without treatment with HIV medicines, HIV usually advances to AIDS in 10 years or longer though it may advance faster in some people.

HIV transmission is possible at any stage of HIV—even if a person with HIV has no symptoms of HIV.

HOW CAN A PERSON REDUCE THE RISK OF GETTING HUMAN IMMUNODEFICIENCY VIRUS?

To reduce your risk of HIV, use condoms correctly every time you have sex, limit your number of sexual partners, and never share injection drug equipment.

Also, talk to your health-care provider about pre-exposure prophylaxis (PrEP). PrEP is an HIV prevention option for people who do not have HIV but who are at high risk of becoming infected with HIV. PrEP involves taking a specific HIV medicine every day.

HIV medicines, given to people with HIV during pregnancy and childbirth and to their babies after birth, reduce the risk of perinatal transmission of HIV. Pregnant women with HIV are encouraged to talk to their medical team about options for feeding their baby after birth. With consistent use of HIV medication and an undetectable viral load during pregnancy and throughout breastfeeding, the risk of transmission to a breastfed baby is low: less than 1 percent, but not zero. Alternatively, properly prepared formula and pasteurized donor human milk from a milk bank are options that eliminate the risk of transmission to a baby after birth. Pregnant women with HIV can speak with their health-care provider to determine what method of feeding their baby is right for them.[3]

---

[3] See footnote [1].

WHAT ARE THE STAGES OF HUMAN IMMUNODEFICIENCY VIRUS?

When people with HIV do not get treatment, they typically progress through three stages. But HIV treatment can slow or prevent the progression of the disease. With advances in HIV treatment, progression to stage 3 (AIDS) is less common nowadays than in the early years of HIV.

- stage 1: acute HIV infection
- stage 2: chronic infection
- stage 3: AIDS[4]

WHAT IS THE TREATMENT FOR HUMAN IMMUNODEFICIENCY VIRUS?

Antiretroviral therapy (ART) is the use of HIV medicines to treat HIV infection. People on ART take a combination of HIV medicines (called an "HIV treatment regimen") every day.

ART is recommended for everyone who has HIV. ART prevents HIV from multiplying, which reduces the amount of HIV in the body (called the "viral load"). Having less HIV in the body protects the immune system and prevents HIV infection from advancing to AIDS. ART cannot cure HIV, but HIV medicines help people with HIV live longer, healthier lives.

ART also reduces the risk of HIV transmission. The main goal of ART is to reduce a person's viral load to an undetectable level. An undetectable viral load means that the level of HIV in the blood is too low to be detected by a viral load test. People with HIV who maintain an undetectable viral load have effectively no risk of transmitting HIV to their HIV-negative partner through sex.

HOW IS ACQUIRED IMMUNODEFICIENCY SYNDROME DIAGNOSED?

Symptoms such as fever, weakness, and weight loss may be a sign that a person's HIV has advanced to AIDS. However, a diagnosis of AIDS is based on the following criteria:

- drop in CD4 count to less than 200 cells/mm^3 (A CD4 count measures the number of CD4 cells in a sample of blood.)
- the presence of certain opportunistic infections

---

[4] See footnote [2].

Although an AIDS diagnosis indicates severe damage to the immune system, HIV medicines can still help people at this stage of HIV infection.[5]

Section 12.2 | The Human Immunodeficiency Virus Life Cycle

WHAT IS THE HUMAN IMMUNODEFICIENCY VIRUS LIFE CYCLE?

Human immunodeficiency virus (HIV) attacks and destroys the CD4 cells (CD4 T lymphocyte) of the immune system. CD4 cells are a type of white blood cell (WBC) that play a major role in protecting the body from infection. HIV uses the machinery of the CD4 cells to multiply and spread throughout the body. This process, which is carried out in seven steps or stages (Figure 12.3), is called the "HIV life cycle."

WHAT ARE THE SEVEN STAGES OF THE HUMAN IMMUNODEFICIENCY VIRUS LIFE CYCLE?

The seven stages of the HIV life cycle are as follows:
- binding
- fusion
- reverse transcription
- integration
- replication
- assembly
- budding[6]

THE STAGES OF HUMAN IMMUNODEFICIENCY VIRUS INFECTION

Without treatment, HIV infection advances in stages, getting worse over time (Figure 12.4). HIV gradually destroys the immune system and eventually causes acquired immunodeficiency syndrome (AIDS).

---

[5] See footnote [1].
[6] HIVinfo, "The HIV Life Cycle," U.S. Department of Health and Human Services (HHS), August 4, 2021. Available online. URL: https://hivinfo.nih.gov/understanding-hiv/fact-sheets/hiv-life-cycle. Accessed May 30, 2023.

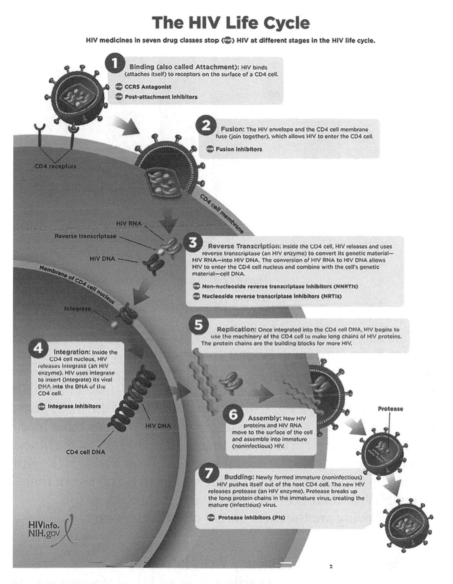

The HIV Life Cycle

HIV medicines in seven drug classes stop (●) HIV at different stages in the HIV life cycle.

1 **Binding (also called Attachment):** HIV binds (attaches itself) to receptors on the surface of a CD4 cell.
- ● CCR5 Antagonist
- ● Post-attachment inhibitors

2 **Fusion:** The HIV envelope and the CD4 cell membrane fuse (join together), which allows HIV to enter the CD4 cell.
- ● Fusion inhibitors

3 **Reverse Transcription:** Inside the CD4 cell, HIV releases and uses reverse transcriptase (an HIV enzyme) to convert its genetic material—HIV RNA—into HIV DNA. The conversion of HIV RNA to HIV DNA allows HIV to enter the CD4 cell nucleus and combine with the cell's genetic material—cell DNA.
- ● Non-nucleoside reverse transcriptase inhibitors (NNRTIs)
- ● Nucleoside reverse transcriptase inhibitors (NRTIs)

4 **Integration:** Inside the CD4 cell nucleus, HIV releases integrase (an HIV enzyme). HIV uses integrase to insert (integrate) its viral DNA into the DNA of the CD4 cell.
- ● Integrase inhibitors

5 **Replication:** Once integrated into the CD4 cell DNA, HIV begins to use the machinery of the CD4 cell to make long chains of HIV proteins. The protein chains are the building blocks for more HIV.

6 **Assembly:** New HIV proteins and HIV RNA move to the surface of the cell and assemble into immature (noninfectious) HIV.

7 **Budding:** Newly formed immature (noninfectious) HIV pushes itself out of the host CD4 cell. The new HIV releases protease (an HIV enzyme). Protease breaks up the long protein chains in the immature virus, creating the mature (infectious) virus.
- ● Protease inhibitors (PIs)

CD4 receptors

HIV RNA

Reverse transcriptase

HIV DNA

Membrane of CD4 cell nucleus

Integrase

HIV DNA

CD4 cell DNA

Protease

CD4 cell membrane

HIVinfo.
NIH.gov

Figure 12.3. The Human Immunodeficiency Virus Life Cycle

HIVinfo, U.S. Department of Health and Human Services (HHS)

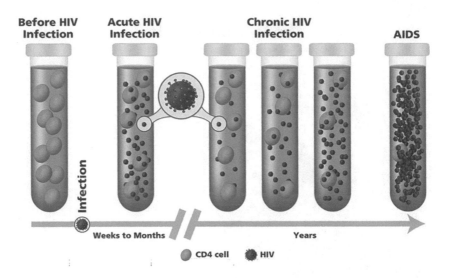

Figure 12.4. Human Immunodeficiency Virus: Progression

HIVinfo, U.S. Department of Health and Human Services (HHS)

There is no cure for HIV, but treatment with HIV medicines (called "antiretroviral therapy" (ART)) can slow or prevent HIV from advancing from one stage to the next. HIV medicines help people with HIV live longer, healthier lives. One of the main goals of ART is to reduce a person's viral load to an undetectable level. An undetectable viral load means that the level of HIV in the blood is too low to be detected by a viral load test. People with HIV who maintain an undetectable viral load have effectively no risk of transmitting HIV to their HIV-negative partner through sex.

The following are the three stages of HIV infection.

Acute Human Immunodeficiency Virus Infection

Acute HIV infection is the earliest stage of HIV infection, and it generally develops within two to four weeks after infection with HIV. During this time, some people have flu-like symptoms, such as fever, headache, and rash. In the acute stage of infection, HIV multiplies rapidly and spreads throughout the body. The virus attacks and destroys the infection-fighting CD4 cells (CD4 T lymphocyte) of the immune system. During the acute HIV infection stage, the level of HIV in the blood is very high, which greatly increases the risk of HIV transmission. A person may experience significant health benefits if they start ART during this stage.

Chronic Human Immunodeficiency Virus Infection

The second stage of HIV infection is chronic HIV infection (also called "asymptomatic HIV infection" or "clinical latency"). During this stage, HIV continues to multiply in the body but at very low levels. People with chronic HIV infection may not have any HIV-related symptoms. Without ART, chronic HIV infection usually advances to AIDS in 10 years or longer, though in some people, it may advance faster. People who are taking ART may be in this stage for several decades. While it is still possible to transmit HIV to others during this stage, people who take ART exactly as prescribed and maintain an undetectable viral load have effectively no risk of transmitting HIV to an HIV-negative partner through sex.

Acquired Immunodeficiency Syndrome

AIDS is the final, most severe stage of HIV infection. Because HIV has severely damaged the immune system, the body cannot fight off opportunistic infections. (Opportunistic infections are infections and infection-related cancers that occur more frequently or are more severe in people with weakened immune systems than in people with healthy immune systems.) People with HIV are diagnosed with AIDS if they have a CD4 count of less than 200 cells/mm^3 or if they have certain opportunistic infections. Once a person is diagnosed with AIDS, they can have a high viral load and are able to transmit HIV to others very easily. Without treatment, people with AIDS typically survive about three years.[7]

---

[7] HIVinfo, "The Stages of HIV Infection," U.S. Department of Health and Human Services (HHS), August 20, 2021. Available online. URL: https://hivinfo.nih.gov/understanding-hiv/fact-sheets/stages-hiv-infection. Accessed May 30, 2023.

WHAT IS THE CONNECTION BETWEEN THE HUMAN IMMUNODEFICIENCY VIRUS LIFE CYCLE AND HUMAN IMMUNODEFICIENCY VIRUS MEDICINES?

Antiretroviral therapy is the use of a combination of HIV medicines to treat HIV infection. People on ART take a combination of HIV medicines (called an "HIV treatment regimen") every day. HIV medicines protect the immune system by blocking HIV at different stages of the HIV life cycle. HIV medicines are grouped into different drug classes according to how they fight HIV. Each class of drugs is designed to target a specific step in the HIV life cycle.

Because an HIV treatment regimen includes HIV medicines from at least two different HIV drug classes, ART is very effective at preventing HIV from multiplying. Having less HIV in the body protects the immune system and prevents HIV from advancing to AIDS.

ART cannot cure HIV, but HIV medicines help people with HIV live longer, healthier lives. HIV medicines also reduce the risk of HIV transmission (the spread of HIV to others).[8]

Section 12.3 | Symptoms of Human Immunodeficiency Virus

HOW CAN YOU TELL IF YOU HAVE HUMAN IMMUNODEFICIENCY VIRUS?

The only way to know for sure if you have human immunodeficiency virus (HIV) is to get tested. You cannot rely on symptoms to tell whether you have HIV.

Knowing your HIV status gives you powerful information, so you can take steps to keep yourself and your partner(s) healthy:

- If you test positive, you can take medicine to treat HIV. People with HIV who take HIV medicine (called "antiretroviral therapy" or "ART") as prescribed and get and keep an undetectable viral load can live long and healthy lives and will not transmit HIV to their

---

[8] See footnote [6].

HIV-negative partners through sex. An undetectable viral load is a level of HIV in the blood so low that it cannot be detected in a standard lab test.

- If you test negative, you have more HIV prevention tools available today than ever before, such as pre-exposure prophylaxis (PrEP), medicine people at risk for HIV take to prevent getting HIV from sex or injection drug use, and postexposure prophylaxis (PEP), HIV medicine taken within 72 hours after a possible exposure to prevent the virus from taking hold.
- If you are pregnant, you should be tested for HIV so that you can begin treatment if you are HIV-positive. If you have HIV and take HIV medicine as prescribed throughout your pregnancy and childbirth and give HIV medicine to your baby for four to six weeks after giving birth, your risk of transmitting HIV to your baby can be less than 1 percent. HIV medicine will protect your own health as well.

WHAT ARE THE SYMPTOMS OF HUMAN IMMUNODEFICIENCY VIRUS?

There are several symptoms of HIV. Not everyone will have the same symptoms. It depends on the person and what stage of the disease they are in.

Below are the three stages of HIV and some of the symptoms people may experience.

Stage 1: Acute Human Immunodeficiency Virus Infection

Within two to four weeks after infection with HIV, about two-thirds of people will have a flu-like illness. This is the body's natural response to HIV infection.

Flu-like symptoms can include:
- fever
- chills
- rash
- night sweats
- muscle aches
- sore throat

- fatigue
- swollen lymph nodes
- mouth ulcers

These symptoms can last anywhere from a few days to several weeks. But some people do not have any symptoms at all during this early stage of HIV.

Do not assume you have HIV just because you have any of these symptoms—they can be similar to those caused by other illnesses. But, if you think you may have been exposed to HIV, get an HIV test. Here is what to do:

- **Find an HIV testing site near you.** You can get an HIV test at your primary care provider's office, your local health department, a health clinic, or many other places. Use the HIV Services Locator to find an HIV testing site near you.
- **Request an HIV test for a recent infection**. Most HIV tests detect antibodies (proteins your body makes as a reaction to HIV), not HIV itself. But it can take a few weeks after you have HIV for your body to produce these antibodies. There are other types of tests that can detect HIV infection sooner. Tell your doctor or clinic if you think you were recently exposed to HIV and ask if their tests can detect early infection.
- **Know your status**. After you get tested, be sure to learn your test results. If you are HIV-positive, see a health-care provider as soon as possible, so you can start treatment with HIV medicine. And be aware: When you are in the early stage of infection, you are at very high risk of transmitting HIV to others. It is important to take steps to reduce your risk of transmission. If you are HIV-negative, there are prevention tools such as PrEP that can help you stay negative.

Stage 2: Clinical Latency

In this stage, the virus still multiplies but at very low levels. People in this stage may not feel sick or have any symptoms. This stage is also called "chronic HIV infection."

Without HIV treatment, people can stay in this stage for 10 or 15 years, but some move through this stage faster.

If you take HIV medicine exactly as prescribed and get and keep an undetectable viral load, you can live a long and healthy life and will not transmit HIV to your HIV-negative partners through sex.

But, if your viral load is detectable, you can transmit HIV during this stage, even when you have no symptoms. It is important to see your health-care provider regularly to get your viral load checked.

Stage 3: Acquired Immunodeficiency Syndrome

If you have HIV and you are not on HIV treatment, eventually, the virus will weaken your body's immune system, and you will progress to acquired immunodeficiency syndrome (AIDS). This is the late stage of HIV infection.

Symptoms of AIDS can include:
- rapid weight loss
- recurring fever or profuse night sweats
- extreme and unexplained tiredness
- prolonged swelling of the lymph glands in the armpits, groin, or neck
- diarrhea that lasts for more than a week
- sores of the mouth, anus, or genitals
- pneumonia
- red, brown, pink, or purplish blotches on or under the skin or inside the mouth, nose, or eyelids
- memory loss, depression, and other neurologic disorders

Each of these symptoms can also be related to other illnesses. The only way to know for sure if you have HIV is to get tested. If you are HIV-positive, a health-care provider will diagnose if your HIV has progressed to stage 3 (AIDS) based on certain medical criteria.

Many of the severe symptoms and illnesses of HIV disease come from the opportunistic infections that occur because your body's immune system has been damaged. See your health-care provider if you are experiencing any of these symptoms.

Thanks to effective treatment, most people in the United States with HIV do not progress to AIDS. If you have HIV and remain in care, take HIV medicine as prescribed, and get and keep an undetectable viral load, you will stay healthy and will not progress to AIDS.[9]

Section 12.4 | Questions and Answers about Human Immunodeficiency Virus Transmission

This section answers some of the most common questions about the risk of human immunodeficiency virus (HIV) transmission for different types of sex, injection drug use (IDU), and other activities.

HOW IS HUMAN IMMUNODEFICIENCY VIRUS PASSED FROM ONE PERSON TO ANOTHER?

Most people get HIV through anal or vaginal sex or sharing needles, syringes, or other drug injection equipment (e.g., cookers). But there are powerful tools to help prevent HIV transmission.

CAN YOU GET HUMAN IMMUNODEFICIENCY VIRUS FROM ANAL SEX?

You can get HIV if you have anal sex with someone who has HIV without using protection (such as condoms or medicine to treat or prevent HIV).

- Anal sex is the riskiest type of sex for getting or transmitting HIV.
- Being the receptive partner (bottom) is riskier than being the insertive partner (top).
- The bottom's risk is higher because the rectum's lining is thin and may allow HIV to enter the body during anal sex.

[9] HIVinfo, "Symptoms of HIV," U.S. Department of Health and Human Services (HHS), June 15, 2022. Available online. URL: www.hiv.gov/hiv-basics/overview/about-hiv-and-aids/symptoms-of-hiv. Accessed May 30, 2023.

- The top is also at risk. HIV can enter the body through the opening at the tip of the penis (urethra), the foreskin if the penis is not circumcised, or small cuts, scratches, or open sores anywhere on the penis.

CAN YOU GET HUMAN IMMUNODEFICIENCY VIRUS FROM VAGINAL SEX?

You can get HIV if you have vaginal sex with someone who has HIV without using protection (such as condoms or medicine to treat or prevent HIV).

- Vaginal sex is less risky for getting HIV than receptive anal sex.
- Either partner can get HIV during vaginal sex.
- HIV can enter a person's body during vaginal sex through the delicate tissue that lines the vagina and cervix.
- Vaginal fluid and blood can carry HIV, which can pass through the opening at the tip of the penis (urethra), the foreskin if the penis is not circumcised, or small cuts, scratches, or open sores anywhere on the penis.

CAN HUMAN IMMUNODEFICIENCY VIRUS BE TRANSMITTED FROM A MOTHER TO HER BABY?

Human immunodeficiency virus can be transmitted from a mother to her baby during pregnancy, birth, or breastfeeding. However, it is less common because of advances in HIV prevention and treatment.

- This is called "perinatal transmission" or "mother-to-child transmission."
- Mother-to-child transmission is the most common way that children get HIV.
- Recommendations to test all pregnant women for HIV and start HIV treatment immediately have lowered the number of babies who are born with HIV.
- If a woman with HIV takes HIV medicine as prescribed throughout pregnancy and childbirth and

gives HIV medicine to her baby for four to six weeks after birth, the risk of transmission can be less than 1 percent.

CAN YOU GET HUMAN IMMUNODEFICIENCY VIRUS FROM SHARING NEEDLES, SYRINGES, OR OTHER DRUG INJECTION EQUIPMENT?

You are at high risk of getting HIV if you share needles, syringes, or other drug injection equipment (e.g., cookers) with someone who has HIV. Never share needles or other equipment to inject drugs, hormones, steroids, or silicone.

- Used needles, syringes, and other injection equipment may have someone else's blood on them that can carry HIV.
- People who inject drugs are also at risk of getting HIV (and other sexually transmitted diseases (STDs)) if they engage in risky sexual behaviors, including having sex without protection (such as condoms or medicine to prevent or treat HIV).
- Sharing needles, syringes, or other injection equipment increases your risk of getting hepatitis B and hepatitis C and other infections.

WHAT ARE SOME RARE WAYS THAT HUMAN IMMUNODEFICIENCY VIRUS HAS BEEN TRANSMITTED?

There is little to no risk of getting HIV from the following activities. For transmission to occur, something very unusual would have to happen.

Oral Sex

- Oral sex involves putting the mouth on the penis (fellatio), vagina or vulva (cunnilingus), or anus (rimming).
- Factors that may affect the risk of getting HIV include:
  - ejaculation in the mouth with oral ulcers, bleeding gums, or genital sores
  - the presence of other STDs

- You can get other STDs from oral sex. If you get feces in your mouth during anilingus, you can get hepatitis A and hepatitis B, parasites such as *Giardia*, and bacteria such as *Shigella*, *Salmonella*, *Campylobacter*, and *Escherichia coli*.

Workplace
- The most likely cause is injury with a contaminated needle or another sharp object.
- Careful practice of standard precautions protects patients and health-care personnel from possible occupational HIV transmission.

Medical Care
- The U.S. blood supply and donated organs and tissues are thoroughly tested. It is very unlikely that you would get HIV from blood transfusions, blood products, or organ and tissue transplants.
- You cannot get HIV from donating blood. Blood collection procedures are highly regulated and safe.

Food Contamination
- The only known cases are among infants. Contamination occurs when blood from a caregiver's mouth mixes with pre-chewed food and an infant eats it.
- You cannot get HIV from consuming food handled by someone with HIV.

Biting and Spitting
- The small number of documented cases have involved severe trauma with extensive tissue damage and the presence of blood. This rare transmission can occur through contact between broken skin, wounds, or mucous membranes and blood or body fluids from a person who has HIV.

- There is no risk of transmission through unbroken skin.
- There are no documented cases of HIV being transmitted through spitting, as HIV is not transmitted through saliva.

Deep, Open-Mouth Kissing
- Very rarely, transmission occurs if both partners have sores or bleeding gums.
- You cannot transmit HIV through closed-mouth or "social" kissing with someone who has HIV.
- You cannot transmit HIV through saliva.

Touching
- Touching involves putting your hands, other body parts, or sex toys on your partner's vagina, penis, or anus.
- The only possible risk would be if body fluids from a person with HIV touch the mucous membranes or damaged tissue of someone without HIV. Mucous membranes are found inside the rectum, vagina, opening of the penis, and mouth. Damaged tissue could include cuts, sores, or open wounds.
- You can get or transmit some other STDs (such as human papillomavirus (HPV), genital herpes, and syphilis) through skin-to-skin contact.
- If you touch someone's anus and get feces on your hands or fingers, you can also get or transmit hepatitis A and hepatitis B. Infection with parasites such as *Giardia* and bacteria such as *Shigella*, *Salmonella*, *Campylobacter*, and *E. coli* can also occur.

Tattoos and Body Piercings
- There are no known cases in the United States of anyone getting HIV this way.
- It is possible to get HIV from tattooing or body piercing if the equipment or ink has someone else's blood in it. This is more likely to happen when the person doing the

procedure is unlicensed because they may use unsterilized needles or ink.

- If you get a tattoo or a body piercing, be sure that the person doing the procedure is properly licensed and uses only new or sterilized equipment.

WHAT BODY FLUIDS TRANSMIT HUMAN IMMUNODEFICIENCY VIRUS?

Only certain body fluids from a person who has HIV can transmit HIV. These fluids include:

- blood
- semen (cum)
- pre-seminal fluid (pre-cum)
- rectal fluids
- vaginal fluids
- breast milk

These fluids must come in contact with a mucous membrane or damaged tissue or be directly injected into the bloodstream (from a needle or syringe) for transmission to occur. Mucous membranes are found inside the rectum, vagina, penis, and mouth.

HOW WELL DOES HUMAN IMMUNODEFICIENCY VIRUS SURVIVE OUTSIDE THE BODY?

Human immunodeficiency virus does not survive long outside the human body (such as on surfaces), and it cannot reproduce outside a human host. It is not transmitted:

- by mosquitoes, ticks, or other insects
- through saliva, tears, or sweat
- by hugging, shaking hands, sharing toilets, sharing dishes, or closed-mouth or "social" kissing with someone who has HIV
- through other sexual activities that do not involve the exchange of body fluids (e.g., touching)
- through the air

HUMAN IMMUNODEFICIENCY VIRUS AND SUBSTANCE USE

Substance use disorders, which are problematic patterns of using alcohol or another substance, such as crack cocaine, methamphetamine ("meth"), amyl nitrite ("poppers"), prescription opioids, and heroin, are closely associated with HIV and other STDs.

IDU can be a direct route of HIV transmission if people share needles, syringes, or other injection materials that are contaminated with HIV. However, drinking alcohol and ingesting, smoking, or inhaling drugs are also associated with increased risk for HIV. These substances alter judgment, which can lead to risky sexual behaviors (e.g., having sex without a condom, having multiple partners) that can make people more likely to get and transmit HIV.

In people living with HIV, substance use can hasten disease progression, affect adherence to antiretroviral therapy (ART; HIV medicine), and worsen the overall consequences of HIV.

Commonly Used Substances and Human Immunodeficiency Virus Risk

- **Alcohol**. Excessive alcohol consumption, notably binge drinking, can be an important risk factor for HIV because it is linked to risky sexual behaviors and, among people living with HIV, can hurt treatment outcomes.
- **Opioids**. Opioids, a class of drugs that reduce pain, include both prescription drugs and heroin. They are associated with HIV risk behaviors such as needle sharing when infected and risky sex and have been linked to an HIV outbreak.
- **Methamphetamine**. "Meth" is linked to risky sexual behavior that places people at greater HIV risk. It can be injected, which also increases HIV risk if people share needles and other injection equipment.
- **Crack cocaine**. Crack cocaine is a stimulant that can create a cycle in which people quickly exhaust their resources and turn to other ways to get the drug, including trading sex for drugs or money, which increases HIV risk.
- **Inhalants**. The use of amyl nitrite ("poppers") has long been linked to risky sexual behaviors, illegal drug use, and STDs among gay and bisexual men.

IF YOU ALREADY HAVE HUMAN IMMUNODEFICIENCY VIRUS, CAN YOU GET ANOTHER KIND OF HUMAN IMMUNODEFICIENCY VIRUS?

When a person with HIV gets another type, or strain, of the virus, it is called "HIV superinfection."

- The new strain of HIV can replace the original strain or remain along with the original strain.
- Superinfection may cause some people to get sicker faster because the new strain of the virus is resistant to the medicine (ART) they are taking to treat the original strain.
- Hard-to-treat superinfection is rare.
- Taking medicine to treat HIV can help protect someone from getting a superinfection.
- If you and your partner have HIV and keep an undetectable viral load, you will not transmit HIV to each other through sex.[10]

Section 12.5 | Acquired Immunodeficiency Syndrome and Opportunistic Infections

WHAT IS ACQUIRED IMMUNODEFICIENCY SYNDROME?

- Acquired immunodeficiency syndrome (AIDS) is the most severe stage of human immunodeficiency virus (HIV; stage 3).
- People with AIDS have badly damaged immune systems. They get an increasing number of severe illnesses called "opportunistic infections" (OIs).
- People receive an AIDS diagnosis when:
  - they develop certain OIs
  - their CD4 cell count drops below 200 cells per milliliter of blood

---

[10] "HIV Transmission," Centers for Disease Control and Prevention (CDC), October 28, 2020. Available online. URL: www.cdc.gov/hiv/basics/transmission.html. Accessed May 30, 2023.

WHAT ARE OPPORTUNISTIC INFECTIONS?

- Opportunistic infections are illnesses that occur more frequently and are more severe in people with HIV. This is because they have damaged immune systems.
- OIs are less common in people with HIV because of effective HIV treatment.
- But some people with HIV still develop OIs because:
  - they may not know they have HIV
  - they may not be on HIV treatment
  - their HIV treatment may not be working properly

HOW CAN YOU PREVENT OPPORTUNISTIC INFECTIONS?

Taking HIV medicine is the best way to prevent getting OIs. HIV medicine can keep your immune system strong and healthy. If you develop an OI, talk to your health-care provider about how to treat it.

The following are a few steps you can take to prevent getting OIs:

- Talk to your health-care provider about medicines and vaccines that prevent certain OIs.
- Prevent exposure to other sexually transmitted diseases (STDs).
- Do not share needles, syringes, or other drug injection equipment (e.g., cookers).
- Limit your exposure to germs that could make you very sick. This includes tuberculosis (TB) or germs found in the stools, in the saliva, or on the skin of animals.
- Do not consume certain foods, including undercooked eggs, raw milk and cheeses, unpasteurized fruit juices, or raw seed sprouts.
- Do not drink untreated water, such as water directly from lakes or rivers. Avoid drinking tap water in foreign countries. Use bottled water or water filters.
- Talk to your health-care provider about things that could expose you to OIs at work, at home, and on vacation.

COMMON OPPORTUNISTIC INFECTIONS
Candidiasis
- Candidiasis is caused by infection with a fungus called "*Candida.*"
- Candidiasis can affect the skin, nails, and mucous membranes throughout the body.
- People with HIV often have trouble with *Candida*, especially in the mouth and vagina.
- Candidiasis is only considered an OI when it causes severe or persistent infections in the mouth or vagina or when it develops in the esophagus (swallowing tube) or lower respiratory tract, such as the trachea and bronchi (breathing tube), or deeper lung tissue.

Invasive Cervical Cancer
- Cervical cancer starts within the cervix (the lower part of the uterus at the top of the vagina) and spreads (becomes invasive) to other parts of the body.
- Cervical cancer can be prevented by having your health-care provider perform regular examinations of the cervix.

Coccidioidomycosis
- This illness is caused by the fungus *Coccidioides.*
- It is sometimes called "valley fever," "desert fever," or "San Joaquin Valley fever."
- People can get it by breathing in fungal spores.
- The disease is especially common in hot, dry regions of the southwestern United States, Central America, and South America.

Cryptococcosis
- This illness is caused by infection with the fungus *Cryptococcus neoformans.*
- The fungus typically enters the body through the lungs and can cause pneumonia.

- Cryptococcosis usually affects the lungs or the central nervous system (the brain and spinal cord), but it can also affect other parts of the body.

Cryptosporidiosis (Crypto)
- Crypto is a diarrheal disease caused by a tiny parasite called "*Cryptosporidium*."
- Symptoms include abdominal cramps and severe, chronic, watery diarrhea.

Cystoisosporiasis
- It is formerly known as "isosporiasis."
- This infection is caused by the parasite *Cystoisospora belli* (formerly known as "*Isospora belli*").
- Cystoisosporiasis can enter the body through contaminated food or water.
- Symptoms include diarrhea, fever, headache, abdominal pain, vomiting, and weight loss.

Cytomegalovirus
- Cytomegalovirus (CMV) can infect multiple parts of the body and cause pneumonia, gastroenteritis (especially abdominal pain caused by infection of the colon), encephalitis (infection) of the brain, and sight-threatening retinitis (infection of the retina at the back of the eye).
- People with CMV retinitis have difficulty with vision that worsens over time. CMV retinitis is a medical emergency because it can cause blindness if not treated promptly.

Encephalopathy Related to Human Immunodeficiency Virus
- This brain disorder can occur as part of acute HIV infection or can result from chronic HIV infection.
- Its exact cause is unknown, but it is thought to be related to infection of the brain with HIV and the resulting inflammation.

Herpes Simplex Virus

- Herpes simplex virus (HSV) is a common virus that causes no major problems for most people.
- HSV is usually acquired sexually or passed from the mother to the child during birth.
- In most people with healthy immune systems, HSV is usually latent (inactive).
- Stress, trauma, other infections, or suppression of the immune system (such as by HIV) can reactivate the latent virus, and symptoms can return.
- HSV can cause painful cold sores (sometimes called "fever blisters") in or around the mouth or painful ulcers on or around the genitals or anus.
- In people with severely damaged immune systems, HSV can also cause infection of the bronchus (breathing tube), pneumonia (infection of the lungs), and esophagitis (infection of the esophagus, or swallowing tube).

Histoplasmosis

- Histoplasmosis is caused by the fungus *Histoplasma*.
- *Histoplasma* most often develops in the lungs and produces symptoms similar to the flu or pneumonia.
- People with severely damaged immune systems can get a very serious form of the disease called "progressive disseminated histoplasmosis." This form of histoplasmosis can last a long time and spread to other parts of the body.

Kaposi Sarcoma

- Kaposi sarcoma (KS) is caused by a virus called "Kaposi sarcoma herpesvirus" (KSHV) or "human herpesvirus 8" (HHV-8).
- KS causes small blood vessels to grow abnormally and can occur anywhere in the body.
- KS appears as firm pink or purple spots on the skin that can be raised or flat.

- KS can be life-threatening when it affects organs inside the body, such as the lung, lymph nodes, or intestines.

Lymphoma
- Lymphoma refers to cancer of the lymph nodes and other lymphoid tissues in the body.
- There are many kinds of lymphomas. Some types, such as non-Hodgkin lymphoma (NHL) and Hodgkin lymphoma (HL), are associated with HIV.

Tuberculosis
- TB is caused by a bacterium called "*Mycobacterium tuberculosis.*"
- TB can spread through the air when a person with TB coughs, sneezes, or speaks. Breathing in the bacteria can lead to infection in the lungs.
- Symptoms of TB in the lungs include cough, tiredness, weight loss, fever, and night sweats.

Mycobacterium avium Complex
- *Mycobacterium avium* complex (MAC) is caused by infection with different types of mycobacterium: *M. avium*, *Mycobacterium intracellulare*, or *Mycobacterium kansasii.*
- These bacteria live in our environment, including in soil and dust particles.
- Infections with these bacteria spread throughout the body and can be life-threatening in people with weakened immune systems.

Pneumocystis Pneumonia
- Pneumocystis pneumonia (PCP) is a lung infection caused by the fungus *Pneumocystis jirovecii.*
- PCP occurs in people with weakened immune systems.
- The first signs of infection are difficulty breathing, high fever, and dry cough.

Pneumonia
- Pneumonia is an infection in one or both lungs.
- Many germs, including bacteria, viruses, and fungi, can cause pneumonia.
- Symptoms include a cough (with mucous), fever, chills, and trouble breathing.
- In people with immune systems severely damaged by HIV, one of the most common and life-threatening causes of pneumonia is an infection with the bacteria *Streptococcus pneumoniae*, also called *"Pneumococcus."* People with HIV should get a vaccine to prevent infection with *S. pneumoniae*.

Progressive Multifocal Leukoencephalopathy
- This rare brain and spinal cord disease is caused by the John Cunningham (JC) virus.
- It is seen almost exclusively in people whose immune systems have been severely damaged by HIV.
- Symptoms may include loss of muscle control, paralysis, blindness, speech problems, and an altered mental state.
- This disease often progresses rapidly and may be fatal.

Salmonella Septicemia
- *Salmonella* is a bacterium that typically enters the body through eating or drinking contaminated food or water.
- Infection with *Salmonella* (called "salmonellosis") can affect anyone and usually causes nausea, vomiting, and diarrhea.
- Salmonella septicemia is a severe form of infection in which the bacteria circulate through the whole body and exceeds the immune system's ability to control it.

Toxoplasmosis
- This infection is caused by the parasite *Toxoplasma gondii*.
- The parasite is carried by warm-blooded animals, including cats, rodents, and birds, and is released in their feces (stool).

- People can develop it by inhaling dust or eating food contaminated with the parasite.
- *Toxoplasma* can also occur in commercial meats, especially red meats and pork, but rarely poultry.
- Infection can occur in the lungs, retina of the eye, heart, pancreas, liver, colon, testes, and brain.
- Although cats can transmit toxoplasmosis, litter boxes can be changed safely by wearing gloves and washing hands thoroughly with soap and water afterward.
- All raw red meats that have not been frozen for at least 24 hours should be cooked through to an internal temperature of at least 150 °F.

Wasting Syndrome due to Human Immunodeficiency Virus
- Wasting is defined as the involuntary loss of more than 10 percent of one's body weight while having experienced diarrhea or weakness and fever for more than 30 days.
- Wasting refers to the loss of muscle mass although part of the weight loss may also be due to the loss of fat.[11]

Section 12.6 | Human Immunodeficiency Virus Testing

The only way to know your human immunodeficiency virus (HIV) status is to get tested. Knowing your status gives you powerful information to keep you and your partner healthy.

This section answers some of the most common questions about HIV testing, including the types of tests available, where to get tested, and what to expect when you get tested.

---

[11] "AIDS and Opportunistic Infections," Centers for Disease Control and Prevention (CDC), May 20, 2021. Available online. URL: www.cdc.gov/hiv/basics/livingwithhiv/opportunisticinfections.html. Accessed May 30, 2023.

HOW DOES TAKING A HUMAN IMMUNODEFICIENCY VIRUS TEST HELP YOU?

Knowing your HIV status gives you powerful information to keep you and your partner healthy.

If your test result is positive, you can take medicine to treat the virus. HIV treatment reduces the amount of HIV in your blood (viral load). Taking HIV treatment as prescribed can make the viral load so low that a test cannot detect it (undetectable viral load). Getting and keeping an undetectable viral load (or staying virally suppressed) is the best way to stay healthy and protect others.

If your test result is negative, you can take actions to prevent HIV.

SHOULD YOU GET TESTED FOR HUMAN IMMUNODEFICIENCY VIRUS?

The Centers for Disease Control and Prevention (CDC) recommends everyone between the ages of 13 and 64 get tested for HIV at least once.

People with certain risk factors should get tested more often. You should get tested at least once a year if:

- you are a man who has had sex with another man
- you have had anal or vaginal sex with someone who has HIV
- you have had more than one sex partner since your last HIV test
- you have shared needles, syringes, or other drug injection equipment (e.g., cookers)
- you have exchanged sex for drugs or money
- you have been diagnosed with or treated for another sexually transmitted disease (STD)
- you have been diagnosed with or treated for hepatitis or tuberculosis (TB)
- you have had sex with someone who has done anything listed above or with someone whose sexual history you do not know

Before having sex for the first time with a new partner, talk about your sexual and drug use history, disclose your HIV status, and consider getting tested for HIV together.

IF YOU ARE A SEXUALLY ACTIVE GAY OR BISEXUAL MAN, HOW OFTEN SHOULD YOU GET TESTED?

If you are a sexually active gay or bisexual man, you may benefit from more frequent testing (every three to six months). Talk to your health-care provider about your risk factors and what testing options are available to you.

SHOULD YOU GET TESTED IF YOU ARE PREGNANT?

All pregnant women should get tested for HIV, so they can take steps to stay healthy and protect their babies.

Testing pregnant women for HIV and treating those who have HIV have decreased the number of babies born with HIV.

HIV treatment is most effective when started as early as possible during pregnancy. However, there are still great health benefits to beginning treatment even during labor or shortly after the baby is born.

If a pregnant person gets HIV treatment early in their pregnancy, the risk of transmitting HIV to their baby is extremely low (1% or less).

Pregnant women who test negative for HIV can talk to their health-care provider about taking pre-exposure prophylaxis (PrEP) to prevent HIV.

SHOULD YOU GET TESTED FOR HUMAN IMMUNODEFICIENCY VIRUS IF YOU DO NOT HAVE ANY RISK FACTORS?

The CDC recommends that everyone between the ages of 13 and 64 gets tested for HIV at least once as part of routine health care and more often if you do things that might increase your chance of getting HIV.

Even if both you and your partner are having sex only with each other, you should both find out your HIV status.

WHO WILL PAY FOR YOUR HUMAN IMMUNODEFICIENCY VIRUS TEST?

Human immunodeficiency virus tests are covered by health insurance without a co-pay, as required by the Affordable Care Act

(ACA). If you do not have medical insurance, some places offer free or low-cost tests.

WHAT SHOULD YOU EXPECT WHEN YOU GO IN FOR A HUMAN IMMUNODEFICIENCY VIRUS TEST?

Your experience may be different depending on the setting.

Health-Care Setting or Lab

If you get an HIV test in a health-care setting or lab, the health-care provider will take a sample of blood or oral fluid.

- With a rapid test (oral fluid or finger stick), you may be able to wait for the results.
- With a lab test, it may take several days for your results to be available.

Your health-care provider may talk with you about your risk factors, answer any questions you might have, and discuss the next steps.

Outside of a Health-Care Setting or Lab

If you are tested outside of a health-care setting or a lab, you will likely receive a rapid test (oral fluid or finger stick). The counselor providing the test should be able to answer questions and provide referrals for follow-up testing if needed.

WHAT TYPES OF TESTS ARE AVAILABLE, AND HOW DO THEY WORK?

There are three types of HIV tests: antibody tests, antigen/antibody tests, and nucleic acid tests (NATs). Antibodies are produced by your immune system when you are exposed to viruses, such as HIV. Antigens are foreign substances that cause your immune system to activate. If you have HIV, an antigen called "p24" is produced even before antibodies develop.

HIV tests are typically performed on blood or oral fluid. They may also be performed on urine.

Antibody Test

An antibody test looks for antibodies to HIV in your blood or oral fluid.

- Most rapid tests and the only HIV self-test approved by the U.S. Food and Drug Administration (FDA) are antibody tests.
- In general, antibody tests that use blood from a vein can detect HIV sooner than tests done with blood from a finger stick or with oral fluid.

Antigen/Antibody Test

An antigen/antibody test looks for both HIV antibodies and antigens.

- Antigen/antibody tests are recommended for testing done in labs and are common in the United States. This lab test involves drawing blood from a vein.
- There is also a rapid antigen/antibody test available that is done with blood from a finger stick.

Nucleic Acid Test

An NAT looks for the actual virus in the blood.

- With an NAT, the health-care provider will draw blood from your vein and send the sample to a lab for testing.
- This test can tell if a person has HIV or how much virus is present in the blood (HIV viral load test).
- An NAT can detect HIV sooner than other types of tests.
- This test should be considered for people who have had a recent exposure or a possible exposure and have early symptoms of HIV and who have tested negative with an antibody or antigen/antibody test.

Talk to your health-care provider about what type of HIV test is right for you.

HOW LONG WILL IT TAKE TO GET YOU HUMAN IMMUNODEFICIENCY VIRUS TEST RESULTS?

It depends on the type of HIV test and where you get tested.

- HIV self-tests provide results within 20 minutes.
- With a rapid antibody test, usually done with blood from a finger stick or with oral fluid, results are ready in 30 minutes or less.
- The rapid antigen/antibody test, done with blood from a finger stick, takes 30 minutes or less.
- It may take several days to receive your test results with an NAT or antigen/antibody lab test.

CAN A HUMAN IMMUNODEFICIENCY VIRUS TEST DETECT THE VIRUS IMMEDIATELY AFTER EXPOSURE?

No HIV test can detect HIV immediately after infection. That is because of the window period—the time between HIV exposure and when a test can detect HIV in your body. The window period depends on the type of HIV test. An NAT can usually detect HIV the soonest (about 10–33 days after exposure).

If you think you have been exposed to HIV in the last 72 hours, talk to a health-care provider, an emergency room doctor, or an urgent care provider about postexposure prophylaxis (PEP) right away.

WHAT IS THE HUMAN IMMUNODEFICIENCY VIRUS WINDOW PERIOD?

The window period for an HIV test refers to the time between HIV exposure and when a test can detect HIV in your body. The window period depends on the type of HIV test used.

WHAT IS THE WINDOW PERIOD FOR THE HUMAN IMMUNODEFICIENCY VIRUS TEST YOU TOOK?

- Antibody tests can usually detect HIV 23–90 days after exposure. Most rapid tests and self-tests are antibody tests.

- A rapid antigen/antibody test done with blood from a finger stick can usually detect HIV 18–90 days after exposure.
- An antigen/antibody lab test using blood from a vein can usually detect HIV 18–45 days after exposure.
- An NAT can usually detect HIV 10–33 days after exposure.

If you get an HIV test after a potential HIV exposure and the result is negative, get tested again after the window period for the test you took.

HOW DO YOU FIND A HUMAN IMMUNODEFICIENCY VIRUS TEST?

Most HIV tests are available for free or at a reduced cost.

Ask your health-care provider for an HIV test. Many medical clinics, substance abuse programs, community health centers, and hospitals offer them too.

You can find a testing site near you by:
- using the CDC's HIV prevention services locator at https://www.cdc.gov/hiv/basics/hiv-testing/finding-tests.html
- visiting gettested.cdc.gov
- calling 800-CDC-INFO (232-4636)

You can also buy an HIV self-test at a pharmacy or online or visit gettested.cdc.gov to see if any organizations in your area are offering free or reduced-cost self-tests.

WHAT IS A HUMAN IMMUNODEFICIENCY VIRUS SELF-TEST?

An HIV self-test (or rapid self-test) is an antibody test that can be used at home or in a private location. With an HIV self-test, you can get your test results within 20 minutes.

HOW DO YOU FIND A HUMAN IMMUNODEFICIENCY VIRUS SELF-TEST?

You can buy an HIV self-test at a pharmacy or online. Your local health department or another organization near you may offer free or low-cost self-tests, which you can find using the locator (https://gettested.cdc.gov). The only HIV self-test approved by the U.S. Food and Drug Administration (FDA) currently available in the United States is an oral fluid test.

HOW DO YOU USE A HUMAN IMMUNODEFICIENCY VIRUS SELF-TEST?

Read the instructions included in the test kit before you start.
- For an HIV self-test, you must swab your gums to collect an oral fluid sample and then test your sample.
- Your results will be ready within 20 minutes.
- If you do not follow the directions as described, the test may not work. There is a phone number included with the HIV self-test if you need help using the test.

You should always interpret HIV self-test results according to the manufacturer's instructions.

If the HIV self-test is invalid, then the test did not work. You will need to use another HIV self-test, use a mail-in HIV test, or find testing at a health-care provider or testing center.

WHAT IS A MAIL-IN HUMAN IMMUNODEFICIENCY VIRUS TEST?

A mail-in HIV test is an antigen/antibody test that includes supplies to collect a small sample of blood from a finger stick. You or your health-care provider can order the test online and send the sample to a lab for testing. If your provider orders the test, they will contact you with the test results.

Mail-in HIV tests are not approved by the FDA. However, under the Clinical Laboratory and Improvement Amendments of 1988, labs that offer this service are required to establish and verify the test's accuracy.

HOW DO YOU FIND A MAIL-IN HUMAN IMMUNODEFICIENCY VIRUS TEST?

You can order a mail-in HIV test online. Your health-care provider can also order a mail-in HIV test for you.

HOW DO YOU USE A MAIL-IN HUMAN IMMUNODEFICIENCY VIRUS TEST?

Read the instructions included in the test kit before you start.

- For a mail-in HIV test, you must prick your finger and collect a very small sample of blood.
- You or your health-care provider will mail the sample to a lab for testing.
- If your health-care provider orders the test, they will contact you when your test results are ready.

You should always follow the manufacturer's instructions to make sure you collect a good sample.

WILL YOUR INSURANCE COVER A HUMAN IMMUNODEFICIENCY VIRUS SELF-TEST OR MAIL-IN TEST?

Human immunodeficiency virus self-tests and mail-in HIV tests may be covered by insurance (Figure 12.5). Be sure to check with your insurance company and health-care provider about reimbursement for tests that you purchase.

WHICH HIV SELF-TEST IS RIGHT FOR YOU?

HIV self-testing allows you to take an HIV test at home or other private location. There are two kinds of HIV self-tests: Rapid and Mail-In. Learn the differences and which may be right for you.

	Rapid self-test	Mail-in test*
Can I order it myself?	✔	✔
Can my health care provider order it for me?	X	✔
Is it available at a pharmacy?	✔	X
Can I order it online?	✔	✔
Does it offer quick results?	✔	X
Can it find HIV soon after exposure?	◯	✔
Does it use an oral swab?	✔	X
Does it use a small blood spot from a finger stick?	X	✔
Is it covered by insurance?	◯	◯
Can I use my Health Savings Account or Flexible Spending Account?	◯	◯

* Not approved by the U. S. Food and Drug Administration. However, labs are required to establish and verify the test's accuracy. ✔ Yes ◯ Sometimes X No

Figure 12.5. Human Immunodeficiency Virus Self-Test Chart

Centers for Disease Control and Prevention (CDC)

WHAT DOES A NEGATIVE HUMAN IMMUNODEFICIENCY VIRUS TEST RESULT MEAN?

A negative result does not necessarily mean that you do not have HIV. That is because of the window period—the time between HIV exposure and when a test can detect HIV in your body.

- If you get an HIV test after a potential HIV exposure and the result is negative, get tested again after the window period for the test you took.
- If you test again after the window period and have no possible HIV exposure during that time and the result is negative, you do not have HIV.

If you are sexually active or use needles to inject drugs, continue to take actions to prevent HIV, such as taking medicines to prevent HIV.

If you have certain risk factors, you should continue getting tested at least once a year.

IF YOU HAVE A NEGATIVE RESULT, DOES THAT MEAN YOUR PARTNER IS HUMAN IMMUNODEFICIENCY VIRUS–NEGATIVE ALSO?

No. Your HIV test result reveals only your HIV status.

HIV is not necessarily transmitted every time you have sex or share needles, syringes, or other drug injection equipment (e.g., cookers). And the chance of getting HIV varies depending on the type of exposure or behavior. Taking an HIV test is not a way to find out if your partner has HIV.

Be open with your partners and ask them to tell you their HIV status. But keep in mind that your partners may not know, may be wrong, or may not tell you about their status. Consider getting tested together, so you can both know your HIV status and take steps to keep yourselves healthy.

WHAT DOES A POSITIVE HUMAN IMMUNODEFICIENCY VIRUS RESULT MEAN?

If you use any type of antibody test and have a positive result, you will need a follow-up test to confirm your results.

- If you test in a community program or take an HIV self-test and it is positive, you should go to a health-care provider for follow-up testing.
- If you test in a health-care setting or a lab and it is positive, the lab will conduct the follow-up testing, usually on the same blood sample as the first test.

If the follow-up test is also positive, it means you have HIV.

WHAT SHOULD YOU DO IF YOU JUST GOT DIAGNOSED WITH HUMAN IMMUNODEFICIENCY VIRUS?

Receiving an HIV diagnosis can be life-changing. You may feel many emotions—sadness, hopelessness, or anger. Allied health-care providers and social service providers can help you work through the early stages of your diagnosis. They can also help you find HIV care and treatment that will help you live a long, healthy life.

- HIV treatment (antiretroviral therapy (ART)) is recommended for all people with HIV, regardless of how long they have had the virus or how healthy they are.
- HIV treatment can make the amount of HIV in the blood (viral load) so low that a test cannot detect it (undetectable viral load). Getting and keeping an undetectable viral load is the best way to stay healthy and protect others.

IF YOU TEST POSITIVE FOR HUMAN IMMUNODEFICIENCY VIRUS, DOES THAT MEAN YOU HAVE ACQUIRED IMMUNODEFICIENCY SYNDROME?

No. Testing positive for HIV does not mean you have acquired immunodeficiency syndrome (AIDS).

- AIDS is the most advanced stage of HIV disease (stage 3).
- HIV can lead to AIDS if a person with HIV does not get treatment or take care of their health. But,

if someone with HIV takes their HIV treatment as prescribed, they can live long, healthy lives and may never develop AIDS.[12]

Section 12.7 | The Affordable Care Act and People Living with Human Immunodeficiency Virus and Acquired Immunodeficiency Syndrome

IMPROVING ACCESS TO COVERAGE

The Affordable Care Act (ACA) provides Americans—including those with and at risk for human immunodeficiency virus (HIV)—better access to health-care coverage and more health insurance options.

Health insurance gives people with HIV access to appropriate HIV medical care, particularly treatment with HIV medicine called "antiretroviral therapy" (ART), which helps people with HIV stay healthy and prevent transmitting HIV to others.

Here are just some of the ways the ACA has improved access to coverage for people with or at risk for HIV:

- **Coverage for people with preexisting conditions.**
  Thanks to the ACA, no American can ever again be dropped or denied coverage because of a preexisting health condition, such as asthma, cancer, HIV, or coronavirus disease 2019 (COVID-19). Insurers also are prohibited from canceling or rescinding coverage because of mistakes made on an application and can no longer impose lifetime caps on insurance benefits. These changes are significant because, prior to the ACA, many people with HIV or other chronic health conditions experienced obstacles in getting health coverage, were dropped from coverage, or avoided

---

[12] "HIV Testing," Centers for Disease Control and Prevention (CDC), June 22, 2022. Available online. URL: www.cdc.gov/hiv/basics/testing.html. Accessed May 31, 2023.

seeking coverage for fear of being denied. Now they can get covered and get the care they need.

- **Broader Medicaid eligibility**. Under the ACA, states have the option, which is fully federally funded for the first three years, to expand Medicaid to generally include those with incomes at or below 138 percent of the federal poverty line, including single adults without children who were previously not generally eligible for Medicaid. (Use www.healthcare.gov/lower-costs to find out if you qualify.) As of September 2022, 39 states (including DC) have expanded Medicaid coverage. Medicaid is the largest payer for HIV care in the United States, and the expansion of Medicaid to low-income childless adults is particularly important for many gay, bisexual, and other men who have sex with men (MSM) who were previously ineligible for Medicaid and yet remain the population most affected by the HIV epidemic. Furthermore, in states that have opted for Medicaid expansion, people with HIV who meet the income threshold no longer have to wait for an AIDS diagnosis in order to become eligible for Medicaid. That means they can get into life-extending care and treatment before the disease has significantly damaged their immune system.

- **More affordable coverage**. To help people access quality, affordable coverage, the ACA created the Healthcare.gov Marketplace (and some state-run Marketplaces, sometimes called "exchanges") that help consumers compare different health plans and determine what savings they may qualify for. The ACA also provides financial assistance for people with low and middle incomes in the form of tax credits that lower the cost of their monthly premiums and lower their out-of-pocket costs. These tax credits depend on a family's household size and income. In addition, Americans can apply for free or low-cost coverage through Medicaid and Children's Health Insurance

Program (CHIP) at any time, all year. If you qualify, coverage can begin immediately.

- **Lower prescription drug costs for Medicare recipients**. In the past, as many as one in four seniors went without a prescription drug every year because they could not afford it. The ACA closed, over time, the Medicare Part D prescription drug coverage gap, once known as the "donut hole"—the gap between when a person's initial Medicare drug coverage ended and when they qualified for catastrophic coverage. Previously, when people reached the donut hole, they had to pay the full cost of their prescription drugs until they reached the catastrophic coverage level, and many struggled to pay for their medications. Under the ACA, the donut hole began shrinking in 2011 and closed in 2020. Now people in the coverage gap will pay no more than 25 percent of the cost of their covered medications. Also, as a result of the ACA, Acquired Immunodeficiency Syndrome (AIDS) Drug Assistance Program (ADAP) spending is now counted as part of Medicare Part D's True Out-of-Pocket ("TrOOP") costs, allowing ADAP clients who are Medicare Part D enrollees to reach the catastrophic coverage level faster, when Medicare starts covering the full cost of medications. (To learn more about your Medicare coverage and choices, visit Medicare.gov.)

ENSURING QUALITY COVERAGE

The ACA also helps all Americans, including those with or at risk for HIV, have access to the best-quality coverage and care. This includes the following:

- **Preventive services**. Under the ACA, most new health insurance plans must cover certain recommended preventive services, including HIV testing for everyone aged 15–65 and other ages at increased risk, without additional cost-sharing, such as co-pays or deductibles. Since about one in eight people with HIV in the United

States (13%) is unaware of their HIV status, improving access to HIV testing will help more people learn their status, so they can be connected to care and treatment. Pre-exposure prophylaxis (PrEP) to prevent HIV is also covered for HIV-negative adults at high risk for getting HIV through sex or injection drug use. This coverage of PrEP includes medications as well as necessary clinic visits and lab tests. Other preventive health services related to HIV risk and/or health outcomes are also covered, such as sexually transmitted infection (STI) counseling, syphilis screening, hepatitis B and hepatitis C screening, and hepatitis A and hepatitis B immunizations.

- **Comprehensive coverage**. The law establishes a minimum set of benefits (called "essential health benefits") that must be covered under health plans offered in the individual and small group markets, both inside and outside of the Health Insurance Marketplace. These include many health services that are important for people with HIV, including prescription drug services, hospital inpatient care, lab tests, services and devices to help you manage a chronic disease, and mental health and substance use disorder services, as well as HIV screening, PrEP, and other preventive services for those at risk for HIV.

- **Coordinated care for those with chronic health conditions**. The law recognizes the value of patient-centered medical homes as an effective way to strengthen the quality of care, especially for people with complex chronic conditions such as HIV. The patient-centered medical home model of care can foster greater patient retention and higher-quality HIV care because of its focus on treating the many needs of the patient at once and better coordination across medical specialties and support services. The Ryan White HIV/AIDS Program has been a pioneer in the development of this model in the HIV health-care system. The ACA also authorized an optional Medicaid State Plan benefit for states to establish Health Homes to coordinate care for Medicaid beneficiaries with certain chronic health conditions. HIV/AIDS is one of the chronic health conditions that states may request approval to cover.

ENHANCING THE CAPACITY OF THE HEALTH-CARE DELIVERY SYSTEM

The ACA expands the capacity of the health-care delivery system to better serve all Americans, including those with and at risk for HIV. The following are a few examples:

- **Expansion of community health centers**. The ACA has made a major investment in expanding the network of community health centers that provide preventive and primary care services to nearly 30 million Americans every year, regardless of their ability to pay. Health centers provide high-quality primary care services and support public health priorities, such as the response to the opioid crisis, the implementation of the National HIV/AIDS Strategy and the Ending the HIV Epidemic in the United States (EHE) initiative, and the response to COVID-19.

- **Delivering culturally competent care**. The ACA expands initiatives to strengthen cultural competency training for all health-care providers and ensure all populations are treated equitably. It also bolsters the federal commitment to reducing health disparities. One effort underway to expand the capacity of health centers to deliver culturally competent care to populations heavily impacted by HIV is the National LGBTQIA+ Health Education Center, funded by Health Resources and Services Administration (HRSA). This center helps health-care organizations better address the needs of lesbian, gay, bisexual, transgender, queer, intersex, asexual, and all sexual and gender minority people, including individuals' needs for HIV prevention, testing, and treatment.

- **Increasing the health-care workforce for underserved communities**. Thanks to the ACA, the National Health Service Corps is providing loan repayment and scholarships to more doctors, nurses, and other health-care providers, a critical health-care workforce expansion to better serve vulnerable populations. This is in line with a key recommendation of the National HIV/AIDS Strategy to increase the number and diversity of available providers of clinical care and related services for people with HIV, many of whom live in underserved communities.[13]

---

[13] HIV.gov, "The Affordable Care Act and HIV/AIDS," U.S. Department of Health and Human Services (HHS), October 7, 2022. Available online. URL: www.hiv.gov/federal-response/policies-issues/the-affordable-care-act-and-hiv-aids. Accessed May 31, 2023.

Chapter 13 | Hepatitis

Chapter Contents

WHAT IS VIRAL HEPATITIS?

Hepatitis means inflammation of the liver. The liver is a vital organ that processes nutrients, filters the blood, and fights infections. When the liver is inflamed or damaged, its function can be affected. Heavy alcohol use, toxins, some medications, and certain medical conditions can cause hepatitis. However, hepatitis is often caused by a virus. In the United States, the most common types of viral hepatitis are hepatitis A, hepatitis B, and hepatitis C.

Many people with hepatitis do not have symptoms and do not know they are infected. If symptoms occur with an acute infection, they can appear anytime from two weeks to six months after exposure. Symptoms of acute hepatitis can include fever, fatigue, loss of appetite, nausea, vomiting, abdominal pain, dark urine, light-colored stools, joint pain, and jaundice. Symptoms of chronic viral hepatitis can take decades to develop.

WHAT CAUSES VIRAL HEPATITIS?

- Hepatitis A is caused by hepatitis A virus (HAV).
- Hepatitis B is caused by hepatitis B virus (HBV).
- Hepatitis C is caused by hepatitis C virus (HCV).

NUMBER OF U.S. CASES

- hepatitis A
  - about 19,900 estimated infections in 2020
- hepatitis B
  - about 14,000 estimated infections in 2020
  - estimated 880,000 adults with chronic hepatitis B
- hepatitis C
  - about 66,700 estimated infections in 2020
  - estimated 2.2 million adults with hepatitis C

KEY FACTS
Hepatitis A

- An effective vaccine is available.
- Outbreaks related to contaminated food or to person-to-person transmission still occur in the United States.
- This is common in many countries, especially those without modern sanitation.

Hepatitis B

- An effective vaccine is available.
- About two in three people with hepatitis B do not know they are infected.
- In 2020, the rate of newly reported cases was almost 12 times higher in Asian Pacific Islander persons than among non-Hispanic White persons.
- Hepatitis B is a leading cause of liver cancer.

Hepatitis C

- Hepatitis C is curable in more than 95 percent of cases.
- Nearly 40 percent of people with hepatitis C do not know they are infected.
- In 2020, the rates of hepatitis C-associated deaths were highest in American Indian/Alaska Native and non-Hispanic Black people.
- Hepatitis C is a leading cause of liver transplants and liver cancer.

HOW LONG DOES VIRAL HEPATITIS LAST?

- Hepatitis A can last from a few weeks to several months.
- Hepatitis B can range from a mild illness lasting a few weeks to a serious, lifelong (chronic) condition.
- Hepatitis C can range from a mild illness lasting a few weeks to a serious, lifelong (chronic) infection. Most people who get infected with the hepatitis C virus develop chronic hepatitis C.

HOW IS VIRAL HEPATITIS SPREAD?
Hepatitis A
Hepatitis A virus is spread when someone ingests the virus (even in microscopic amounts too small to see) through close, personal contact with an infected person or through eating contaminated food or drink.

Hepatitis B
Hepatitis B is primarily spread when blood, semen, or certain other body fluids—even in microscopic amounts—from a person infected with the hepatitis B virus enters the body of someone who is not infected. The hepatitis B virus can also be transmitted by:
- birth to an infected pregnant person
- sex with an infected person
- sharing equipment that has been contaminated with blood from an infected person, such as needles, syringes, and even medical equipment, such as glucose monitors
- sharing personal items such as toothbrushes or razors (which is less common)
- direct contact with the blood or open sores of a person who has hepatitis B
- poor infection control in health-care facilities

Although the virus can be found in saliva, it is not spread through kissing or sharing utensils. Hepatitis B is not spread through sneezing, coughing, hugging, breastfeeding, or food or water.

Hepatitis C
Hepatitis C is spread when blood from a person infected with the hepatitis C virus—even in microscopic amounts—enters the body of someone who is not infected. The hepatitis C virus can also be transmitted by:
- sharing equipment that has been contaminated with blood from an infected person, such as needles and syringes

- poor infection control, which has resulted in outbreaks in health-care facilities
- unregulated tattoos or body piercings with contaminated instruments
- receiving a blood transfusion or organ transplant before 1992 (when widespread screening eliminated hepatitis C from the blood supply)
- birth to an infected pregnant person
- sexual contact with an infected person

Hepatitis C is not spread by sharing eating utensils, breastfeeding, hugging, kissing, holding hands, coughing, or sneezing or through food or water.

HOW SERIOUS IS VIRAL HEPATITIS?
Hepatitis A
- People can be sick for a few weeks to a few months.
- Most recover with no lasting liver damage.
- Although very rare, death can occur.

Hepatitis B
- Acute hepatitis B is a short-term illness that occurs within the first six months after someone is exposed to the hepatitis B virus. Some people with acute hepatitis B have no symptoms at all or only mild illness. For others, acute hepatitis B causes a more severe illness that requires hospitalization.
- Approximately 25 percent of people who become chronically infected during childhood and 15 percent of those who become chronically infected after childhood die prematurely from cirrhosis or liver cancer, and most remain asymptomatic until the onset of cirrhosis or end-stage liver disease.

Hepatitis C
- About half of adults who get infected with the hepatitis C virus develop a chronic infection.

- Approximately 5–25 percent of people with chronic hepatitis C develop cirrhosis over 10–20 years.

WHO SHOULD BE TESTED?
Hepatitis A

- Screening for prior hepatitis A is not routinely recommended.
- People should only be tested for hepatitis A if they have symptoms and think they might have been infected.

Hepatitis B

- all adults aged 18 and older at least once in their lifetime
- all pregnant women early during each pregnancy
- infants born to pregnant women with HBV infection
- any person who requests hepatitis B testing

Anyone with ongoing risk of exposure should be tested periodically, including:
- people born in countries with 2 percent or higher HBV prevalence
- people not vaccinated as infants with parents born in countries with 8 percent or higher HBV prevalence
- people who inject or have used injection drugs
- people incarcerated in jail, prison, or detention setting
- men who have sex with men (MSM)
- people with HIV
- people with hepatitis C
- people with a sexually transmitted infection (STI) or multiple sex partners
- people who share needles or are in sexual contact with people with hepatitis B
- household contacts of people with hepatitis B
- people requiring immunosuppressive therapy
- people on kidney dialysis
- people with elevated liver enzymes without knowing the cause

- people who donate blood, plasma, organs, tissues, or semen

Hepatitis C
- universal screening for:
  - all adults aged 18 years and older at least once in their lifetime
  - all pregnant women early during each pregnancy
- at least one-time testing for:
  - people with HIV
  - people who ever injected drugs and shared needles, syringes, or other drug equipment, including those who injected once or a few times many years ago
  - people with persistently abnormal liver enzymes
  - people who received clotting factor concentrates produced before 1987
  - people who received an organ transplant or a transfusion of blood or blood components before July 1992
  - people who were notified that they received blood from a donor who later tested positive for HCV infection
  - health-care, emergency medical, and public safety personnel after needle sticks, sharps, or mucosal exposures to HCV-positive blood
  - children born to people with HCV infection
- regular or routine testing for:
  - people with ongoing risk factors, including people who currently inject and share needles, syringes, or other drug equipment
  - people with certain medical conditions, including those who ever received maintenance hemodialysis
  - any person who requests hepatitis C testing

TREATMENT FOR HEPATITIS A
- People who test positive for hepatitis A are usually treated through supportive care (rest, adequate nutrition, and fluids) to help relieve symptoms.

TREATMENT FOR HEPATITIS B

- People who test positive for acute hepatitis B are usually treated through supportive care (rest, adequate nutrition, and fluids) to help relieve symptoms. There is no specific medication available.
- People with chronic hepatitis B can be treated with antiviral drugs and should be monitored regularly for signs of liver disease progression.

TREATMENT FOR HEPATITIS C

- People who test positive for hepatitis C should be treated with medication right away.
- Treatment is typically taking pills for 8–12 weeks. The pills can cure more than 95 percent of people, and side effects are minimal.
- The sooner the treatment starts, the better it will be at preventing liver damage and further spread.

Experts recommend not waiting until a person already has liver damage.[1]

Section 13.2 | Hepatitis and Human Immunodeficiency Virus Coinfection

HUMAN IMMUNODEFICIENCY VIRUS AND HEPATITIS B AND HEPATITIS C COINFECTION

Hepatitis B and hepatitis C are liver infections caused by a virus. Because these infections can be spread in the same ways as human immunodeficiency virus (HIV), people with HIV in the United States are often also affected by chronic viral hepatitis.

---

[1] "What Is Viral Hepatitis?" Centers for Disease Control and Prevention (CDC), March 9, 2023. Available online. URL: www.cdc.gov/hepatitis/abc/index.htm. Accessed May 30, 2023.

Viral hepatitis progresses faster and causes more liver-related health problems among people with HIV than among those who do not have HIV. Liver disease, much of which is related to hepatitis B virus (HBV) or hepatitis C virus (HCV), is a major cause of deaths related to non–acquired immunodeficiency syndrome (AIDS) among people with HIV.

Given the risks of hepatitis B or hepatitis C coinfection to the health of people with HIV, it is important to understand these risks, take steps to prevent infection, know your status, and, if necessary, get medical care from a health-care provider who is experienced in treating people who are coinfected with HIV and HBV or HIV and HCV.

HOW ARE HEPATITIS B AND HEPATITIS C SPREAD FROM PERSON TO PERSON?

Like HIV, HBV and HCV spread in the following ways:

- **By sharing**. These viruses spread by sharing needles, syringes, and other injection equipment.
- **Perinatally**. Pregnant women can pass these infections to their infants. HIV–HCV coinfection increases the risk of passing on hepatitis C to the baby.
- **Sexually**. Both viruses can also be transmitted sexually, but HBV is much more likely than HCV to be transmitted sexually. Sexual transmission of HCV is most likely to happen among gay and bisexual men who have HIV.

Viral hepatitis screening and care prevention are important parts of HIV care.[2]

PEOPLE WITH HUMAN IMMUNODEFICIENCY VIRUS AND HEPATITIS A

People with HIV who have underlying liver disease are at risk of severe disease from hepatitis A infection, and widespread

[2] HIV.gov, "Hepatitis B & C," U.S. Department of Health and Human Services (HHS), September 20, 2022. Available online. URL: www.hiv.gov/hiv-basics/staying-in-hiv-care/other-related-health-issues/hepatitis-b-and-c. Accessed May 30, 2023.

hepatitis A outbreaks associated with person-to-person transmission have been occurring in the United States since 2016. Therefore, the Centers for Disease Control and Prevention (CDC) and the Advisory Committee on Immunization Practices (ACIP) recommend hepatitis A vaccination for this population. Because the response to the vaccine might be reduced in people with HIV infection who are immunosuppressed, postvaccination serologic testing (PVST) should be performed for all people with HIV infection one month or over after completing the hepatitis A vaccine series. All people with HIV infection who receive the hepatitis A vaccine, regardless of PVST results, should be counseled that the vaccine might not provide long-term protection against hepatitis A. Therefore, they might need to receive immune globulin (IG) after a high-risk exposure (e.g., a sexual or household contact).

PEOPLE WITH HUMAN IMMUNODEFICIENCY VIRUS AND HEPATITIS B

Hepatitis B virus and HIV are blood-borne viruses (BBVs) transmitted primarily through sexual contact and injection drug use. Because of these shared modes of transmission, a high proportion of adults at risk for HIV infection are also at risk for HBV infection. People with HIV who become infected with HBV are at increased risk for liver-related morbidity and mortality. To prevent HBV infection in people with HIV, the ACIP recommends universal hepatitis B vaccination for all susceptible people infected with HIV. The first vaccine dose can be administered immediately after collection of blood for prevaccination serologic testing and regardless of CD4+ lymphocyte cell count. To confirm adequate immune response, PVST for protective concentrations of antibodies to hepatitis B surface antigen should be conducted one to two months after completion of the hepatitis B vaccine series. People with HIV who test positive for HBV should receive HIV antiviral medication with activity against HBV (e.g., tenofovir and entecavir). For the structure of the HBV, see Figure 13.1.

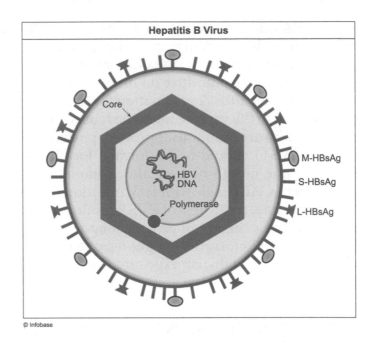

Figure 13.1. Hepatitis B Virus

Infobase

PEOPLE WITH HUMAN IMMUNODEFICIENCY VIRUS AND HEPATITIS C

According to the CDC, approximately 21 percent of adults with HIV who were tested for past or present HCV infection tested positive although coinfection prevalence varies substantially according to risk group (e.g., men who have sex with men (MSM), high-risk heterosexuals, and people who inject drugs). As HCV is a BBV transmitted through direct contact with the blood of an infected person, coinfection with HIV and HCV is common (62–80%) among injection drug users who have HIV. Although transmission via injection drug use remains the most common mode of HCV acquisition in the United States, sexual transmission is an important mode of acquisition among MSM with HIV who also have risk factors, including those who participate in unprotected anal intercourse, use sex toys, and use non–injection drugs. HCV is one of the primary causes of chronic liver disease (CLD) in the United States, and HCV-related liver injury progresses more rapidly among people coinfected with HIV. HCV infection may also affect the management of HIV infection. The CDC now recommends one-time hepatitis C testing of all adults (18 years of age and older), including those with HIV. The CDC continues to recommend people with risk factors, like people who inject drugs, be tested regularly. The American Association for the Study of Liver Disease (AASLD) and the Infectious Diseases Society of America (IDSA) also recommend that people who are coinfected with HIV and HCV be provided with curative, direct-acting antiviral medications to treat their HCV infection. For the structure of the hepatitis C virus, see Figure 13.2.[3]

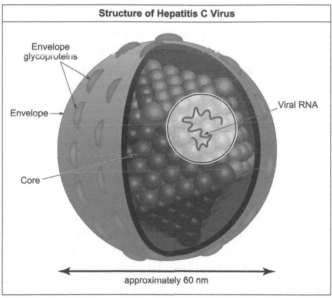

© Infobase

Figure 13.2. Hepatitis C Virus

Infobase

---

[3] "People Coinfected with HIV and Viral Hepatitis," Centers for Disease Control and Prevention (CDC), September 21, 2020. Available online. URL: www.cdc.gov/hepatitis/populations/hiv.htm. Accessed May 30, 2023.

IS HEPATITIS TESTING RECOMMENDED FOR PEOPLE WITH HUMAN IMMUNODEFICIENCY VIRUS?

Yes. Everyone with HIV should be tested for HBV and HCV when they are first diagnosed with HIV and begin treatment. People with HIV who have ongoing risk factors for getting hepatitis B or hepatitis C should be tested annually.

In addition, HCV screening recommendations from the CDC call for:

- one-time screening for all adults aged 18 and over
- screening of all pregnant women during every pregnancy
- testing for all persons with risk factors, with testing continued for those with ongoing risk

HOW CAN YOU PREVENT HEPATITIS B AND HEPATITIS C?

- **Hepatitis B.** Vaccination is the best way to prevent all the ways that hepatitis B is transmitted. People with HIV who do not have active HBV infection should be vaccinated against it. The hepatitis B vaccine is now recommended for all infants, children, and adults aged 19–59, as well as adults aged 60 and over at high risk for infection. There are a three-dose series of hepatitis B vaccine given over six months and a two-dose series given over one month. Additionally, there is a two-dose combination vaccine that protects against both hepatitis A and hepatitis B.
- **Hepatitis C.** No vaccine exists for HCV, and no effective pre- or post-exposure prophylaxis is available. Injection drug use is one of the risk factors for hepatitis C. For people who inject drugs, the best way to prevent hepatitis C infection is to always use new, sterile needles or syringes and never reuse or share needles or syringes, water, or other drug preparation equipment. Community-based prevention programs, such as medication-assisted treatment (MAT) and syringe services programs (SSPs), provide support and services aimed at preventing and reducing the transmission of HCV. Although the risk of sexual transmission of HCV is considered to be

low, avoiding unprotected sexual exposure by using condoms has been shown to reduce the chance of sexually transmitted infections.

TREATMENT FOR HUMAN IMMUNODEFICIENCY VIRUS–HEPATITIS COINFECTIONS

The coinfections of HIV–HBV and HIV–HCV can be effectively treated in most people. But medical treatment can be complex, and people with coinfection should look for health-care providers with expertise in the management of both HIV infection and viral hepatitis.

- **Hepatitis B.** For hepatitis B, treatment can delay or limit liver damage by suppressing the virus. Like treatment for HIV, hepatitis B treatment may need to be taken for the rest of your life. Some HIV medications can also treat hepatitis B. If you are diagnosed with hepatitis B, your health-care provider will go over which treatment regimen is best for you.
- **Hepatitis C.** Hepatitis C is a curable disease. Left untreated, it can cause severe liver damage, liver cancer, or death. However, new treatments for hepatitis C have been approved in recent years. These direct-acting antiviral treatments are much better than the previously available treatment because they have few side effects and do not need to be injected. These treatments for HCV infection cure about 97 percent of people, including those living with HIV, with just 8–12 weeks of oral therapy (pills).[4]

---

[4] See footnote [2].

Chapter 14 | Human Papillomavirus

Section 14.1 | **What Is Human Papillomavirus?**

Human papillomavirus (HPV) is the most common sexually transmitted infection (STI). There are many different types of HPV. Some types can cause health problems, including genital warts and cancers. But there are vaccines that can stop these health problems from happening. HPV is a different virus than human immunodeficiency virus (HIV) and herpes simplex virus (HSV). For the structure of the HPV, see Figure 14.1.

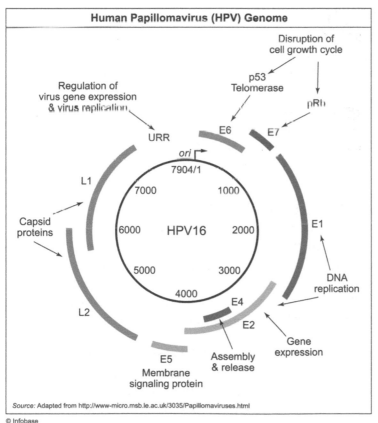

Human Papillomavirus (HPV) Genome

Source: Adapted from http://www-micro.msb.le.ac.uk/3035/Papillomaviruses.html

© Infobase

Figure 14.1. Human Papillomavirus Genome

Infobase

HOW IS HUMAN PAPILLOMAVIRUS SPREAD?

You can get HPV by having vaginal, anal, or oral sex with someone who has the virus. It is most commonly spread during vaginal or anal sex. It also spreads through close skin-to-skin touching during sex. A person with HPV can pass the infection to someone even when they have no signs or symptoms.

If you are sexually active, you can get HPV, even if you have had sex with only one person. You can also develop symptoms years after having sex with someone who has the infection. This makes it hard to know when you first got it.

DOES HUMAN PAPILLOMAVIRUS CAUSE HEALTH PROBLEMS?

In most cases (9 out of 10), HPV goes away on its own within two years without health problems. But, when HPV does not go away, it can cause health problems such as genital warts and cancer.

Genital warts usually appear as a small bump or group of bumps in the genital area. They can be small or large, raised or flat, or shaped like a cauliflower. A health-care provider can usually diagnose warts by looking at the genital area.

DOES HUMAN PAPILLOMAVIRUS CAUSE CANCER?

Human papillomavirus can cause cervical and other cancers, including cancer of the vulva, vagina, penis, or anus. It can also cause cancer in the back of the throat (called "oropharyngeal cancer"). This can include the base of the tongue and tonsils.

Cancer often takes years, even decades, to develop after a person gets HPV. Genital warts and cancers result from different types of HPV.

There is no way to know who will develop cancer or other health problems from HPV. People with weak immune systems (including those with HIV) may be less able to fight off HPV. They may also be more likely to develop health problems from HPV.

HOW CAN YOU AVOID HUMAN PAPILLOMAVIRUS AND THE HEALTH PROBLEMS IT CAN CAUSE?

You can do the following things to lower your chances of getting HPV:

- **Get vaccinated.** The HPV vaccine is safe and effective. It can protect against diseases (including cancers) caused by HPV when given in the recommended age groups.
- **Get screened for cervical cancer.** Routine screening for women aged 21–65 can prevent cervical cancer.

If you are sexually active, do the following:

- Use condoms the right way every time you have sex. This can lower your chances of getting HPV. But HPV can infect areas the condom does not cover. So condoms may not fully protect against getting HPV.
- Be in a mutually monogamous relationship or have sex only with someone who only has sex with you.

WHO SHOULD GET THE HUMAN PAPILLOMAVIRUS VACCINE?

The Centers for Disease Control and Prevention (CDC) recommends HPV vaccination for:

- all preteens (including boys and girls) at the age of 11 or 12 (or can start at age 9)
- everyone through the age of 26, if not vaccinated already

Vaccination is not recommended for everyone over the age of 26. However, some adults aged 27–45 who are not already vaccinated may decide to get the HPV vaccine after speaking with their health-care provider about their risk for new HPV infections and the possible benefits of vaccination. HPV vaccination in this age range provides less benefit. Most sexually active adults have already been exposed to HPV although not necessarily all of the HPV types targeted by vaccination.

At any age, having a new sex partner is a risk factor for getting a new HPV infection. People who are already in a long-term,

227

mutually monogamous relationship are not likely to get a new HPV infection.

HOW DO YOU KNOW IF YOU HAVE HUMAN PAPILLOMAVIRUS?

There is no test to find out a person's "HPV status." Also, there is no approved HPV test to find HPV in the mouth or throat.

There are HPV tests that can screen for cervical cancer. Healthcare providers only use these tests for screening women aged 30 and older. HPV tests are not recommended to screen men, adolescents, or women under the age of 30.

Most people with HPV do not know they have the infection. They never develop symptoms or health problems from it. Some people find out they have HPV when they get genital warts. Women may find out they have HPV when they get an abnormal Pap test result (during cervical cancer screening). Others may only find out once they have developed more serious problems from HPV, such as cancers.

HOW COMMON ARE HUMAN PAPILLOMAVIRUS AND HEALTH PROBLEMS THAT DEVELOP FROM HUMAN PAPILLOMAVIRUS?

The Centers for Disease Control and Prevention (CDC) estimates that there were 43 million HPV infections in 2018. In that same year, there were 13 million new infections. HPV is so common that almost every sexually active person will get HPV at some point if they do not get vaccinated.

Health problems related to HPV include genital warts and cervical cancer:

- **Genital warts**: Prior to HPV vaccines, genital warts caused by HPV affected roughly 340,000–360,000 people yearly.* About 1 in 100 sexually active adults in the United States has genital warts at any given time.
- **Cervical cancer**: Every year, nearly 12,000 women living in the United States will have cervical cancer. More than 4,000 women die from cervical cancer— even with screening and treatment.

There are other conditions and cancers caused by HPV that occur in people living in the United States. Every year, about 19,400 women and 12,100 men experience cancers caused by HPV.

These figures only look at the number of people who sought care for genital warts. This could be less than the actual number of people who get genital warts.

DOES HAVING HUMAN PAPILLOMAVIRUS AFFECT PREGNANCY?

Pregnant women with HPV can get genital warts or develop abnormal cell changes on the cervix. Routine cervical cancer screening can help find abnormal cell changes. A woman should get routine cervical cancer screening even when she is pregnant.

IS THERE TREATMENT FOR HUMAN PAPILLOMAVIRUS OR HEALTH PROBLEMS THAT DEVELOP FROM HUMAN PAPILLOMAVIRUS?

There is no treatment for the virus itself. However, there are treatments for the health problems that HPV can cause:

- Genital warts can go away with treatment from your health-care provider or with prescription medicine. If left untreated, genital warts may go away, stay the same, or grow in size or number.
- Cervical precancer treatment is available. Women who get routine Pap tests and follow-ups as needed can find problems before cancer develops. Prevention is always better than treatment.
- Other HPV-related cancers are also more treatable when found and treated early.[1]

---

[1] "Genital HPV Infection," Centers for Disease Control and Prevention (CDC), April 12, 2022. Available online. URL: www.cdc.gov/std/hpv/stdfact-hpv.htm. Accessed June 5, 2023.

Section 14.2 | Cancers Associated with Human Papillomavirus

Cancer is a disease in which cells in the body grow out of control. Cancer is always named for the part of the body where it starts, even if it spreads to other body parts later.

Genital human papillomavirus (HPV) is the most common sexually transmitted infection (STI) in the United States. More than 40 HPV types can infect the genital areas of men and women, including the skin of the penis, vulva (area outside the vagina), anus, and the linings of the vagina, cervix, and rectum. These types can also infect the lining of the mouth and throat.

HIGH- AND LOW-RISK HUMAN PAPILLOMAVIRUS TYPES

Human papillomavirus types are often referred to as "non-oncogenic" (wart-causing) or "oncogenic" (cancer-causing) based on whether they put a person at risk for cancer. The International Agency for Research on Cancer (IARC) found that 13 HPV types can cause cervical cancer and at least one of these types can cause cancers of the vulva, vagina, penis, anus, and certain head and neck cancers (specifically, the oropharynx, which includes the back of the throat, base of the tongue, and tonsils). The types of HPV that can cause genital warts are not the same as the types that can cause cancer.

Most people who become infected with HPV do not know they have it. Usually, the body's immune system gets rid of the HPV infection naturally within two years. This is true of both oncogenic and non-oncogenic HPV types. By age 50, at least four out of every five women will have been infected with HPV at one point in their lives. HPV is also very common in men and often has no symptoms.

HOW CAN A HUMAN PAPILLOMAVIRUS INFECTION LEAD TO CANCER?

When the body's immune system cannot get rid of an HPV infection with oncogenic HPV types, it can linger over time and turn normal cells into abnormal cells and then cancer. About 10 percent of women with HPV infection on their cervix will develop long-lasting HPV infections that put them at risk for cervical cancer. Similarly, when high-risk HPV lingers and infects the cells of the vulva, vagina, penis, or anus, it can cause cell changes called "precancers." These may eventually develop into cancer if they are not found and removed in time. These cancers are much less common than cervical cancer. Much less is known about how many people with HPV will develop cancer in these areas.

CANCERS ASSOCIATED WITH HUMAN PAPILLOMAVIRUS

Almost all cervical cancer is caused by HPV. Some cancers of the vulva, vagina, penis, anus, and oropharynx (back of the throat, including the base of the tongue and tonsils) are also caused by HPV. Research is still being done to understand how and to what extent HPV causes these cancers.

In general, HPV is thought to be responsible for more than 90 percent of anal and cervical cancers, about 70 percent of vaginal and vulvar cancers, and 60 percent of penile cancers. Cancers in the back of the throat (oropharynx) traditionally have been caused by tobacco and alcohol, but studies show that about 60–70 percent of cancers of the oropharynx may be linked to HPV. Many of these may be caused by a combination of tobacco, alcohol, and HPV.

Most of the time, HPV goes away by itself within two years and does not cause health problems. It is thought that the immune system fights off HPV naturally. It is only when HPV stays in the body for many years that it can cause these cancers. It is not known why HPV goes away in most, but not all, cases.

HUMAN PAPILLOMAVIRUS AND OROPHARYNGEAL CANCER

Human papillomavirus can infect the mouth and throat and cause cancers of the oropharynx (back of the throat, including the base of the tongue and tonsils). This is called "oropharyngeal cancer." HPV is thought to cause 70 percent of oropharyngeal cancers in the United States.

It usually takes years after being infected with HPV for cancer to develop. It is unclear if having HPV alone is enough to cause oropharyngeal cancers or if other factors (such as smoking or chewing tobacco) interact with HPV to cause these cancers. HPV is not

231

known to cause other head and neck cancers, including those in the mouth, larynx, lip, nose, or salivary glands.

SYMPTOMS OF OROPHARYNGEAL CANCER

Symptoms of oropharyngeal cancer may include a long-lasting sore throat, earaches, hoarseness, swollen lymph nodes, pain when swallowing, and unexplained weight loss. Some people have no symptoms. If you have any symptoms that worry you, be sure to see your doctor right away.

CAN THE HUMAN PAPILLOMAVIRUS VACCINE PREVENT OROPHARYNGEAL CANCERS?

The HPV vaccine was developed to prevent cervical and other cancers of the reproductive system. The vaccine protects against the types of HPV that can cause oropharyngeal cancers, so it may also prevent oropharyngeal cancers.

The Centers for Disease Control and Prevention (CDC) recommends HPV vaccination for 11- to 12-year-olds. The CDC also recommends HPV vaccination for everyone through age 26 if not vaccinated already.

Vaccination is not recommended for everyone older than age 26. However, some adults aged 27–45 years who are not already vaccinated may decide to get the HPV vaccine after speaking with their doctor about their risk for new HPV infections and the possible benefits of vaccination. HPV vaccination in this age range provides less benefit, as more people have already been exposed to HPV.

HPV vaccination prevents new HPV infections but does not treat existing infections or diseases. This is why the HPV vaccine works best when given before any exposure to HPV.

WHAT ARE OTHER WAYS TO LOWER YOUR RISK OF GETTING HUMAN PAPILLOMAVIRUS OR OROPHARYNGEAL CANCER?
Condoms and Dental Dams

When used consistently and correctly, condoms and dental dams can lower the chance that HPV is passed from one person to another.

Alcohol and Tobacco

Alcohol and tobacco products may contribute to oropharyngeal cancers. Do not smoke or use smokeless tobacco products and avoid smoke from other people's cigarettes. Limit the amount of alcohol you drink.

PREVENTING CANCERS ASSOCIATED WITH HUMAN PAPILLOMAVIRUS

Vaccines protect against the types of HPV that most often cause cervical, vaginal, vulvar, penile, and anal precancers and cancers, as well as the types of HPV that cause most oropharyngeal cancers. The vaccine used in the United States also protects against the HPV types that cause most genital warts.

Cervical cancer can also be prevented or found early through regular screening and follow-up treatment.

- The Pap test (or Pap smear) looks for precancers (cell changes on the cervix that might become cervical cancer if they are not treated appropriately).
- The HPV test looks for the virus that can cause these cell changes.

If your doctor finds any abnormal results from a cervical cancer screening test, make sure to follow up in case you need treatment or further tests.

Screening tests for other types of HPV-associated cancers are not recommended.[2]

---

[2] "HPV and Cancer," Centers for Disease Control and Prevention (CDC), October 3, 2022. Available online. URL: www.cdc.gov/cancer/hpv/basic_info/index.htm. Accessed June 5, 2023.

Section 14.3 | **Recurrent Respiratory Papillomatosis and Human Papillomavirus**

WHAT IS RECURRENT RESPIRATORY PAPILLOMATOSIS?

Recurrent respiratory papillomatosis (RRP) is a disease in which benign (noncancerous) tumors called "papillomas" grow in the air passages leading from the nose and mouth into the lungs (respiratory tract). Although the tumors can grow anywhere in the respiratory tract, they most commonly grow in the larynx (voice box)—a condition called "laryngeal papillomatosis." The papillomas may vary in size and grow very quickly. They often grow back after they have been removed.

WHAT CAUSES RECURRENT RESPIRATORY PAPILLOMATOSIS?

Recurrent respiratory papillomatosis is caused by two types of human papillomavirus (HPV): HPV 6 and HPV 11. There are more than 150 types of HPV, and they do not have all the same symptoms.

Most people who encounter HPV never develop a related illness. However, in a small number of people exposed to the HPV 6 or 11 virus, respiratory-tract papillomas and genital warts can form. Although scientists do not fully understand why some people develop the disease and others do not, the virus is thought to be spread through sexual contact or when a mother with genital warts passes the HPV 6 or 11 virus to her baby during childbirth. See Figure 14.2 to understand which parts can be affected by RRP.

WHO IS AFFECTED BY RECURRENT RESPIRATORY PAPILLOMATOSIS?

Recurrent respiratory papillomatosis may occur in adults (adult-onset RRP) as well as in infants and small children (juvenile-onset RRP) who may have contracted the virus during childbirth. The RRP Foundation estimates that there are roughly 20,000 active cases in the United States. According to the Centers for Disease Control and Prevention (CDC), estimates of the incidence of juvenile-onset RRP are imprecise but range from two or fewer cases per 100,000 children under age 18. Even less is known about the incidence of

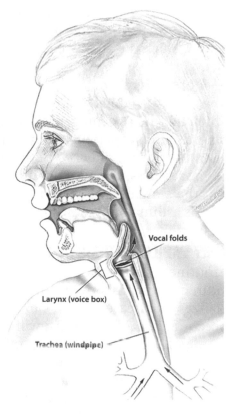

Figure 14.2. Parts of the Respiratory Tract Affected by Recurrent Respiratory Papillomatosis

National Institute on Deafness and Other Communication Disorders (NIDCD)

the adult form of RRP. Estimates of the incidence of adult-onset RPP range between two and three cases per 100,000 adults in the United States.

WHAT ARE THE SYMPTOMS OF RECURRENT RESPIRATORY PAPILLOMATOSIS?

Normally, the human voice is produced when air from the lungs is pushed through two side-by-side specialized muscles—called "vocal folds"—with enough pressure to cause them to vibrate.

Hoarseness, the most common RRP symptom, is caused when RRP papillomas interfere with the normal vibrations of the vocal folds. Eventually, RRP tumors may block the airway passage and cause difficulty breathing.

RRP symptoms tend to be more severe in children than in adults. Because the tumors grow quickly, young children with the disease may find it difficult to breathe when sleeping, or they may have difficulty swallowing. Some children experience some relief or remission of the disease when they begin puberty. Both children and adults may experience hoarseness, chronic coughing, or breathing problems. Because of the similarity of the symptoms, RRP is sometimes misdiagnosed as asthma or chronic bronchitis.

HOW IS RECURRENT RESPIRATORY PAPILLOMATOSIS DIAGNOSED?

Health professionals use two routine tests for RRP: indirect and direct laryngoscopy. In an indirect laryngoscopy, an otolaryngologist—a doctor who specializes in diseases of the ear, nose, throat, head, and neck—or speech-language pathologist will typically insert a fiber optic telescope, called an "endoscope," into a patient's nose or mouth and then view the larynx on a monitor. Some medical professionals use a video camera attached to this endoscope to view and record the exam. An older, less common method is for the otolaryngologist to place a small mirror in the back of the throat and angle the mirror down toward the larynx to inspect it for papillomas.

A direct laryngoscopy is conducted in the operating room with the use of general anesthesia. This method allows the otolaryngologist to view the vocal folds and other parts of the larynx under high magnification. This procedure is usually used to minimize discomfort, especially with children, or to enable the doctor to biopsy tissue samples from the larynx or other parts of the throat to obtain a diagnosis of RRP.

HOW IS RECURRENT RESPIRATORY PAPILLOMATOSIS PREVENTED OR TREATED?

Vaccination with the HPV vaccine could prevent the development of RRP. The CDC currently recommends that all children receive the HPV vaccine at age 11 or 12. Ask your child's doctor whether the type of HPV vaccine your child will receive will protect against HPV 6 and 11. As more young people receive the vaccine, future research will reveal its effectiveness in preventing HPV-associated diseases such as RRP.

Once RRP develops, there is currently no cure. Surgery is the primary method for removing tumors from the larynx or airway. Because traditional surgery can cause problems due to scarring of the larynx tissue, many surgeons now use laser surgery. Carbon dioxide (CO_2) or potassium titanyl phosphate (KTP) lasers are frequently used for this purpose. Surgeons also commonly use a device called a "microdebrider," which uses suction to hold the tumor in place while a small internal rotary blade removes the growth.

Once the tumors have been removed, they can still return. It is common for patients to require multiple surgeries. With some patients, surgery may be required every few weeks in order to keep the breathing passage open, while others may require surgery only once a year or even less frequently.

In the most extreme cases of aggressive tumor growth, a tracheotomy may be performed. A tracheotomy is a surgical procedure in which an incision is made in the front of the patient's neck and a breathing tube (trach tube) is inserted through an opening, called a "stoma," into the trachea (windpipe). Rather than breathing through the nose and mouth, the patient will now breathe through the trach tube. Although the trach tube keeps the breathing passage open, doctors try to remove it as soon as possible.

Some patients may be required to keep a trach tube indefinitely in order to keep the breathing passage open. Because the trach tube reroutes all or some of the exhaled air away from the vocal folds, the patient may find it difficult to use his or her voice. With the help of a voice specialist or speech-language pathologist who specializes in voice, the patient can learn to use his or her voice with the use of a speaking valve.

In severe cases of RRP, therapies in addition to surgery may be used. Drug treatments may include antivirals such as interferon and cidofovir, which block the virus from making copies of itself; indole-3-carbinol, a cancer-fighting compound found in cruciferous vegetables such as broccoli and brussels sprouts; or bevacizumab, which targets the blood vessel growth of papilloma. To date, the results of these and other nonsurgical therapies have been mixed or not yet fully proven.[3]

[3] "Recurrent Respiratory Papillomatosis or Laryngeal Papillomatosis," National Institute on Deafness and Other Communication Disorders (NIDCD), November 28, 2017. Available online. URL: www.nidcd.nih.gov/health/recurrent-respiratory-papillomatosis. Accessed June 19, 2023.

Chapter 15 | Lymphogranuloma Venereum

Lymphogranuloma venereum (LGV) is caused by *Chlamydia trachomatis* serovars L1, L2, or L3. LGV can cause severe inflammation and invasive infection, in contrast with *C. trachomatis* serovars A–K that cause mild or asymptomatic infection. Clinical manifestations of LGV can include genital ulcer disease (GUD), lymphadenopathy, or proctocolitis. Rectal exposure among men who have sex with men (MSM) or women can result in proctocolitis, which is the most common presentation of LGV infection and can mimic inflammatory bowel disease (IBD) with clinical findings of mucoid or hemorrhagic rectal discharge, anal pain, constipation, fever, or tenesmus. Outbreaks of LGV proctocolitis have been reported among MSM with high rates of human immunodeficiency virus (HIV) infection. LGV proctocolitis can be an invasive, systemic infection and, if it is not treated early, can lead to chronic colorectal fistulas and strictures; reactive arthropathy has also been reported. However, reports indicate that rectal LGV can also be asymptomatic. A common clinical manifestation of LGV among heterosexuals is tender inguinal or femoral lymphadenopathy that is typically unilateral. A self-limited genital ulcer or papule sometimes occurs at the site of inoculation. However, by the time persons seek care, the lesions have often disappeared. LGV-associated lymphadenopathy can be severe, with bubo formation from fluctuant or suppurative inguinal or femoral lymphadenopathy. Oral ulceration can

239

occur and might be associated with cervical adenopathy. Persons with genital or colorectal LGV lesions can also experience secondary bacterial infection or can be infected with other sexually and nonsexually transmitted pathogens.

DIAGNOSTIC CONSIDERATIONS FOR LYMPHOGRANULOMA VENEREUM

A definitive LGV diagnosis can be made only with LGV-specific molecular testing (e.g., polymerase chain reaction or PCR-based genotyping). These tests can differentiate LGV from non-LGV *C. trachomatis* in rectal specimens. However, these tests are not widely available, and results are not typically available in a time frame that would influence clinical management. Therefore, diagnosis is based on clinical suspicion, epidemiologic information, and a *C. trachomatis* nucleic acid amplification test (NAAT) at the symptomatic anatomic site, along with the exclusion of other etiologies for proctocolitis, inguinal lymphadenopathy, or genital, oral, or rectal ulcers. Genital or oral lesions, rectal specimens, and lymph node specimens (i.e., lesion swab or bubo aspirate) can be tested for *C. trachomatis* by NAAT or culture. The NAAT is the preferred approach for testing because it can detect both LGV strains and non–LGV *C. trachomatis* strains. Therefore, all persons presenting with proctocolitis should be tested for chlamydia with an NAAT performed on rectal specimens. Severe symptoms of proctocolitis (e.g., bloody discharge, tenesmus, and rectal ulcers) indicate LGV. A rectal Gram stain with more than 10 white blood cells (WBCs) has also been associated with rectal LGV.

Chlamydia serology (complement fixation or microimmuno-fluorescence) should not be used routinely as a diagnostic tool for LGV because the utility of these serologic methods has not been established, interpretation has not been standardized, and validation for clinical proctitis presentation has not been done. It might support an LGV diagnosis in cases of isolated inguinal or femoral lymphadenopathy for which diagnostic material for *C. trachomatis* NAAT cannot be obtained.

TREATMENT FOR LYMPHOGRANULOMA VENEREUM

At the time of the initial visit (before diagnostic NAATs for chlamydia are available), persons with a clinical syndrome consistent with LGV should be presumptively treated. Presumptive treatment for LGV is indicated among patients with symptoms or signs of proctocolitis (e.g., bloody discharge, tenesmus, or ulceration); in cases of severe inguinal lymphadenopathy with bubo formation, particularly if the patient has a recent history of a genital ulcer; or in the presence of a genital ulcer if other etiologies have been ruled out. The goal of treatment is to cure the infection and prevent ongoing tissue damage although tissue reaction to the infection can result in scarring. Buboes might require aspiration through intact skin or incision and drainage to prevent the formation of inguinal or femoral ulcerations.

Recommended Regimen for Lymphogranuloma Venereum

The following regimen can be used:
- doxycycline: 100 mg orally two times a day for 21 days

Alternative Regimens for Lymphogranuloma Venereum

One of the following regimens can be used:
- azithromycin: 1 g orally once weekly for three weeks*
- erythromycin base: 500 mg orally four times a day for 21 days

Because this regimen has not been validated, a test of cure with C. trachomatis NAAT four weeks after completion of treatment can be considered.

The optimal treatment duration for symptomatic LGV has not been studied in clinical trials. The recommended 21-day course of doxycycline is based on long-standing clinical practice and is highly effective, with an estimated cure rate of more than 98.5 percent. Shorter courses of doxycycline might be effective on the basis of a small retrospective study of MSM with rectal LGV, 50 percent of whom were symptomatic, who received a 7- to 14-day course of doxycycline and had a 97 percent cure rate. Randomized prospective studies of shorter-course doxycycline for treating LGV are needed. Longer courses of therapy might be required in the setting of fistulas, buboes, and other forms of severe disease.

A small nonrandomized study from Spain involving patients with rectal LGV demonstrated cure rates of 97 percent with a regimen of azithromycin 1 g once weekly for three weeks. Pharmacokinetic data support this dosing strategy; however, this regimen has not been validated. Fluoroquinolone-based treatments might also be effective; however, the optimal duration of treatment has not been evaluated. The clinical significance of asymptomatic LGV is unknown, and it is effectively treated with a seven-day course of doxycycline.

OTHER MANAGEMENT CONSIDERATIONS
Patients should be followed clinically until signs and symptoms have resolved. Persons who receive an LGV diagnosis should be tested for other sexually transmitted infections (STIs), especially HIV, gonorrhea, and syphilis. Those whose HIV test results are negative should be offered HIV pre-exposure prophylaxis (PrEP).

FOLLOW-UP
All persons who have been treated for LGV should be retested for chlamydia approximately three months after treatment. If retesting at three months is not possible, providers should retest at the patient's next visit for medical care within the 12-month period after initial treatment.

MANAGEMENT OF SEX PARTNERS
Persons who have had sexual contact with a patient who has LGV within the 60 days before the onset of the patient's symptoms should be evaluated, examined, and tested for chlamydial infection, depending on the anatomic site of exposure. Asymptomatic partners should be presumptively treated with a chlamydia regimen (doxycycline: 100 mg orally two times a day for seven days).

SPECIAL CONSIDERATIONS
Pregnancy

The use of doxycycline in pregnancy might be associated with discoloration of teeth; however, the risk is not well-defined. Doxycycline is compatible with breastfeeding. Azithromycin might prove useful for LGV treatment during pregnancy at a presumptive dose of 1 g weekly for three weeks; no published data are available regarding an effective dose and duration of treatment. Pregnant and lactating women with LGV can be treated with erythromycin although this regimen is associated with frequent gastrointestinal side effects. Pregnant women treated for LGV should have a test of cure performed four weeks after the initial *C. trachomatis* NAAT-positive test.

Human Immunodeficiency Virus Infection

Persons with LGV and HIV infection should receive the same regimens as those who do not have HIV. Prolonged therapy might be required because a delay in resolution of symptoms might occur.[1]

---

[1] "Lymphogranuloma Venereum (LGV)," Centers for Disease Control and Prevention (CDC), July 22, 2021. Available online. URL: www.cdc.gov/std/treatment-guidelines/lgv.htm. Accessed May 22, 2023.

Chapter 16 | Syphilis

WHAT IS SYPHILIS?
Syphilis is a sexually transmitted infection (STI) that can cause serious health problems without treatment. Infection develops in stages (primary, secondary, latent, and tertiary). Each stage can have different signs and symptoms.

HOW IS SYPHILIS SPREAD?
You can get syphilis by direct contact with a syphilis sore during vaginal, anal, or oral sex.

Syphilis can spread from a mother with syphilis to her unborn baby.

You cannot get syphilis through casual contact with objects such as:
- toilet seats
- doorknobs
- swimming pools
- hot tubs
- bathtubs
- sharing clothing or eating utensils

HOW CAN YOU REDUCE YOUR RISK OF GETTING SYPHILIS?
The only way to completely avoid sexually transmitted diseases (STDs) is not to have vaginal, anal, or oral sex.

If you are sexually active, you can do the following things to lower your chances of getting syphilis:
- being in a long-term, mutually monogamous relationship with a partner who has been tested and does not have syphilis
- using condoms the right way every time you have sex

Condoms prevent the spread of syphilis by preventing contact with a sore. Sometimes, sores occur in areas not covered by a condom. Contact with these sores can still transmit syphilis.

ARE YOU AT RISK FOR SYPHILIS?

Sexually active people can get syphilis through vaginal, anal, or oral sex without a condom with a partner who has syphilis. If you are sexually active, have an honest and open talk with your healthcare provider. Ask them if you should get tested for syphilis or other STDs.

You should get tested regularly for syphilis if you are sexually active and:

- are a gay or bisexual man
- have human immunodeficiency virus (HIV)
- are taking pre-exposure prophylaxis (PrEP) for HIV prevention
- have partner or partners who have tested positive for syphilis

All pregnant women should receive syphilis testing at their first prenatal visit. Some pregnant women need to receive syphilis testing again during the third trimester at 28 weeks and at delivery.

IF YOU ARE PREGNANT, HOW DOES SYPHILIS AFFECT YOUR BABY?

If you are pregnant and have syphilis, you can give the infection to your unborn baby. Having syphilis can lead to a low-birth-weight baby. It can make it more likely you will deliver your baby too early or stillborn (a baby born dead). To protect your baby, you should receive syphilis testing at least once during your pregnancy. Receive treatment right away if you test positive.

At birth, a baby with a syphilis infection may not have signs or symptoms of the disease. However, if the baby does not receive treatment right away, the baby may develop serious problems within a few weeks. These babies can have health problems, such as cataracts, deafness, or seizures, and can die.

WHAT ARE THE SIGNS AND SYMPTOMS OF SYPHILIS?

The following are the four stages of syphilis (primary, secondary, latent, and tertiary). Each stage has different signs and symptoms.

Primary Stage

During the first (primary) stage of syphilis, you may notice a single sore or multiple sores. The sore is the location where syphilis entered your body. These sores usually occur in, on, or around the:
- penis
- vagina
- anus
- rectum
- lips or mouth

Sores are usually (but not always) firm, round, and painless. Because the sore is painless, you may not notice it. The sore usually lasts three to six weeks and heals regardless of whether you receive treatment. Even after the sore goes away, you must still receive treatment. This will stop your infection from moving to the secondary stage.

Secondary Stage

During the secondary stage, you may have skin rashes and/or sores in your mouth, vagina, or anus. This stage usually starts with a rash on one or more areas of your body. The rash can show up when your primary sore is healing or several weeks after the sore has healed. The rash can be on the palms of your hands and/or the bottoms of your feet and look:
- rough
- red
- reddish-brown

The rash usually would not itch, and it is sometimes so faint that you would not notice it. Other symptoms may include:
- fever
- swollen lymph glands

- sore throat
- patchy hair loss
- headaches
- weight loss
- muscle aches
- fatigue (feeling very tired)

The symptoms from this stage will go away whether you receive treatment. Without the right treatment, your infection will move to the latent and possibly tertiary stages of syphilis.

Latent Stage

The latent stage of syphilis is a period when there are no visible signs or symptoms. Without treatment, you can continue to have syphilis in your body for years.

Tertiary Stage

Most people with untreated syphilis do not develop tertiary syphilis. However, when it does happen, it can affect many different organ systems. These include the heart and blood vessels and the brain and nervous system. Tertiary syphilis is very serious and would occur 10–30 years after your infection began. In tertiary syphilis, the disease damages your internal organs and can result in death. A health-care provider can usually diagnose tertiary syphilis with the help of multiple tests.

Neurosyphilis, Ocular Syphilis, and Otosyphilis

Without treatment, syphilis can spread to the brain and nervous system (neurosyphilis), the eye (ocular syphilis), or the ear (otosyphilis). This can happen during any of the stages described above.
Signs and symptoms of neurosyphilis can include:
- severe headache
- muscle weakness and/or trouble with muscle movements
- changes to your mental state (trouble focusing, confusion, and personality change) and/or

dementia (problems with memory, thinking, and/or decision-making)

Signs and symptoms of ocular syphilis can include:
- eye pain and/or redness
- changes in your vision or even blindness

Signs and symptoms of otosyphilis may include:
- hearing loss
- ringing, buzzing, roaring, or hissing in the ears (tinnitus)
- dizziness or vertigo (feeling like you or your surroundings are moving or spinning)

HOW WILL YOU OR YOUR HEALTH-CARE PROVIDERS KNOW IF YOU HAVE SYPHILIS?

Most of the time, health-care providers will use a blood test to test for syphilis. Some will diagnose syphilis by testing fluid from a syphilis sore.

IS THERE A CURE FOR SYPHILIS?

Yes, syphilis is curable with the right antibiotics from your health-care provider. However, treatment might not undo any damage the infection can cause.

CAN YOU GET SYPHILIS AGAIN AFTER RECEIVING TREATMENT?

Having syphilis once does not protect you from getting it again. Even after successful treatment, you can get syphilis again. Only laboratory tests can confirm whether you have syphilis. Follow-up testing by your health-care provider is necessary to make sure your treatment is successful.

It may not be obvious that a sex partner has syphilis. Syphilis sores in the vagina, anus, mouth, or under the foreskin of the penis can be hard to see. You may get syphilis again if your sex partner or partners do not receive testing and treatment.[1]

---

[1] "Syphilis," Centers for Disease Control and Prevention (CDC), February 10, 2022. Available online. URL: www.cdc.gov/std/syphilis/stdfact-syphilis.htm. Accessed May 22, 2023.

Chapter 17 | **Trichomoniasis**

WHAT IS TRICHOMONIASIS?

Trichomoniasis (trich) is a very common sexually transmitted disease (STD) caused by infection with *Trichomonas vaginalis* (a protozoan parasite). Although symptoms vary, most people who have trich cannot tell they have it.

HOW COMMON IS TRICHOMONIASIS?

In the United States, the Centers for Disease Control and Prevention (CDC) estimates that there were more than 2 million trichomoniasis infections in 2018. However, only about 30 percent develop any symptoms of trich. Infection is more common in women than in men. Older women are more likely than younger women to have the infection.

HOW IS TRICHOMONIASIS SPREAD?

Sexually active people can get trich by having sex without a condom with a partner who has trich.

In women, the infection is most commonly found in the lower genital tract (vulva, vagina, cervix, or urethra). In men, the infection is most commonly found inside the penis (urethra). During sex, the parasite usually spreads from a penis to a vagina or from a vagina to a penis. It can also spread from one vagina to another vagina.

It is not common for the parasite to infect other body parts, such as the hands, mouth, or anus. It is unclear why some people with the infection get symptoms while others do not. It probably depends on factors such as a person's age and overall health. People with trich can pass the infection to others, even if they do not have symptoms.

WHAT ARE THE SIGNS AND SYMPTOMS OF TRICHOMONIASIS?
About 70 percent of people with the infection do not have any signs or symptoms. When trich does cause symptoms, they can range from mild irritation to severe inflammation. Some people get symptoms within 5–28 days after getting the infection. Others do not develop symptoms until much later. Symptoms can come and go.

Men with trich may notice:
- itching or irritation inside the penis
- burning after peeing or ejaculating
- discharge from the penis

Women with trich may notice:
- itching, burning, redness, or soreness of the genitals
- discomfort when peeing
- a clear, white, yellowish, or greenish vaginal discharge (i.e., thin discharge or increased volume) with a fishy smell

Having trich can make sex feel unpleasant. Without treatment, the infection can last for months or even years.

WHAT ARE THE COMPLICATIONS OF TRICHOMONIASIS?
Trichomoniasis can increase the risk of getting or spreading other sexually transmitted infections. For example, trich can cause genital inflammation, making it easier to get human immunodeficiency virus (HIV) or pass it to a sex partner.

HOW DOES TRICHOMONIASIS AFFECT A PREGNANT WOMAN AND HER BABY?
Pregnant women with trich are more likely to have their babies early. Also, their babies are more likely to have a low birth weight (less than 5.5 pounds).

HOW DO HEALTH-CARE PROVIDERS DIAGNOSE TRICHOMONIASIS?

It is not possible to diagnose trich based on symptoms alone. Your health-care provider can examine you, and a laboratory test will confirm the diagnosis.

WHAT IS THE TREATMENT FOR TRICHOMONIASIS?

Trichomoniasis is the most common curable STD. A health-care provider can treat the infection with medication (pills) taken by mouth. This treatment is also safe for pregnant women.

If you receive and complete treatment for trich, you can still get it again. Reinfection occurs in about one in five people within three months after receiving treatment. This can happen if you have sex without a condom with a person who has trich. To avoid reinfection, your sex partners should receive treatment at the same time.

You should not have sex again until you and your sex partner(s) complete treatment. You should receive testing again about three months after your treatment, even if your sex partner(s) received treatment.

HOW CAN YOU PREVENT TRICHOMONIASIS?

The only way to avoid STDs is to avoid vaginal, anal, or oral sex.

If you are sexually active, you can do the following things to lower your chances of getting trich:

- being in a long-term mutually monogamous relationship with a partner who has been tested and does not have trich
- using condoms the right way every time you have sex

Also, talk about the potential risk of STDs before having sex with a new partner. This can help inform the choices you are comfortable taking with your sex life.

If you are sexually active, have an honest and open talk with your health-care provider. Ask them if you should get tested for trich or other STDs.[1]

---

[1] "Trichomoniasis," Centers for Disease Control and Prevention (CDC), April 25, 2022. Available online. URL: www.cdc.gov/std/trichomonas/stdfact-trichomoniasis.htm. Accessed May 23, 2023.

Part 3 | Health Complications That May Co-occur with Sexually Transmitted Diseases

Chapter 18 | Infections and Syndromes That Develop after Sexual Contact

Chapter Contents

Section 18.1 | Bacterial Vaginosis

WHAT IS BACTERIAL VAGINOSIS?

Bacterial vaginosis (BV) is a condition caused by changes in the amount of certain types of bacteria in your vagina. BV can develop when your vagina has more harmful bacteria than good bacteria.

WHO GETS BACTERIAL VAGINOSIS?

Bacterial vaginosis is the most common vaginal condition in women aged 15–44. But women of any age can get it, even if they have never had sex.

You may be more at risk for BV if you:

- have a new sex partner
- have multiple sex partners
- douche
- do not use condoms or dental dams
- are pregnant (BV is common during pregnancy. About one in four pregnant women gets BV. The risk for BV is higher for pregnant women because of the hormonal changes that happen during pregnancy.)
- are African American (BV is twice as common in African American women as in White women.)
- have an intrauterine device (IUD), especially if you also have irregular bleeding

HOW DO YOU GET BACTERIAL VAGINOSIS?

Researchers are still studying how women get BV. You can get BV without having sex, but BV is more common in women who are sexually active. Having a new sex partner or multiple sex partners, as well as douching, can upset the balance of good and harmful bacteria in your vagina. This raises your risk of getting BV.

WHAT ARE THE SYMPTOMS OF BACTERIAL VAGINOSIS?

Many women have no symptoms. If you do have symptoms, they may include:

- unusual vaginal discharge (The discharge can be white (milky) or gray. It may also be foamy or watery. Some

women report a strong fish-like odor, especially after sex.)
- burning when urinating
- itching around the outside of the vagina
- vaginal irritation

These symptoms may be similar to vaginal yeast infections and other health problems. Only your doctor or nurse can tell you for sure whether you have BV.

WHAT IS THE DIFFERENCE BETWEEN BACTERIAL VAGINOSIS AND A VAGINAL YEAST INFECTION?

Bacterial vaginosis and vaginal yeast infections are both common causes of vaginal discharge. They have similar symptoms, so it can be hard to know if you have BV or a yeast infection. Only your doctor or nurse can tell you for sure if you have BV.

With BV, your discharge may be white or gray but may also have a fishy smell. Discharge from a yeast infection may also be white or gray but may look like cottage cheese.

HOW IS BACTERIAL VAGINOSIS DIAGNOSED?

There are tests to find out if you have BV. Your doctor or nurse takes a sample of vaginal discharge. Your doctor or nurse may then look at the sample under a microscope, use an in-office test, or send it to a lab to check for harmful bacteria. Your doctor or nurse may also see signs of BV during an exam.

Before you see a doctor or nurse for a test, do the following:
- Do not douche or use vaginal deodorant sprays. They might cover odors that can help your doctor diagnose BV. They can also irritate your vagina.
- Make an appointment for a day when you do not have your period.

HOW IS BACTERIAL VAGINOSIS TREATED?

Bacterial vaginosis is treated with antibiotics prescribed by your doctor.

If you get BV, your male sex partner will not need to be treated. But, if you are female and have a female sex partner, she might also have BV. If your current partner is female, she needs to see her doctor. She may also need treatment.

It is also possible to get BV again.

BV and vaginal yeast infections are treated differently. BV is treated with antibiotics prescribed by your doctor. Yeast infections can be treated with over-the-counter (OTC) medicines. But you cannot treat BV with OTC yeast infection medicine.

WHAT CAN HAPPEN IF BACTERIAL VAGINOSIS IS NOT TREATED?

If BV is untreated, possible problems may include the following:

- **Higher risk of getting sexually transmitted infections (STIs), including human immunodeficiency virus (HIV).** Having BV can raise your risk of getting HIV, genital herpes, chlamydia, pelvic inflammatory disease (PID), and gonorrhea. Women with HIV who get BV are also more likely to pass HIV to a male sexual partner.
- **Pregnancy problems.** BV can lead to premature birth or a low-birth-weight baby (smaller than 5½ pounds at birth). All pregnant women with symptoms of BV should be tested and treated if they have it.

WHAT SHOULD YOU DO IF YOU HAVE BACTERIAL VAGINOSIS?

Bacterial vaginosis is easy to treat. If you think you have BV, do the following:

- See a doctor or nurse. Antibiotics will treat BV.
- Take all of your medicine. Even if symptoms go away, you need to finish all of the antibiotics.
- Tell your sex partner(s) if she is female so that she can be treated.
- Avoid sexual contact until you finish your treatment.

See your doctor or nurse again if you have symptoms that do not go away within a few days after finishing the antibiotic.

IS IT SAFE TO TREAT PREGNANT WOMEN WHO HAVE BACTERIAL VAGINOSIS?

Yes. The medicine used to treat BV is safe for pregnant women. All pregnant women with symptoms of BV should be tested and treated if they have it.

If you do have BV, you can be treated safely at any stage of your pregnancy. You will get the same antibiotic given to women who are not pregnant.

HOW CAN YOU LOWER YOUR RISK OF BACTERIAL VAGINOSIS?

Researchers do not know exactly how BV spreads. Steps that might lower your risk of BV include the following:

- **Keeping your vaginal bacteria balanced**. Use warm water only to clean the outside of your vagina. You do not need to use soap. Even mild soap can irritate your vagina. Always wipe front to back from your vagina to your anus. Keep the area cool by wearing cotton or cotton-lined underpants.
- **Not douching**. Douching upsets the balance of good and harmful bacteria in your vagina. This may raise your risk of BV. It may also make it easier to get BV again after treatment. Doctors do not recommend douching.
- **Not having sex**. Researchers are still studying how women get BV. You can get BV without having sex, but BV is more common in women who have sex.
- **Limiting your number of sex partners**. Researchers think that your risk of getting BV goes up with the number of partners you have.

HOW CAN YOU PROTECT YOURSELF IF YOU ARE A FEMALE AND YOUR FEMALE PARTNER HAS BACTERIAL VAGINOSIS?

If your partner has BV, you might be able to lower your risk by using protection during sex.

- Use a dental dam every time you have sex. A dental dam is a thin piece of latex that is placed over the vagina before oral sex.

- Cover sex toys with condoms before use. Remove the condom and replace it with a new one before sharing the toy with your partner.[1]

Section 18.2 | Cytomegalovirus

WHAT IS CYTOMEGALOVIRUS?

Cytomegalovirus (CMV) is a common virus for people of all ages; however, a healthy person's immune system usually keeps the virus from causing illness.

In the United States, nearly one in three children is already infected with CMV by the age of five. Over half of adults have been infected with CMV by the age of 40. Once CMV is in a person's body, it stays there for life and can reactivate. A person can also be reinfected with a different strain (variety) of the virus. Most people with CMV infection have no symptoms and are not aware that they have been infected.

Signs and Symptoms of Cytomegalovirus

In some cases, infection in healthy people can cause mild illness that may include:
- fever
- sore throat
- fatigue
- swollen glands

Occasionally, CMV can cause mononucleosis or hepatitis (liver problem).

People with weakened immune systems who get CMV can have more serious symptoms affecting the eyes, lungs, liver, esophagus, stomach, and intestines.

---

[1] Office on Women's Health (OWH), "Bacterial Vaginosis," U.S. Department of Health and Human Services (HHS), May 31, 2022. Available online. URL: www.womenshealth.gov/a-z-topics/bacterial-vaginosis. Accessed June 7, 2023.

Babies born with CMV can have brain, liver, spleen, lung, and growth problems. The most common long-term health problem in babies born with congenital CMV infection is hearing loss, which may be detected soon after birth or may develop later in childhood.

Transmission of Cytomegalovirus

People with CMV may pass the virus in body fluids, such as saliva, urine, blood, tears, semen, and breast milk. CMV is spread from an infected person in the following ways:

- from direct contact with saliva or urine, especially from babies and young children
- through sexual contact
- from breast milk to nursing infants
- through transplanted organs and blood transfusions

Diagnosis and Treatment of Cytomegalovirus

Blood tests can be used to diagnose CMV infection in adults who have symptoms. However, blood is not the best fluid to test newborns with suspected CMV infection. Tests of saliva or urine are preferred for newborns.

Healthy people who are infected with CMV usually do not require medical treatment. Medications are available to treat CMV infection in people who have weakened immune systems and babies with signs of congenital CMV.[2]

Most people have been infected with CMV but do not have symptoms. If a pregnant woman is infected with CMV, she can pass it on to her developing baby. This is called "congenital CMV," and it can cause birth defects and other health problems.

CYTOMEGALOVIRUS FACTS FOR PREGNANT WOMEN
You Can Pass Cytomegalovirus to Your Baby

If you are pregnant and have CMV, the virus in your blood can cross through your placenta and infect your developing baby. This

---

[2] "About Cytomegalovirus (CMV)," Centers for Disease Control and Prevention (CDC), August 18, 2020. Available online. URL: www.cdc.gov/cmv/overview.html. Accessed June 7, 2023.

is more likely to happen if you have a first-time CMV infection while pregnant but can also happen if you have a subsequent infection during pregnancy.

You Are Not Likely to Be Tested for Cytomegalovirus

It is not recommended that doctors routinely test pregnant women for CMV infection. This is because laboratory tests cannot predict which developing babies will become infected with CMV or have long-term health problems.

You May Be Able to Reduce Your Risk

You may be able to lessen your risk of getting CMV by reducing contact with saliva and urine from babies and young children. The saliva and urine of children with CMV have high amounts of the virus. You can avoid getting a child's saliva in your mouth by, for example, not sharing food, utensils, or cups with a child. Also, you should wash your hands after changing diapers. These cannot eliminate your risk of getting CMV but may lessen the chances of getting it.[3]

BABIES BORN WITH CONGENITAL CYTOMEGALOVIRUS

When a baby is born with CMV infection, it is called "congenital CMV." Most babies with congenital CMV never show signs or have health problems. However, some babies have health problems at birth or that develop later.

CMV is the most common infectious cause of birth defects in the United States. About one out of 200 babies is born with congenital CMV.

One out of five babies with congenital CMV will have symptoms or long-term health problems, such as hearing loss.

---

[3] "Cytomegalovirus (CMV) and Congenital CMV Infection—CMV Fact Sheet for Pregnant Women and Parents," Centers for Disease Control and Prevention (CDC), September 27, 2018. Available online. URL: www.cdc.gov/cmv/fact-sheets/parents-pregnant-women.html. Accessed June 7, 2023.

Signs and Symptoms of Congenital Cytomegalovirus

Some babies with congenital CMV infection have signs at birth, such as:

- rash
- jaundice (yellowing of the skin or whites of the eyes)
- microcephaly (small head)
- low birth weight
- hepatosplenomegaly (enlarged liver and spleen)
- seizures
- retinitis (damaged eye retina)

Some babies with signs of congenital CMV infection at birth can have long-term health problems, such as:

- hearing loss
- developmental and motor delay
- vision loss
- microcephaly (small head)
- seizures

Some babies can have hearing loss at birth or can develop it later, even babies who passed the newborn hearing test or did not have any other signs at birth.

In the most severe cases, CMV can cause pregnancy loss.

How Does Cytomegalovirus Spread?

Most people with CMV infection have no symptoms and are not aware that they have been infected. If you are pregnant and get infected with CMV, you can pass the virus to your baby during pregnancy. This can happen when you are infected with CMV for the first time or again during pregnancy.

Young children are a common source of CMV.

By the age of five years, one in three children has been infected with CMV but usually does not have symptoms. The virus can stay in a child's body fluids such as saliva and urine for months after the infection. People who are around young children a lot are at a greater risk of CMV infection.

Parents and childcare providers can lower their risk of getting CMV by reducing contact with saliva (spit) and urine from babies and young children.

- Do not share food, utensils, or cups with a child.
- Wash your hands with soap and water after changing diapers or helping a child to use the toilet.

Diagnosis of Congenital Cytomegalovirus

Congenital CMV infection can be diagnosed by testing a newborn baby's urine (preferred specimen), saliva, or blood. These specimens must be collected for testing within two to three weeks after the baby is born to confirm a diagnosis of congenital CMV infection.

Treatment for Congenital Cytomegalovirus

For babies with signs of congenital CMV infection at birth, antiviral medications (primarily valganciclovir) might improve hearing and developmental outcomes. Valganciclovir can have serious side effects and has only been studied in babies with signs of congenital CMV infection. There is limited information on the effectiveness of valganciclovir to treat infants with hearing loss alone.[4]

Section 18.3 | Yeast Infection

WHAT IS A VAGINAL YEAST INFECTION?

A vaginal yeast infection is an infection of the vagina that causes itching and burning of the vulva, the area around the vagina. Vaginal yeast infections are caused by an overgrowth of the fungus *Candida*.

---

[4] "Babies Born with Congenital CMV," Centers for Disease Control and Prevention (CDC), May 27, 2022. Available online. URL: www.cdc.gov/cmv/congenital-infection.html. Accessed June 7, 2023.

WHO GETS VAGINAL YEAST INFECTIONS?

Women and girls of all ages can get vaginal yeast infections. Three out of four women will have a yeast infection at some point in their life. Almost half of women have two or more infections.

Vaginal yeast infections are rare before puberty and after menopause.

ARE SOME WOMEN MORE AT RISK FOR YEAST INFECTIONS?

Yes. Your risk for yeast infections is higher if:
- you are pregnant
- you have diabetes and your blood sugar is not under control
- you use a type of hormonal birth control that has higher doses of estrogen
- you douche or use vaginal sprays
- you recently took antibiotics such as amoxicillin or steroid medicines
- you have a weakened immune system, such as from human immunodeficiency virus (HIV)

WHAT CAUSES YEAST INFECTIONS?

Yeast infections are caused by an overgrowth of the microscopic fungus *Candida*.

Your vagina may have small amounts of yeast at any given time without causing any symptoms. However, when too much yeast grows, you can get an infection.

WHAT ARE THE SYMPTOMS OF VAGINAL YEAST INFECTIONS?

The most common symptom of a vaginal yeast infection is extreme itchiness in and around the vagina.

Other signs and symptoms include:
- burning, redness, and swelling of the vagina and the vulva
- pain when urinating
- pain during sex
- soreness

- a thick, white vaginal discharge that looks like cottage cheese and does not have a bad smell

You may have only a few of these symptoms. They may be mild or severe.

CAN YOU GET A YEAST INFECTION FROM HAVING SEX?

Yes. A yeast infection is not considered a sexually transmitted infection (STI) because you can get a yeast infection without having sex. But you can get a yeast infection from your sexual partner. Condoms and dental dams may help prevent getting or passing yeast infections through vaginal, oral, or anal sex.

SHOULD YOU CALL YOUR DOCTOR OR NURSE IF YOU THINK YOU HAVE A YEAST INFECTION?

Yes. Seeing your doctor or nurse is the only way to know for sure if you have a yeast infection and not a more serious type of infection.

The signs and symptoms of a yeast infection are a lot like symptoms of other more serious infections, such as STIs and bacterial vaginosis (BV). If left untreated, STIs and BV raise your risk of getting other STIs, including HIV, and can lead to problems getting pregnant. BV can also lead to problems during pregnancy, such as premature delivery.

HOW IS A YEAST INFECTION DIAGNOSED?

Your doctor will do a pelvic exam to look for swelling and discharge. Your doctor may also use a cotton swab to take a sample of the discharge from your vagina. A lab technician will look at the sample under a microscope to see whether there is an overgrowth of the fungus *Candida* that causes a yeast infection.

HOW IS A YEAST INFECTION TREATED?

Yeast infections are usually treated with antifungal medicine. See your doctor or nurse to make sure that you have a vaginal yeast infection and not another type of infection.

You can then buy antifungal medicine for yeast infections at a store, without a prescription. Antifungal medicines come in the form of creams, tablets, ointments, or suppositories that you insert into your vagina. You can apply treatment in one dose or daily for up to seven days, depending on the brand you choose.

Your doctor or nurse can also give you a single dose of antifungal medicine taken by mouth, such as fluconazole. If you get more than four vaginal yeast infections a year or if your yeast infection does not go away after using over-the-counter (OTC) treatment, you may need to take regular doses of antifungal medicine for up to six months.

IS IT SAFE TO USE OVER-THE-COUNTER MEDICINES FOR YEAST INFECTIONS?

Yes, but always talk with your doctor or nurse before treating yourself for a vaginal yeast infection because of the following reasons:

- You may be trying to treat an infection that is not a yeast infection. Studies show that two out of three women who buy yeast infection medicine do not really have a yeast infection. Instead, they may have an STI or BV. STIs and BV require different treatments than yeast infections and, if left untreated, can cause serious health problems.
- Using treatment when you do not actually have a yeast infection can cause your body to become resistant to the yeast infection medicine. This can make actual yeast infections harder to treat in the future.
- Some yeast infection medicine may weaken condoms and diaphragms, increasing your chance of getting pregnant or an STI when you have sex. Talk to your doctor or nurse about what is best for you and always read and follow the directions on the medicine carefully.

HOW DO YOU TREAT A YEAST INFECTION IF YOU ARE PREGNANT?

During pregnancy, it is safe to treat a yeast infection with vaginal creams or suppositories that contain miconazole or clotrimazole.

Do not take the oral fluconazole tablet to treat a yeast infection during pregnancy. It may cause birth defects.

CAN YOU GET A YEAST INFECTION FROM BREASTFEEDING?

Yes. Yeast infections can happen on your nipples or in your breast (commonly called "thrush") from breastfeeding. Yeast thrives on milk and moisture. A yeast infection you get while breastfeeding is different from a vaginal yeast infection. However, it is caused by an overgrowth of the same fungus.

Symptoms of thrush during breastfeeding include:

- sore nipples that last more than a few days, especially after several weeks of pain-free breastfeeding
- flaky, shiny, itchy, or cracked nipples
- deep pink and blistered nipples
- achy breast
- shooting pain in the breast during or after feedings

If you have any of these signs or symptoms or think your baby might have thrush in his or her mouth, call your doctor.

IF YOU HAVE A YEAST INFECTION, DOES YOUR SEXUAL PARTNER NEED TO BE TREATED?

Maybe. Yeast infections are not STIs. But it is possible to pass yeast infections to your partner during vaginal, oral, or anal sex.

- If your partner is a man, the risk of infection is low. About 15 percent of men get an itchy rash on the penis if they have unprotected sex with a woman who has a yeast infection. If this happens to your partner, he should see a doctor. Men who have not been circumcised and men with diabetes are at a higher risk.
- If your partner is a woman, she may be at risk. She should be tested and treated if she has any symptoms.

HOW CAN YOU PREVENT A YEAST INFECTION?

You can take the following steps to lower your risk of getting yeast infections:

- Do not douche. Douching removes some of the normal bacteria in the vagina that protect you from infection.
- Do not use scented feminine products, including bubble baths, sprays, pads, and tampons.

- Change tampons, pads, and panty liners often.
- Do not wear tight underwear, pantyhose, pants, or jeans. These can increase body heat and moisture in your genital area.
- Wear underwear with a cotton crotch. Cotton underwear helps keep you dry and does not hold in warmth and moisture.
- Change out of wet swimsuits and workout clothes as soon as you can.
- After using the bathroom, always wipe from front to back.
- Avoid hot tubs and very hot baths.

If you have diabetes, be sure your blood sugar is under control.

DOES YOGURT PREVENT OR TREAT YEAST INFECTIONS?

Maybe. Studies suggest that eating 8 ounces of yogurt with "live cultures" daily or taking *Lactobacillus acidophilus* capsules can help prevent infection.

But more research studies still need to be done to say for sure if yogurt with *Lactobacillus* or other probiotics can prevent or treat vaginal yeast infections. If you think you have a yeast infection, see your doctor or nurse to make sure before taking any OTC medicine.

WHAT SHOULD YOU DO IF YOU GET REPEATED YEAST INFECTIONS?

If you get four or more yeast infections in a year, talk to your doctor or nurse.

About 5 percent of women get four or more vaginal yeast infections in one year. This is called "recurrent vulvovaginal candidiasis" (RVVC). RVVC is more common in women with diabetes or weak immune systems, such as with HIV, but it can also happen in otherwise healthy women.

Doctors most often treat RVVC with antifungal medicine for up to six months. Researchers also are studying the effects of a vaccine to help prevent RVVC.[5]

---

[5] Office on Women's Health (OWH), "Vaginal Yeast Infections," U.S. Department of Health and Human Services (HHS), February 22, 2021. Available online. URL: www.womenshealth.gov/a-z-topics/vaginal-yeast-infections. Accessed June 7, 2023.

Section 18.4 | **Intestinal Infections**

GIARDIASIS
What Is Giardiasis?

Giardiasis is a diarrheal disease caused by the microscopic parasite *Giardia duodenalis* ("*Giardia*" for short). Once a person or animal has been infected with *Giardia,* the parasite lives in the intestines and is passed in stool (poop). Once outside the body, *Giardia* can sometimes survive for weeks or even months. *Giardia* can be found in every region of the United States and around.the world.

How Do You Get Giardiasis, and How Is It Spread?

You can get giardiasis if you swallow the *Giardia* parasite (germ). *Giardia*—or poop from people or animals infected with *Giardia*—can contaminate anything it touches. *Giardia* spreads very easily; even getting tiny amounts of poop in your mouth could make you sick.

Giardiasis can be spread by:

- swallowing unsafe food or water contaminated with *Giardia* germs
- having close contact with someone who has giardiasis, particularly in childcare settings
- traveling within areas that have poor sanitation
- exposure to poop through sexual contact from someone who is sick or recently sick with *Giardia*
- transferring *Giardia* germs picked up from contaminated surfaces (such as bathroom handles, changing tables, diaper pails, or toys) into your mouth
- having contact with infected animals or animal environments contaminated with poop

What Are the Symptoms of Giardiasis?

Giardia infection (giardiasis) can cause a variety of intestinal symptoms, which include:

- diarrhea
- gas

- foul-smelling, greasy poop that can float
- stomach cramps or pain
- upset stomach or nausea
- dehydration

Symptoms of giardiasis generally begin by having two to five loose stools (poop) per day and progressively increasing fatigue. Other less common symptoms include fever, itchy skin, hives, and swelling of the eyes and joints. Over time, giardiasis can also cause weight loss and keep the body from absorbing the nutrients it needs, such as fat, lactose, vitamin A, and vitamin B_{12}. Some people with *Giardia* infections have no symptoms at all.

How Long after Infection Do Symptoms Appear?
Symptoms of giardiasis normally begin one to two weeks after becoming infected.

How Long Will Symptoms Last?
Symptoms generally last anywhere from two to six weeks. In people with weakened immune systems (e.g., due to illnesses, such as human immunodeficiency virus (HIV)), symptoms may last longer. Health-care providers can prescribe the appropriate antiparasitic medications to help reduce the amount of time symptoms last.

Who Is Most at Risk of Getting Giardiasis?
Anyone can become infected with *Giardia*. However, those at greatest risk are:
- people in childcare settings
- people who are in close contact with someone who has the disease
- travelers within areas that have poor sanitation
- people who have contact with poop during sexual activity
- backpackers or campers who drink untreated water from springs, lakes, or rivers
- swimmers who swallow water from swimming pools, hot tubs, splash pads, or untreated recreational water from springs, lakes, or rivers

- people who get their household water from a shallow well
- people with weakened immune systems
- people who have contact with infected animals or animal environments contaminated with poop

How Is Giardiasis Diagnosed?

Contact your health-care provider if you think you may have giardiasis. Your health-care provider will ask you to submit stool (poop) samples to see if you are infected. Because it can be difficult to detect *Giardia*, you may be asked to submit several stool specimens collected over several days to see if you are infected.

What Is the Treatment for Giardiasis?

Many prescription drugs are available to treat giardiasis. Although *Giardia* can infect all people, infants and pregnant women may be more likely to experience dehydration from diarrhea caused by giardiasis. To prevent dehydration, infants and pregnant women should drink a lot of fluids while sick. Dehydration can be life-threatening for infants, so it is especially important that parents talk to their health-care providers about treatment options for their infants.

Your Child Does Not Have Diarrhea but Was Recently Diagnosed with Giardiasis. Your Health-Care Provider Says Treatment Is Not Necessary. Is This Correct?

Your child may not need treatment if they have no symptoms though it is important to consider that their poop may remain a source of infection for other household members for an uncertain period of time. However, if your child does not have diarrhea but does have other symptoms, such as nausea or upset stomach, tiredness, weight loss, or a lack of hunger, you and your health-care provider may need to consider treatment. The same is true if many family members are sick or if a family member is pregnant and unable to take the most effective medications to treat *Giardia*. Contact your health-care provider for specific treatment recommendations.

Can You Get Giardiasis from Your Private Well?

Giardia-contaminated poop can enter groundwater in different ways, including sewage overflows, sewage systems that are not working properly, and polluted stormwater. Wells may be more likely to be contaminated by poop after flooding, particularly if the wells are shallow, have been dug or bored, or have been covered by floodwater for long periods of time. Overused, leaky, or poorly maintained septic systems could contaminate nearby wells with germs from poop, including *Giardia*.

What Can You Do to Prevent and Control Giardiasis?

To prevent and control *Giardia* infection, it is important to:
- wash your hands with soap and water during key times, especially:
  - before preparing food or eating
  - after using the bathroom or changing diapers
- avoid eating food and drinking water that might be contaminated with Giardia germs:
  - Properly treat water from springs, lakes, or rivers (surface water) while backpacking or camping if no other source of safe water is available.
  - Avoid swallowing water from swimming pools, hot tubs, splash pads, and untreated water from springs, lakes, or rivers (surface water) while swimming.
  - Store, clean, and prepare fruits and vegetables properly.
- practice safe sex by reducing your contact with poop during sex or avoid having sex several weeks after you or your partner has recovered from giardiasis

Can You Get Giardiasis from Your Pet?

The chances of people getting a *Giardia* infection from dogs or cats are small. The type of *Giardia* that infects humans is usually not the same type that infects dogs and cats.[6]

---

[6] "Parasites - *Giardia*," Centers for Disease Control and Prevention (CDC), February 26, 2021. Available online. URL: www.cdc.gov/parasites/giardia/general-info.html. Accessed June 7, 2023.

CRYPTOSPORIDIOSIS
What Is Cryptosporidiosis?

Cryptosporidiosis is a disease that causes watery diarrhea. It is caused by microscopic germs—parasites called "*Cryptosporidium.*" *Cryptosporidium* (Crypto for short) can be found in water, food, or soil or on surfaces or dirty hands that have been contaminated with the feces of humans or animals infected with the parasite. The parasite is found in every region of the United States and throughout the world.

How Is Cryptosporidiosis Spread?

Cryptosporidium lives in the gut of infected humans or animals. An infected person or animal sheds *Cryptosporidium* parasites in their poop. An infected person can shed 10,000,000–100,000,000 Crypto germs in a single bowel movement. Shedding of Crypto in poop begins when symptoms, such as diarrhea, begin and can last for weeks after symptoms stop. Swallowing as few as 10 *Cryptosporidium* germs can cause infection.

Crypto can be spread by:

- swallowing recreational water (e.g., the water in swimming pools, fountains, lakes, rivers) contaminated with Crypto
  - Crypto's high tolerance to chlorine enables the parasite to survive for long periods of time in chlorinated drinking and swimming pool water.
- drinking untreated water from a lake or river that is contaminated with Crypto
- swallowing water, ice, or beverages contaminated with poop from infected humans or animals
- eating undercooked food or drinking unpasteurized/raw apple cider or milk that gets contaminated with Crypto
- touching your mouth with contaminated hands
  - Hands can become contaminated through a variety of activities, such as touching surfaces or objects (e.g., toys, bathroom fixtures, changing tables, diaper pails) that have been contaminated by poop from

an infected person, changing diapers, caring for an infected person, and touching an infected animal.
- exposure to poop from an infected person through oral–anal sexual contact

Crypto is not spread through contact with blood.

What Are the Symptoms of Cryptosporidiosis, When Do They Begin, and How Long Do They Last?

Symptoms of Crypto generally begin 2–10 days (average of seven days) after becoming infected with the parasite. Symptoms include:
- watery diarrhea
- stomach cramps or pain
- dehydration
- nausea
- vomiting
- fever
- weight loss

Symptoms usually last about one to two weeks (with a range of a few days to four or more weeks) in people with healthy immune systems.

The most common symptom of cryptosporidiosis is watery diarrhea. Some people with Crypto will have no symptoms at all.

Who Is Most at Risk for Cryptosporidiosis?

People who are most likely to become infected with *Cryptosporidium* include:
- children who attend childcare centers, including diaper-aged children
- childcare workers
- parents of infected children
- older adults (ages 75 years and older)
- people who take care of other people with Crypto
- international travelers
- backpackers, hikers, and campers who drink unfiltered, untreated water

- people who drink from untreated shallow, unprotected wells
- people, including swimmers, who swallow water from contaminated sources
- people who handle infected calves or other ruminants, such as sheep
- people exposed to human poop through sexual contact

Contaminated water might include water that has not been boiled or filtered, as well as contaminated recreational water sources (e.g., swimming pools, lakes, rivers, ponds, and streams). Several community-wide outbreaks have been linked to drinking tap water or recreational water contaminated with *Cryptosporidium*. Crypto's high tolerance to chlorine enables the parasite to survive for long periods of time in chlorinated drinking and swimming pool water. This means anyone swallowing contaminated water could get ill.

Note: Although Crypto can infect all people, some groups are likely to develop more serious illnesses.

- Young children and pregnant women may be more likely to get dehydrated because of their diarrhea, so they should drink plenty of fluids while ill.
- People with severely weakened immune systems are at risk for more serious diseases. Symptoms may be more severe and could lead to serious or life-threatening illness. Examples of people with weakened immune systems include those with HIV/ acquired immunodeficiency syndrome (AIDS), those with inherited diseases that affect the immune system, and cancer and transplant patients who are taking certain immunosuppressive drugs.

How Is Cryptosporidiosis Diagnosed?

Cryptosporidiosis is a diarrheal disease that is spread through contact with the stool of an infected person or animal. The disease is diagnosed by examining stool samples. People infected with Crypto can shed the parasite irregularly in their poop (e.g., one day they shed the parasite, the next day they do not, and the third day they do), so patients may need to give three samples collected on three different days to help make sure that a negative test result is accurate and really means they do not have Crypto. Health-care providers should specifically request testing for Crypto. Routine ova and parasite testing does not normally include Crypto testing.

What Is the Treatment for Cryptosporidiosis?

Most people with healthy immune systems will recover from cryptosporidiosis without treatment. The following actions may help relieve symptoms:

- Drink plenty of fluids to remain well-hydrated and avoid dehydration. Serious health problems can occur if the body does not maintain proper fluid levels. For some people, diarrhea can be severe, resulting in hospitalization due to dehydration.
- Maintain a well-balanced diet. Doing so may help speed recovery.
- Avoid beverages that contain caffeine, such as tea, coffee, and many soft drinks.
- Avoid alcohol, as it can lead to dehydration.

Over-the-counter (OTC) antidiarrheal medicine might help slow down diarrhea, but a health-care provider should be consulted before such medicine is taken.

A drug called "nitazoxanide" has been approved by the U.S. Food and Drug Administration (FDA) for the treatment of diarrhea caused by *Cryptosporidium* in people with healthy immune systems and is available by prescription. Consult with your health-care provider for more information about the potential advantages and disadvantages of taking nitazoxanide.

Individuals who have health concerns should talk to their health-care provider.

Note: Infants, young children, and pregnant women may be more likely than others to suffer from dehydration. Losing a lot of fluids from diarrhea can be dangerous—and especially life-threatening in infants. These people should drink extra fluids when they are sick. Severe dehydration may require hospitalization for treatment with fluids given through your vein (intravenous (IV) fluids). If you are pregnant or a parent and you suspect you or your child are severely dehydrated, contact a health-care provider about fluid replacement options.

How Should You Clean Your House to Help Prevent the Spread of Cryptosporidiosis?

No cleaning method is guaranteed to be completely effective against Crypto. However, you can lower the chance of spreading Crypto by taking the following precautions:

- Wash linens, clothing, dishwasher- or dryer-safe soft toys, and so on soiled with poop or vomit as soon as possible.
  - Flush excess vomit or poop on clothes or objects down the toilet.
  - Use laundry detergent and wash in hot water: 113 °F (45 °C) or hotter for at least 20 minutes or at 122 °F (50 °C) or hotter for at least five minutes.
  - Machine-dry on the highest heat setting.
- For other household objects and surfaces (e.g., diaper-change areas), do the following:
  - Remove all visible poop.
  - Clean with soap and water.
  - Let dry completely for at least four hours.
  - If possible, expose to direct sunlight for four hours.
- Wash your hands with soap and water after cleaning objects or surfaces that could be contaminated with Crypto.

Note: The best way to prevent the spread of *Cryptosporidium* in the home is by practicing good hygiene. Wash your hands frequently with soap and water, especially after using the toilet, after changing diapers, and before eating or preparing food. Alcohol-based hand sanitizers are not effective against Crypto.[7]

---

[7] "Parasites - *Cryptosporidium* (Also Known as 'Crypto')," Centers for Disease Control and Prevention (CDC), February 8, 2021. Available online. URL: www.cdc.gov/parasites/crypto/general-info.html. Accessed June 7, 2023.

SHIGELLA INFECTIONS AMONG GAY, BISEXUAL, AND OTHER MEN WHO HAVE SEX WITH MEN

Gay, bisexual, and other men who have sex with men are among the groups at high risk for infection with *Shigella* germs. This infection is called "shigellosis." *Shigella* germs spread easily and rapidly among people, including during sexual activity.

Men who have sex with men are particularly at risk for infections with antimicrobial-resistant *Shigella*. Antimicrobial resistance happens when germs such as bacteria and fungi develop the ability to defeat the drugs designed to kill them. That means the germs are not killed and continue to grow. *Shigella* germs are increasingly resistant to antibiotic treatment.

Antimicrobial-Resistant *Shigella*

Infections with antimicrobial-resistant *Shigella* have been on the rise in the United States since 2013. Most people with *Shigella* infection—including those infected with antimicrobial-resistant *Shigella*—recover within five to six days without antibiotics. However, some people need antibiotics, including people who have a severe or long-lasting infection or are at risk of one.

People at risk of a severe or long-lasting infection include those with a weakened immune system due to certain medical conditions (such as infection with HIV) or treatments (such as chemotherapy for cancer). These people are also at increased risk of the infection spreading into the blood, which can be life-threatening.

Shigella Germs Can Spread during Sexual Activity

Shigella germs pass from the poop (stool) or unclean fingers of one person to the mouth of another person. This can happen during sexual activity in the following ways:

- **Direct sexual contact**. Anal or oral sex or anal play (rimming or fingering).
- **Indirect sexual contact**. Handling contaminated objects, such as sex toys, used condoms or barriers, and douching materials.

Symptoms typically start one to two days after swallowing the germs and include diarrhea, fever, and abdominal pain. However, not everyone with a *Shigella* infection has symptoms.

Shigella germs can be found in the poop of people with diarrhea and can continue to be found in their poop for up to two weeks after the diarrhea has gone away.

Protect Yourself and Your Partner

Take steps to reduce oral contact with poop during sex:
- Wash your hands, genitals, and anus with soap and water before and after sexual activity. Wash hands, especially after touching sex toys, used condoms or barriers, and douching materials.
- Use barriers such as condoms or dental dams during oral sex and oral-anal sex.
  - Use condoms the right way every time you have anal sex or oral sex. Condoms will also help prevent other sexually transmitted diseases (STDs).
- Use latex gloves during anal fingering or fisting.
- Wash sex toys with soap and water after each use and wash hands after touching used sex toys.

If you or your partner has been diagnosed with shigellosis, do not have sex. To reduce the chance of *Shigella* germs spreading, wait at least two weeks after the diarrhea ends to have sex.

Talk with Your Doctor

Talk with your doctor if you think you might have a *Shigella* infection (shigellosis). Your doctor can test your poop to determine if you are sick with shigellosis. They can also order an additional test at the same time to check whether your type of infection is resistant to antibiotics.

If You Have Been Diagnosed with *Shigella* Infection

If you have been diagnosed with *Shigella* infection (shigellosis), take the following steps to prevent spreading it to others.

- Wash hands often, especially:
  - before eating or preparing food
  - after using the bathroom
- Do not prepare food if you are sick or share food with anyone.
- Do not swim.
- Do not have sex for at least two weeks after you no longer have diarrhea.
- Stay home from school or from health-care, food service, or childcare jobs while sick or until your health department says it is safe to return.[8]

Section 18.5 | Molluscum Contagiosum

Molluscum contagiosum is an infection caused by a poxvirus (molluscum contagiosum virus (MCV)). The result of the infection is usually a benign, mild skin disease characterized by lesions (growths) that may appear anywhere on the body. Within 6–12 months, molluscum contagiosum typically resolves without scarring but may take as long as four years.

The lesions, known as "mollusca," are small, raised, and usually white, pink, or flesh-colored with a dimple or pit in the center. They often have a pearly appearance. They are usually smooth and firm. In most people, the lesions range from about the size of a pinhead to as large as a pencil eraser (2–5 millimeters in diameter). They may become itchy, sore, red, and/or swollen.

Mollusca may occur anywhere on the body, including the face, neck, arms, legs, abdomen, and genital area, alone or in groups. The lesions are rarely found on the palms of the hands or the soles of the feet.

---

[8] "*Shigella* Infection among Gay, Bisexual, and Other Men Who Have Sex with Men," Centers for Disease Control and Prevention (CDC), March 8, 2023. Available online. URL: www.cdc.gov/shigella/msm.html. Accessed June 7, 2023.

TRANSMISSION OF MOLLUSCUM CONTAGIOSUM

The virus that causes molluscum spreads from direct person-to-person physical contact and through contaminated fomites. Fomites are inanimate objects that can become contaminated with virus; in the instance of molluscum contagiosum, this can include linens, such as clothing and towels, bathing sponges, pool equipment, and toys. Although the virus might be spread by sharing swimming pools, baths, saunas, or other wet and warm environments, this has not been proven. Researchers who have investigated this idea think it is more likely the virus is spread by sharing towels and other items around a pool or sauna than through water.

Someone with molluscum can spread it to other parts of their body by touching or scratching a lesion and then touching their body somewhere else. This is called "autoinoculation." Shaving and electrolysis can also spread mollusca to other parts of the body.

Molluscum can spread from one person to another by sexual contact. Many, but not all, cases of molluscum in adults are caused by sexual contact.

Conflicting reports make it unclear whether the disease may be spread by simple contact with seemingly intact lesions or if the breaking of a lesion and the subsequent transferring of core material is necessary to spread the virus.

The MCV remains in the top layer of the skin (epidermis) and does not circulate throughout the body; therefore, it cannot spread through coughing or sneezing.

Since the virus lives only in the top layer of skin, once the lesions are gone, the virus is gone, and you cannot spread it to others. Molluscum contagiosum is not like herpes viruses, which can remain dormant (sleeping) in your body for long periods and then reappear.

RISK FACTORS FOR MOLLUSCUM CONTAGIOSUM

Molluscum contagiosum is common enough that you should not be surprised if you see someone with it or if someone in your family becomes infected. Although not limited to children, it is most common in children aged 1–10.

People at increased risk for getting the disease include the following:

- People with weakened immune systems (i.e., persons infected with human immunodeficiency virus (HIV) or persons being treated for cancer) are at a higher risk of getting molluscum contagiosum. Their growths may look different, be larger, and be more difficult to treat.
- Atopic dermatitis may also be a risk factor for getting molluscum contagiosum due to frequent breaks in the skin. People with this condition may also be more likely to spread molluscum contagiosum to other parts of their body for the same reason.
- People who live in warm, humid climates where living conditions are crowded are at a higher risk.

In addition, there is evidence that molluscum infections have been on the rise in the United States since 1966, but these infections are not routinely monitored because they are seldom serious and routinely disappear without treatment.

TREATMENT OPTIONS FOR MOLLUSCUM CONTAGIOSUM

Because molluscum contagiosum is self-limited in healthy individuals, treatment may be unnecessary. Nonetheless, issues such as lesion visibility, underlying atopic disease, and the desire to prevent transmission may prompt therapy.

Treatment for molluscum is usually recommended if lesions are in the genital area (on or near the penis, vulva, vagina, or anus). If lesions are found in this area, it is a good idea to visit your healthcare provider as there is a possibility that you may have another disease spread by sexual contact.

Be aware that some treatments available through the Internet may not be effective and may even be harmful.

Physical Removal

Physical removal of lesions may include cryotherapy (freezing the lesion with liquid nitrogen), curettage (the piercing of the core and scraping of caseous or cheesy material), and laser therapy. These options are rapid and require a trained health-care provider, may require local anesthesia, and can result in postprocedural pain, irritation, and scarring.

It is not a good idea to try and remove lesions or the fluid inside of lesions yourself. By removing lesions or lesion fluid by yourself, you may unintentionally autoinoculate other parts of the body or risk spreading it to others. By scratching or scraping the skin, you could cause a bacterial infection.

Oral Therapy

Gradual removal of lesions may be achieved by oral therapy. This technique is often desirable for pediatric patients because it is generally less painful and may be performed by parents at home in a less threatening environment. Oral cimetidine has been used as an alternative treatment for small children who are either afraid of the pain associated with cryotherapy, curettage, and laser therapy or because the possibility of scarring is to be avoided. While cimetidine is safe, painless, and well-tolerated, facial mollusca do not respond as well as lesions elsewhere on the body.

Topical Therapy

Podophyllotoxin cream (0.5%) is reliable as a home therapy for men but is not recommended for pregnant women because of presumed toxicity to the fetus. Each lesion must be treated individually as the therapeutic effect is localized. Other options for topical therapy include iodine and salicylic acid, potassium hydroxide, tretinoin, cantharidin (a blistering agent usually applied in an office setting), and imiquimod (T cell modifier). Imiquimod has not been proven effective for the treatment of molluscum contagiosum in children and is not recommended for children due to possible adverse events. These treatments must be prescribed by a health-care professional.

Therapy for Immunocompromised Persons

Most therapies are effective in immunocompetent patients; however, patients with HIV infection/acquired immune deficiency syndrome (AIDS) or other immunosuppressive conditions often do not respond to traditional treatments. In addition, these treatments are largely ineffective in achieving long-term control in HIV patients.

Low CD4 cell counts have been linked to widespread facial mollusca and, therefore, have become a marker for severe HIV disease. Thus far, therapies targeted at boosting the immune system have proven the most effective therapy for molluscum contagiosum in immunocompromised persons. In extreme cases, intralesional interferon has been used to treat facial lesions in these patients. However, the severe and unpleasant side effects of interferon, such as influenza-like symptoms, site tenderness, depression, and lethargy, make it a less-than-desirable treatment. Furthermore, interferon therapy proved most effective in otherwise healthy persons. Radiation therapy is also of little benefit.

PREVENTION OF MOLLUSCUM CONTAGIOSUM
The best way to avoid getting molluscum is by following good hygiene habits. Remember that the virus lives only in the skin, and once the lesions are gone, the virus is gone, and you cannot spread the virus to others.

Wash Your Hands
There are ways to prevent the spread of molluscum contagiosum. The best way is to follow good hygiene (cleanliness) habits. Keeping your hands clean is the best way to avoid molluscum infection, as well as many other infections. Handwashing removes germs that may have been picked up from other people or from surfaces that have germs on them.

Do Not Scratch or Pick at Molluscum Lesions
It is important not to touch, pick, or scratch skin that has lesions, which includes not only your own skin but anyone else's. Picking and scratching can spread the virus to other parts of the body and make it easier to spread the disease to other people, too.

Keep Molluscum Lesions Covered

It is important to keep the area with molluscum lesions clean and covered with clothing or a bandage so that others do not touch the lesions and become infected. Do remember to keep the affected skin clean and dry.

Any time there is no risk of others coming into contact with your skin, such as at night when you sleep, uncover the lesions to help keep your skin healthy.

Be Careful during Sports Activities

- Do not share towels, clothing, or other personal items.
- People with molluscum should not take part in contact sports such as wrestling, basketball, and football unless all lesions can be covered by clothing or bandages.
- Activities that use shared gear such as helmets, baseball gloves, and balls should also be avoided unless all lesions can be covered.
- Swimming should also be avoided unless all lesions can be covered by watertight bandages. Personal items such as towels, goggles, and swimsuits should not be shared. Other items and equipment such as kickboards and water toys should be used only when all lesions are covered by clothing or watertight bandages.

Other Ways to Avoid Sharing Your Infection

- Do not shave or have electrolysis on areas with lesions.
- Do not share personal items such as unwashed clothes, hairbrushes, wristwatches, and bar soap with others.
- If you have lesions on or near the penis, vulva, vagina, or anus, avoid sexual activities until you see a health-care provider.

LONG-TERM EFFECTS OF MOLLUSCUM CONTAGIOSUM

Recovery from one molluscum infection does not prevent future infections. Molluscum contagiosum is not like herpes viruses that can remain dormant (sleeping) in your body for long periods of time and then reappear. If you get new molluscum contagiosum lesions after you are cured, it means you have come in contact with an infected person or object again.

Complications of Molluscum Contagiosum

The lesions caused by molluscum are usually benign and resolve without scarring. However, scratching at the lesion, or using scraping and scooping to remove the lesion, can cause scarring. For this reason, physically removing the lesion is not often recommended in otherwise healthy individuals.

The most common complication is a secondary infection caused by bacteria. Secondary infections may be a significant problem in immunocompromised patients, such as those with HIV/AIDS or those taking immunosuppressive drug therapies. In these cases, treatment to prevent further spread of the infection is recommended.[9]

Section 18.6 | Proctitis, Proctocolitis, and Enteritis

Sexually transmitted gastrointestinal syndromes include proctitis, proctocolitis, and enteritis. Evaluation for these syndromes should include recommended diagnostic procedures, including anoscopy or sigmoidoscopy, stool examination for white blood cells (WBCs), and microbiologic workup (e.g., gonorrhea, chlamydia (lymphogranuloma venereum polymerase chain reaction (LGV PCR) if available), herpes simplex nucleic acid amplification test (NAAT), and syphilis serology). For those with enteritis, stool culture or LGV PCR is also recommended.

Proctitis is inflammation of the rectum (i.e., the distal 10–12 cm) that can be associated with anorectal pain, tenesmus, or rectal

---

[9] "Molluscum Contagiosum," Centers for Disease Control and Prevention (CDC), May 11, 2015. Available online. URL: www.cdc.gov/poxvirus/molluscum-contagiosum/index.html. Accessed June 7, 2023.

discharge. Fecal leukocytes are common. Proctitis occurs predominantly among persons who have receptive anal exposures (oral-anal, digital-anal, or genital-anal). *Neisseria gonorrhoeae, Chlamydia trachomatis* (including LGV serovars), herpes simplex virus (HSV), and *Treponema pallidum* are the most common sexually transmitted infection (STI) pathogens. Genital HSV and LGV proctitis are more prevalent among persons with human immunodeficiency virus (HIV) infection. *Mycoplasma genitalium* has been detected in certain cases of proctitis and might be more common among persons with HIV infection. *Neisseria meningitidis* has been identified as an etiology of proctitis among men who have sex with men (MSM) with HIV infection.

Proctocolitis is associated with symptoms of proctitis, diarrhea or abdominal cramps, and inflammation of the colonic mucosa extending to 12 cm above the anus. Fecal leukocytes might be detected on stool examination, depending on the pathogen. Proctocolitis can be acquired through receptive anal intercourse or by oral-anal contact, depending on the pathogen.

Pathogenic organisms include *Campylobacter* species, *Shigella* species, *E. histolytica*, LGV serovars of *C. trachomatis*, and *T. pallidum*. Among immunosuppressed persons with HIV infection, cytomegalovirus (CMV) or other opportunistic agents should be considered. The clinical presentation can be mistaken for inflammatory bowel disease (IBD) or malignancy, resulting in a delayed diagnosis.

Enteritis usually results in diarrhea and abdominal cramping without signs of proctitis or proctocolitis. Fecal leukocytes might be detected on stool examination, depending on the pathogen. When outbreaks of gastrointestinal illness occur among social or sexual networks of MSM, clinicians should consider sexual transmission as a mode of spread and provide counseling accordingly. Sexual practices that can facilitate the transmission of enteric pathogens include oral-anal contact or, in certain instances, direct genital-anal contact. *Giardia lamblia* is the most frequently implicated parasite, and bacterial pathogens include *Shigella* species, *Salmonella*, *Escherichia coli*, *Campylobacter* species, and *Cryptosporidium*. Outbreaks of *Shigella* species, *Campylobacter*, *Cryptosporidium*, and microsporidiosis have been reported among MSM. Multiple enteric pathogens and concurrent STIs have also been reported. Among immunosuppressed persons with HIV infection, CMV or other opportunistic pathogens should be considered.

DIAGNOSTIC AND TREATMENT CONSIDERATIONS FOR ACUTE PROCTITIS
Diagnosis
Persons with symptoms of acute proctitis should be examined by anoscopy. A Gram-stained smear of any anorectal exudate from anoscopic or anal examination should be examined for polymorphonuclear leukocytes (PMNs). All persons should be evaluated for herpes simplex (preferably by NAAT of rectal lesions), *N. gonorrhoeae* (NAAT or culture), *C. trachomatis* (NAAT), and *T. pallidum* (darkfield of lesion if available and serologic testing). If the *C. trachomatis* NAAT test is positive on a rectal swab and severe symptoms associated with LGV are present (including rectal ulcers, anal discharge, bleeding, greater than or equal to 10 WBCs on Gram stain, and tenesmus), patients should be treated empirically for LGV. Molecular testing for LGV is not widely available or not U.S. Food and Drug Administration (FDA) cleared, and results are not typically available in time for clinical decision-making. However, if available, molecular PCR testing for *C. trachomatis* serovars L1, L2, or L3 can be considered for confirming LGV.

The pathogenic role of *M. genitalium* in proctitis is unclear. For persons with persistent symptoms after the standard treatment, providers should consider testing for *M. genitalium* with NAAT and treat if positive.

Treatment
Acute proctitis among persons who have anal exposure through oral, genital, or digital contact is usually sexually acquired. Presumptive therapy should be initiated while awaiting the results of laboratory tests for persons with anorectal exudate detected on examination or PMNs detected on a Gram-stained smear of anorectal exudate or secretions. Such therapy should also be initiated

when anoscopy or Gram stain is not available and when the clinical presentation is consistent with acute proctitis for persons reporting receptive anal exposures.

Bloody discharge, perianal ulcers, or mucosal ulcers among persons with acute proctitis and rectal chlamydia (NAAT) should receive presumptive treatment for LGV with an extended course of doxycycline 100 mg orally two times per day for three weeks. If painful perianal ulcers are present or mucosal ulcers are detected on anoscopy, presumptive therapy should also include a regimen for genital herpes.

DIAGNOSTIC AND TREATMENT CONSIDERATIONS FOR PROCTOCOLITIS OR ENTERITIS

Treatment for proctocolitis or enteritis should be directed to the specific enteric pathogen identified. Multiple stool examinations might be necessary for detecting *Giardia*, and special stool preparations are required for diagnosing cryptosporidiosis and microsporidiosis. Diagnostic and treatment recommendations for all enteric infections are beyond the scope of these guidelines. Providers should be aware of the potential for antimicrobial-resistant pathogens, particularly during outbreaks of *Shigella* and *Campylobacter* among sexual networks of MSM, where increased resistance to azithromycin, fluoroquinolones, and isolates resistant to multiple antibiotics has been described.

OTHER MANAGEMENT CONSIDERATIONS

To minimize transmission and reinfection, patients treated for acute proctitis should be instructed to abstain from sexual intercourse until they and their partners have been treated (i.e., until completion of a seven-day regimen and symptoms have resolved). Studies have reported that behaviors that facilitate enteric pathogen transmission might be associated with the acquisition of other STIs, including HIV infection. All persons with acute proctitis and concern for sexually transmitted proctocolitis or enteritis should be tested for HIV, syphilis, gonorrhea, and chlamydia (at other exposed sites). Postexposure prophylaxis (PEP) should be considered for exposures that present a risk for HIV acquisition. For ongoing risk for HIV acquisition, pre-exposure prophylaxis (PrEP) should be considered.

Evidence-based interventions for preventing the acquisition of sexually transmitted enteric pathogens are not available. However, extrapolating from general infection control practices for communicable diseases and established STI prevention practices, recommendations include avoiding contact with feces during sex, using barriers, and washing hands after handling materials that have been in contact with the anal area (i.e., barriers and sex toys) and after touching the anus or rectal area.

FOLLOW-UP
Follow-up should be based on specific etiology and severity of clinical symptoms. For proctitis associated with gonorrhea or chlamydia, retesting for the respective pathogen should be performed three months after the treatment.

MANAGEMENT OF SEX PARTNERS
Partners who have had sexual contact with persons treated for gonorrhea or chlamydia less than 60 days before the onset of the person's symptoms should be evaluated, tested, and presumptively treated for the respective infection. Partners of persons with proctitis should be evaluated for any diseases diagnosed in the index partner. Sex partners should abstain from sexual contact until they and their partners are treated. No specific recommendations are available for screening or treating sex partners of persons with diagnosed sexually transmitted enteric pathogens; however, partners should seek care if symptomatic.

SPECIAL CONSIDERATIONS
Drug Allergy, Intolerance, and Adverse Reactions
Allergic reactions with third-generation cephalosporins (e.g., ceftriaxone) are uncommon among persons with a history of penicillin allergy.

Human Immunodeficiency Virus Infection

Persons with HIV infection and acute proctitis might present with bloody discharge, painful perianal ulcers, or mucosal ulcers, and LGV and herpes proctitis are more prevalent among this population. Presumptive treatment in such cases should include a regimen for genital herpes and LGV.[10]

Section 18.7 | Pubic Lice

WHAT ARE PUBIC LICE?

Also called "crab lice" or "crabs," pubic lice are parasitic insects found primarily in the pubic or genital area of humans. Pubic lice infestation is found worldwide and occurs in all races, ethnic groups, and levels of society.

WHAT DO PUBIC LICE LOOK LIKE?

Pubic lice have three forms: the egg (also called a "nit"), the nymph, and the adult.

- **Nit.** Nits are lice eggs. They can be hard to see and are found firmly attached to the hair shaft. They are oval and usually yellow to white. Pubic lice nits take about 6–10 days to hatch.
- **Nymph.** The nymph is an immature louse that hatches from the nit (egg). A nymph looks like an adult pubic louse, but it is smaller. Pubic lice nymphs take about two to three weeks after hatching to mature into adults capable of reproducing. To live, a nymph must feed on blood.

---

[10] "Proctitis, Proctocolitis, and Enteritis," Centers for Disease Control and Prevention (CDC), July 22, 2021. Available online. URL: www.cdc.gov/std/treatment-guidelines/proctitis.htm. Accessed June 7, 2023.

- **Adult**. The adult pubic louse resembles a miniature crab when viewed through a strong magnifying glass. Pubic lice have six legs; their two front legs are very large and look like the pincher claws of a crab. This is how they got the nickname "crabs." Pubic lice are tan to grayish-white in color. Females lay nits and are usually larger than males. To live, lice must feed on blood. If the louse falls off a person, it dies within one or two days.

WHERE ARE PUBIC LICE FOUND?

Pubic lice are usually found in the genital area on pubic hair, but they may occasionally be found on other coarse body hair, such as hair on the legs, armpits, mustache, beard, eyebrows, or eyelashes. Pubic lice on the eyebrows or eyelashes of children may be a sign of sexual exposure or abuse. Lice found on the head generally are head lice, not pubic lice. Animals do not get or spread pubic lice.

WHAT ARE THE SIGNS AND SYMPTOMS OF PUBIC LICE?

Signs and symptoms of pubic lice include the following:
- itching in the genital area
- visible nits (lice eggs) or crawling lice

HOW DO PUBIC LICE SPREAD?

Pubic lice are usually spread through sexual contact and are most common in adults. Pubic lice found on children may be a sign of sexual exposure or abuse. Occasionally, pubic lice may be spread by close personal contact or contact with articles such as clothing, bed linens, or towels that have been used by an infested person. A common misconception is that pubic lice are spread easily by sitting on a toilet seat. This would be extremely rare because lice cannot live long away from a warm human body, and they do not have feet designed to hold onto or walk on smooth surfaces such as toilet seats.

HOW IS A PUBIC LICE INFESTATION DIAGNOSED?

A pubic lice infestation is diagnosed by finding a "crab" louse or egg (nit) on hair in the pubic region or, less commonly, elsewhere on the body (eyebrows, eyelashes, beard, mustache, armpit, perianal area, groin, trunk, scalp). Pubic lice may be difficult to find because there may be only a few. Pubic lice often attach themselves to more than one hair and generally do not crawl as quickly as head and body lice. If crawling lice are not seen, finding nits in the pubic area strongly suggests that a person is infested and should be treated. If you are unsure about infestation or if treatment is not successful, see a health-care provider for a diagnosis. Persons infested with pubic lice should be investigated for the presence of other sexually transmitted diseases (STDs).

Although pubic lice and nits can be large enough to be seen with the naked eye, a magnifying lens may be necessary to find lice or eggs.

HOW IS A PUBIC LICE INFESTATION TREATED?

A lice killing lotion containing 1 percent permethrin or a mousse containing pyrethrins and piperonyl butoxide can be used to treat pubic ("crab") lice. These products are available over-the-counter without a prescription at a local drug store or pharmacy. These medications are safe and effective when used exactly according to the instructions in the package or on the label. Also, to treat pubic lice infestations, do the following:

- Wash the infested area; towel dry.
- Carefully follow the instructions in the package or on the label. Thoroughly saturate the pubic hair and other infested areas with lice medication. Leave the medication on hair for the time recommended in the instructions. After waiting the recommended time, remove the medication by following carefully the instructions on the label or in the box.
- Following treatment, most nits will still be attached to hair shafts. Nits may be removed with fingernails or by using a fine-toothed comb.

- Put on clean underwear and clothing after treatment.
- To kill any lice or nits remaining on clothing, towels, or bedding, machine-wash and machine-dry those items that the infested person used during the two to three days before treatment. Use hot water (at least 130 °F (54.44 °C)) and the hot dryer cycle.
- Items that cannot be laundered can be dry-cleaned or stored in a sealed plastic bag for two weeks.
- All sex partners from within the previous month should be informed that they are at risk for infestation and should be treated.
- Persons should avoid sexual contact with their sex partner(s) until both they and their partners have been successfully treated and reevaluated to rule out persistent infestation.
- Repeat treatment in 9–10 days if live lice are still found.
- Persons with pubic lice should be evaluated for other STDs.[11]

Section 18.8 | Scabies

WHAT IS SCABIES?

Scabies is an infestation of the skin by the human itch mite (*Sarcoptes scabiei* var. *hominis*). The microscopic scabies mite burrows into the upper layer of the skin where it lives and lays its eggs. The most common symptoms of scabies are intense itching and a pimple-like skin rash. The scabies mite is usually spread by direct, prolonged, skin-to-skin contact with a person who has scabies.

Scabies is found worldwide and affects people of all races and social classes. Scabies can spread rapidly under crowded conditions

---

[11] "Pubic 'Crab' Lice," Centers for Disease Control and Prevention, June 15, 2023. Available online. URL: www.cdc.gov/parasites/lice/pubic/index.html. Accessed July 7, 2023.

where close body and skin contact is frequent. Institutions such as nursing homes, extended-care facilities, and prisons are often sites of scabies outbreaks. Childcare facilities also are a common site of scabies infestations.

WHAT IS CRUSTED (NORWEGIAN) SCABIES?

Crusted scabies is a severe form of scabies that can occur in some persons who are immunocompromised (have a weak immune system), elderly, disabled, or debilitated. It is also called "Norwegian scabies." Persons with crusted scabies have thick crusts of skin that contain large numbers of scabies mites and eggs. Persons with crusted scabies are very contagious to other persons and can spread the infestation easily both by direct skin-to-skin contact and by contamination of items such as their clothing, bedding, and furniture. Persons with crusted scabies may not show the usual signs and symptoms of scabies, such as the characteristic rash or itching (pruritus). Persons with crusted scabies should receive quick and aggressive medical treatment for their infestation to prevent outbreaks of scabies.

HOW SOON AFTER INFESTATION DO SYMPTOMS OF SCABIES BEGIN?

If a person has never had scabies before, symptoms may take four to eight weeks to develop. It is important to remember that an infested person can spread scabies during this time, even if he/she does not have symptoms yet.

In a person who has had scabies before, symptoms usually appear much sooner (one to four days) after exposure.

WHAT ARE THE SIGNS AND SYMPTOMS OF SCABIES INFESTATION?

The most common signs and symptoms of scabies are intense itching (pruritus), especially at night, and a pimple-like (papular) itchy rash. The itching and rash may affect much of the body or be limited to common sites such as the wrist, elbow, armpit, webbing between the fingers, nipple, penis, waist, beltline, and buttocks. The rash can also include tiny blisters (vesicles) and scales.

Scratching the rash can cause skin sores; sometimes, these sores become infected by bacteria.

Tiny burrows sometimes are seen on the skin; these are caused by the female scabies mite tunneling just beneath the surface of the skin. These burrows appear as tiny, raised, and crooked (serpiginous) grayish-white or skin-colored lines on the skin surface. Because mites are often few in number (only 10–15 mites per person), these burrows may be difficult to find. They are found most often in the webbing between the fingers; in the skin folds on the wrist, elbow, or knee; and on the penis, breast, or shoulder blades.

The head, face, neck, palms, and soles are often involved in infants and very young children but usually not in adults and older children.

Persons with crusted scabies may not show the usual signs and symptoms of scabies, such as the characteristic rash or itching (pruritus).

HOW CAN YOU GET SCABIES?

Scabies is usually spread by direct, prolonged, skin-to-skin contact with a person who has scabies. Contact generally must be prolonged; a quick handshake or hug usually will not spread scabies. Scabies is spread easily to sexual partners and household members. Scabies in adults is frequently sexually acquired. Scabies is sometimes spread indirectly by sharing articles such as clothing, towels, or bedding used by an infested person; however, such indirect spread can occur much more easily when the infested person has crusted scabies.

HOW IS SCABIES INFESTATION DIAGNOSED?

Diagnosis of a scabies infestation is usually made based on the customary appearance and distribution of the rash and the presence of burrows. Whenever possible, the diagnosis of scabies should be confirmed by identifying the mite, mite eggs, or mite fecal matter (scybala). This can be done by carefully removing a mite from the end of its burrow using the tip of a needle or by obtaining skin scraping to examine under a microscope for mites, eggs, or mite fecal matter. It is important to remember that a person can still be infested even if mites, eggs, or fecal matter cannot be found; typically, fewer than 10–15 mites can be present on the entire body of an infested person who is otherwise healthy. However, persons with crusted scabies can be infested with thousands of mites and should be considered highly contagious.

HOW LONG CAN SCABIES MITES LIVE?

On a person, scabies mites can live for as long as one to two months. Off a person, scabies mites usually do not survive more than 48–72 hours. Scabies mites will die if exposed to a temperature of 122 °F (50 °C) for 10 minutes.

CAN SCABIES BE TREATED?

Yes. Products used to treat scabies are called "scabicides" because they kill scabies mites; some also kill eggs. Scabicides to treat human scabies are available only with a doctor's prescription; no over-the-counter (OTC) or nonprescription products have been tested and approved for humans.

Always follow carefully the instructions provided by the doctor and pharmacist, as well as those contained in the box or printed on the label. When treating adults and older children, scabicide cream or lotion is applied to all areas of the body, from the neck down to the feet and toes; when treating infants and young children, the cream or lotion is also applied to the head and neck. The medication should be left on the body for the recommended time before it is washed off. Clean clothes should be worn after treatment.

In addition to the infested person, the treatment is also recommended for household members and sexual contacts, particularly those who have had prolonged skin-to-skin contact with the infested person. All persons should be treated at the same time in order to prevent reinfestation. Retreatment may be necessary if itching continues more than two to four weeks after treatment or if new burrows or rashes continue to appear.

Never use a scabicide intended for veterinary or agricultural use to treat humans.

WHO SHOULD BE TREATED FOR SCABIES?

Anyone who is diagnosed with scabies, as well as his or her sexual partners and other contacts who have had prolonged skin-to-skin contact with the infested person, should be treated. Treatment is recommended for members of the same household as the person with scabies, particularly those persons who have had prolonged skin-to-skin contact with the infested person. All persons should be treated at the same time to prevent reinfestation.

Retreatment may be necessary if itching continues more than two to four weeks after treatment or if new burrows or rashes continue to appear.

HOW SOON AFTER TREATMENT WILL YOU FEEL BETTER?

If itching continues more than two to four weeks after initial treatment or if new burrows or rashes continue to appear (if initial treatment includes more than one application or dose, then the two to four time period begins after the last application or dose), retreatment with scabicide may be necessary; seek the advice of a physician.

CAN YOU GET SCABIES FROM YOUR PET?

No. Animals do not spread human scabies. Pets can become infested with a different kind of scabies mite that does not survive or reproduce on humans but causes "mange" in animals. If an animal with "mange" has close contact with a person, the animal mite can get under the person's skin and cause temporary itching and skin irritation. However, the animal mite cannot reproduce on a person and will die on its own in a couple of days. Although the person does not need to be treated, the animal should be treated because its mites can continue to burrow into the person's skin and cause symptoms until the animal has been treated successfully.

CAN SCABIES BE SPREAD BY SWIMMING IN A PUBLIC POOL?

Scabies is spread by prolonged skin-to-skin contact with a person who has scabies. Scabies sometimes can also be spread through contact with items, such as clothing, bedding, or towels, that have been used by a person with scabies, but such spread is very uncommon unless the infested person has crusted scabies.

Scabies is very unlikely to be spread by water in a swimming pool. Except for a person with crusted scabies, only about 10–15 scabies mites are present in an infested person; it is extremely unlikely that any would emerge from under wet skin.

Although uncommon, scabies can be spread by sharing a towel or item of clothing that has been used by a person with scabies.

HOW CAN YOU REMOVE SCABIES MITES FROM YOUR HOUSE OR CARPET?

Scabies mites do not survive more than two to three days away from human skin. Items such as bedding, clothing, and towels used by a person with scabies can be decontaminated by machine-washing in hot water and drying using the hot cycle or by dry-cleaning. Items that cannot be washed or dry-cleaned can be decontaminated by removing from any body contact for at least 72 hours.

Because persons with crusted scabies are considered very infectious, careful vacuuming of furniture and carpets in rooms used by these persons is recommended.

Fumigation of living areas is unnecessary.

YOUR SPOUSE AND YOU WERE DIAGNOSED WITH SCABIES. AFTER SEVERAL TREATMENTS, HE/SHE STILL HAS SYMPTOMS WHILE YOU ARE CURED. WHY?

The rash and itching of scabies can persist for several weeks to a month after treatment, even if the treatment was successful and all the mites and eggs have been killed. Your health-care provider may prescribe additional medication to relieve itching if it is severe. Symptoms that persist for longer than two weeks after treatment can be due to a number of reasons, including:

- incorrect diagnosis of scabies (Many drug reactions can mimic the symptoms of scabies and cause a skin rash and itching; the diagnosis of scabies should be confirmed by a skin scraping that includes observing the mite, eggs, or mite feces (scybala) under a microscope. If you are sleeping in the same bed with your spouse and have not become reinfested and you have not retreated yourself for at least 30 days, then it is unlikely that your spouse has scabies.)

- reinfestation with scabies from a family member or other infested person if all patients and their contacts are not treated at the same time (Infested persons and their contacts must be treated at the same time to prevent reinfestation.)
- treatment failure caused by resistance to medication, faulty application of topical scabicides, or failure to do a second application when necessary (No new burrows should appear 24–48 hours after effective treatment.)
- treatment failure of crusted scabies because of poor penetration of scabicide into thick, scaly skin containing large numbers of scabies mites (Repeated treatment with a combination of both topical and oral medication may be necessary to treat crusted scabies successfully.)
- reinfestation from items (fomites) such as clothing, bedding, or towels that were not appropriately washed or dry-cleaned (This is mainly of concern for items used by persons with crusted scabies. Potentially contaminated items (fomites) should be machine-washed in hot water and dried using the hot temperature cycle, dry-cleaned, or removed from skin contact for at least 72 hours.)
- an allergic skin rash (dermatitis) exposure to household mites that cause symptoms to persist because of cross-reactivity between mite antigens

If itching continues for more than two to four weeks or if new burrows or rashes continue to appear, seek the advice of a physician; retreatment with the same or a different scabicide may be necessary.

IF YOU COME IN CONTACT WITH A PERSON WHO HAS SCABIES, SHOULD YOU TREAT YOURSELF?

No. If a person thinks he or she might have scabies, he/she should contact a doctor. The doctor can examine the person, confirm the diagnosis of scabies, and prescribe an appropriate treatment. Products used to treat scabies in humans are available only with a doctor's prescription.

Sleeping with or having sex with any scabies-infested person presents a high risk of transmission. The longer a person has skin-to-skin exposure, the greater the likelihood for transmission to occur. Although briefly shaking hands with a person who has non-crusted scabies could be considered as presenting a relatively low risk, holding the hand of a person with scabies for 5–10 minutes could be considered to present a relatively high risk of transmission. However, transmission can occur even after brief skin-to-skin contact, such as a handshake, with a person who has crusted scabies. In general, a person who has skin-to-skin contact with a person who has crusted scabies would be considered a good candidate for treatment.

To determine when prophylactic treatment should be given to reduce the risk of transmission, early consultation should be sought with a health-care provider who understands:

- the type of scabies (i.e., noncrusted versus crusted) to which a person has been exposed
- the degree and duration of skin exposure that a person has had to the infested patient
- whether the exposure occurred before or after the patient was treated for scabies
- whether the exposed person works in an environment where he/she would be likely to expose other people during the asymptomatic incubation period (e.g., a nurse or caretaker who works in a nursing home or hospital would often be treated prophylactically to reduce the risk of further scabies transmission in the facility.)[12]

[12] "Scabies Frequently Asked Questions (FAQs)," Centers for Disease Control and Prevention (CDC), September 1, 2020. Available online. URL: www.cdc.gov/parasites/scabies/gen_info/faqs.html. Accessed June 7, 2023.

Chapter 19 | **Urethritis and Cervicitis**

URETHRITIS

Urethritis, as characterized by urethral inflammation, can result from either infectious or noninfectious conditions. Symptoms, if present, include dysuria, urethral pruritis, and mucoid, muco-purulent, or purulent discharge. Signs of urethral discharge on examination can also be present among persons without symptoms. Although *Chlamydia trachomatis* and *Neisseria gonorrhoeae* are well established as clinically important infectious causes of ure-thritis, *Mycoplasma genitalium* has been strongly associated with urethritis and, less commonly, prostatitis. If point-of-care (POC) diagnostic tools (e.g., Gram, methylene blue (MB), or gentian violet (GV) stain microscopy) are unavailable, drug regimens effective against both gonorrhea and chlamydia should be administered. Further testing to determine the specific etiology is recommended for preventing complications, reinfection, and transmission because a specific diagnosis might improve treatment compliance, deliv-ery of risk-reduction interventions, and partner services. Both chlamydia and gonorrhea are reportable to health departments. Nucleic acid amplification tests (NAATs) are preferred for detect-ing *C. trachomatis* and *N. gonorrhoeae*, and urine is the preferred specimen for males. NAAT-based tests for diagnosing *Trichomonas vaginalis* among men with urethritis have not been cleared by the U.S. Food and Drug Administration (FDA); however, laboratories have performed the validation studies complied with the Clinical Laboratory Improvement Amendments (CLIA).

Diagnostic Considerations of Urethritis

Clinicians should attempt to obtain objective evidence of urethral inflammation. If POC diagnostic tests (e.g., Gram stain or MB or GV microscopy) are unavailable, urethritis can be documented on the basis of any of the following signs or laboratory tests:

- mucoid, mucopurulent, or purulent discharge on examination
- Gram stain, a POC diagnostic test for evaluating urethritis that is highly sensitive and specific for documenting both urethritis and the presence or absence of gonococcal infection (MB or GV stain of urethral secretions is an alternative POC diagnostic test with performance characteristics similar to Gram stain; thus, the cutoff number for white blood cells (WBCs) per oil immersion field should be the same.)
    - Presumed gonococcal infection is established by documenting the presence of WBCs containing the presence of Gram-negative intracellular diplococci (GNID) in Gram stain or intracellular purple diplococci in MB or GV smears; men should be tested for *C. trachomatis* and *N. gonorrhoeae* by NAATs and presumptively treated and managed accordingly for gonococcal infection.
    - If no intracellular Gram-negative or purple diplococci are present, men should receive NAATs for *C. trachomatis* and *N. gonorrhoeae* and can be managed for nongonococcal urethritis (NGU) as recommended.
    - Gram stains of urethral secretions exist that demonstrate greater than or equal to two WBCs per oil immersion field. The microscopy diagnostic cutoff might vary, depending on background prevalence (greater than or equal to two WBCs/high power field (HPF) in high-prevalence settings (STI clinics) or greater than or equal to five WBCs/HPF in lower-prevalence settings).
- positive leukocyte esterase test on first-void urine or microscopic examination of sediment from a spun

first-void urine demonstrating greater than or equal to 10 WBCs/HPF

Men evaluated in settings in which Gram stain or MB or GV smear is unavailable who meet at least one criterion for urethritis (i.e., urethral discharge, positive leukocyte esterase test on first-void urine, or microscopic examination of first-void urine sediment with greater than or equal to 10 WBCs/HPF) should be tested for *C. trachomatis* and *N. gonorrhoeae* by NAATs and treated with regimens effective against gonorrhea and chlamydia.

If symptoms are present, but no evidence of urethral inflammation is present, NAATs for *C. trachomatis* and *N. gonorrhoeae* might identify infections. Persons with chlamydia or gonorrhea should receive recommended treatment, and sex partners should be referred for evaluation and treatment. If none of these clinical criteria are present, empiric treatment of men with symptoms of urethritis is recommended only for those at high risk for infection who are unlikely to return for a follow-up evaluation or test results. Such men should be treated with drug regimens effective against gonorrhea and chlamydia.

CERVICITIS

The following are the two major diagnostic signs that characterize cervicitis:

- a purulent or mucopurulent endocervical exudate visible in the endocervical canal or on an endocervical swab specimen (commonly referred to as "mucopurulent cervicitis")
- sustained endocervical bleeding easily induced by gentle passage of a cotton swab through the cervical os

Either or both signs might be present. Cervicitis frequently is asymptomatic; however, certain women might report an abnormal vaginal discharge and intermenstrual vaginal bleeding (e.g., especially after sexual intercourse). The criterion of using an increased number of WBCs on endocervical Gram stain in the diagnosis of cervicitis has not been standardized; it is not sensitive, has a low positive predictive value for *C. trachomatis* and *N. gonorrhoeae* infections, and is not available in most clinical settings. Leukorrhea, defined as more than 10 WBCs/HPF on microscopic examination of vaginal fluid, might be a sensitive indicator of cervical inflammation with a high negative predictive value (i.e., cervicitis is unlikely in the absence of leukorrhea). Finally, although the presence of Gram-negative intracellular diplococci on Gram stain of endocervical exudate might be specific for diagnosing gonococcal cervical infection when evaluated by an experienced laboratorian, it is not a sensitive indicator of infection.

Diagnostic Considerations of Cervicitis

Because cervicitis might be a sign of upper genital tract infection (e.g., endometritis), women should be assessed for signs of pelvic inflammatory disease (PID) and tested for *C. trachomatis* and *N. gonorrhoeae* with NAAT on vaginal, cervical, or urine samples. Women with cervicitis should also be evaluated for concomitant BV and trichomoniasis. Because the sensitivity of microscopy for detecting *T. vaginalis* is relatively low (approximately 50%), symptomatic women with cervicitis and negative wet-mount microscopy for trichomonads should receive further testing (i.e., NAAT, culture, or other FDA-cleared diagnostic tests). Testing for *M. genitalium* with the FDA-cleared NAAT can be considered. Although HSV-2 infection has been associated with cervicitis, the utility of specific testing (i.e., polymerase chain reaction (PCR) or culture) for HSV-2 is unknown. Testing for *U. parvum*, *U. urealyticum*, *Mycoplasma hominis*, or genital culture for group B streptococcus is not recommended.

Treatment of Cervicitis

Multiple factors should affect the decision to provide presumptive therapy for cervicitis. Presumptive treatment with antimicrobials for *C. trachomatis* and *N. gonorrhoeae* should be provided for women at increased risk (e.g., those who are younger than 25 years of age and women with a new sex partner, a sex partner with concurrent partners, or a sex partner who has an STI) if follow-up cannot be ensured or if testing with NAAT is not possible. Trichomoniasis and BV should be treated if detected. For women at lower risk for STIs, deferring treatment until the results of diagnostic tests are available is an option. If treatment is deferred and *C. trachomatis* and *N. gonorrhoeae* NAATs are negative, a follow-up visit to determine whether the cervicitis has resolved can be considered.

RECOMMENDED REGIMEN*
- doxycycline: 100 mg orally two times a day for seven days

Consider concurrent treatment for gonococcal infection if the patient is at risk for gonorrhea or lives in a community where the prevalence of gonorrhea is high.

ALTERNATIVE REGIMEN
- azithromycin: 1 g orally in a single dose

Other Management Considerations of Cervicitis
To minimize transmission and reinfection, women treated for cervicitis should be instructed to abstain from sexual intercourse until they and their partners have been treated (i.e., until completion of a seven-day regimen or for seven days after single-dose therapy) and symptoms have resolved. Women who receive a cervicitis diagnosis should be tested for syphilis and HIV in addition to other recommended diagnostic tests.

Management of Sex Partners
Management of sex partners of women treated for cervicitis should be tailored for the specific infection identified or suspected. All sex partners during the previous 60 days should be referred for evaluation, testing, and presumptive treatment if chlamydia, gonorrhea, or trichomoniasis is identified. EPT and other effective partner referral strategies are alternative approaches for treating male partners of women who have a chlamydial or gonococcal

infection. To avoid reinfection, sex partners should abstain from sexual intercourse until they and their partners are treated.

Special Considerations
HUMAN IMMUNODEFICIENCY VIRUS INFECTION
Women with cervicitis and HIV infection should receive the same treatment regimen as those who do not have HIV. Cervicitis can increase cervical HIV shedding, and treatment reduces HIV shedding from the cervix and thereby might reduce HIV transmission to susceptible sex partners.

PREGNANCY
Diagnosis and treatment of cervicitis for pregnant women should follow treatment recommendations for chlamydia and gonorrhea.

CONTRACEPTIVE MANAGEMENT
According to the U.S. *Medical Eligibility Criteria for Contraceptive Use, 2016*, leaving an intrauterine device (IUD) in place during treatment for cervicitis is advisable. However, there are recommendations that specify that an IUD should not be placed if active cervicitis is diagnosed.[1]

---

[1] "Diseases Characterized by Urethritis and Cervicitis," Centers for Disease Control and Prevention (CDC), September 21, 2022. Available online. URL: www.cdc.gov/std/treatment-guidelines/urethritis-and-cervicitis. htm. Accessed June 12, 2023.

Chapter 20 | **Epididymitis**

Acute epididymitis is a clinical syndrome causing pain, swelling, and inflammation of the epididymis and lasting less than six weeks. Sometimes, a testicle is also involved, a condition referred to as "epididymo-orchitis." A high index of suspicion for the spermatic cord (testicular) torsion should be maintained among men who have a sudden onset of symptoms associated with epididymitis because this condition is a surgical emergency.

Acute epididymitis can be caused by sexually transmitted infections (STIs; e.g., *Chlamydia trachomatis, Neisseria gonorrhoeae, Mycoplasma genitalium*) or enteric organisms (i.e., *Escherichia coli*). Acute epididymitis caused by an STI is usually accompanied by urethritis, which is frequently asymptomatic. Acute epididymitis caused by sexually transmitted enteric organisms might also occur among men who are insertive partners during anal sex. Nonsexually transmitted acute epididymitis caused by genitourinary pathogens typically occurs with bacteriuria secondary to bladder outlet obstruction (e.g., benign prostatic hyperplasia). Among older men, nonsexually transmitted acute epididymitis is also associated with prostate biopsy, urinary tract instrumentation or surgery, systemic disease, or immunosuppression. Uncommon infectious causes of nonsexually transmitted acute epididymitis (e.g., Fournier gangrene) should be managed in consultation with a urologist.

Chronic epididymitis is characterized by six or more weeks of history of symptoms of discomfort or pain in the scrotum, testicle, or epididymis. Chronic infectious epididymitis is most frequently observed with conditions associated with a granulomatous reaction. Mycobacterium tuberculosis (TB) is the most common granulomatous disease affecting the epididymis and should be suspected, especially among men with a known history of or recent exposure to TB. The differential diagnosis of chronic noninfectious epididymitis, sometimes termed orchialgia or epididymalgia, is broad (e.g., trauma, cancer, autoimmune conditions, or idiopathic conditions). Men with this diagnosis should be referred to a urologist for clinical management.

DIAGNOSTIC CONSIDERATIONS FOR EPIDIDYMITIS

Men who have acute epididymitis typically have unilateral testicular pain and tenderness, hydrocele, and palpable swelling of the epididymis. Although inflammation and swelling usually begin in the tail of the epididymis, it can spread to the rest of the epididymis and testicle. The spermatic cord is usually tender and swollen. Spermatic cord (testicular) torsion, a surgical emergency, should be considered in all cases; however, it occurs more frequently among adolescents and men without evidence of inflammation or infection. For men with severe unilateral pain with sudden onset, for those whose test results do not support a diagnosis of urethritis or urinary tract infection (UTI), or for whom the diagnosis of acute epididymitis is questionable, immediate referral to a urologist for evaluation for testicular torsion is vital because testicular viability might be compromised.

Bilateral symptoms should increase suspicion of other causes of testicular pain. Radionuclide scanning of the scrotum is the most accurate method for diagnosing epididymitis, but it is not routinely available. Ultrasound should be used primarily for ruling out torsion of the spermatic cord in cases of acute, unilateral, painful scrotal swelling. However, because partial spermatic cord torsion can mimic epididymitis on scrotal ultrasound, differentiation between spermatic cord torsion and epididymitis when torsion is not ruled out by ultrasound should be made on the basis of clinical evaluation. Although ultrasound can demonstrate epididymal hyperemia and swelling associated with epididymitis, it provides minimal diagnostic usefulness for men with a clinical presentation consistent with epididymitis. A negative ultrasound does not rule out epididymitis and thus does not alter clinical management. Ultrasound should be reserved for men if torsion of the spermatic cord is suspected or for those with scrotal pain who cannot receive an accurate diagnosis by history, physical examination, and objective laboratory findings.

All suspected cases of acute epididymitis should be evaluated for objective evidence of inflammation by one of the following point-of-care (POC) tests:

- Gram, methylene blue (MB), or gentian violet (GV) stain of urethral secretions demonstrating greater than or equal to two white blood counts (WBC) per oil immersion field (These stains are preferred POC diagnostic tests for evaluating urethritis because they are highly sensitive and specific for documenting both urethral inflammation and the presence or absence of gonococcal infection. Gonococcal infection is established by documenting the presence of WBC-containing intracellular Gram-negative or purple diplococci on urethral Gram, MB, or GV stain.)
- positive leukocyte esterase test on first-void urine
- microscopic examination of sediment from a spun first-void urine demonstrating greater than or equal to 10 WBCs/HPF (high-power field)

All suspected cases of acute epididymitis should be tested for *C. trachomatis* and *N. gonorrhoeae* by nucleic acid amplification testing (NAAT). Urine is the preferred specimen for NAAT for men. Urine cultures for chlamydial and gonococcal epididymitis are insensitive and are not recommended. Urine bacterial cultures should also be performed for all men to evaluate the presence of genitourinary organisms and to determine antibiotic susceptibility.

TREATMENT FOR EPIDIDYMITIS

To prevent complications and transmission of STIs, presumptive therapy for all sexually active men is indicated at the time of the visit before all laboratory test results are available. The selection of presumptive therapy is based on risk for chlamydial and gonococcal infections or enteric organisms.

Treatment goals for acute epididymitis are:
- microbiologic infection cure
- improvement of signs and symptoms
- prevention of transmission of chlamydia and gonorrhea to others
- decreased potential for chlamydial or gonococcal epididymitis complications (e.g., infertility or chronic pain)

Although the majority of men with acute epididymitis can be treated on an outpatient basis, referral to a specialist and hospitalization should be considered when severe pain or fever indicates other diagnoses (e.g., torsion, testicular infarction, abscess, or necrotizing fasciitis) or when men are unable to comply with an antimicrobial regimen. Age, history of diabetes, fever, and elevated C-reactive protein can indicate more severe disease requiring hospitalization.

OTHER MANAGEMENT CONSIDERATIONS

Men who have acute epididymitis confirmed or suspected to be caused by *N. gonorrhoeae* or *C. trachomatis* should be advised to abstain from sexual intercourse until they and their partners have been treated and symptoms have resolved. All men with acute epididymitis should be tested for human immunodeficiency virus (HIV) and syphilis.

FOLLOW-UP

Men should be instructed to return to their health-care providers if their symptoms do not improve less than 72 hours after treatment. Signs and symptoms of epididymitis that do not subside in less than three days require reevaluation of the diagnosis and therapy. Men who experience swelling and tenderness that persist after completion of antimicrobial therapy should be evaluated for alternative diagnoses, including tumor, abscess, infarction, testicular cancer, TB, and fungal epididymitis.

MANAGEMENT OF SEX PARTNERS

Men who have acute sexually transmitted epididymitis confirmed or suspected to be caused by *N. gonorrhoeae* or *C. trachomatis* should be instructed to refer all sex partners during the previous 60 days before symptom onset for evaluation, testing, and presumptive treatment. If the last sexual intercourse was more than 60 days before the onset of symptoms or diagnosis, the most recent sex partner should be evaluated and treated. Arrangements should be made to link sex partners to care. Expedited partner therapy (EPT) is an effective strategy for treating sex partners of men who have or are suspected of having chlamydia or gonorrhea for whom linkage to care is anticipated to be delayed. Partners should be instructed to abstain from sexual intercourse until they and their sex partners are treated and symptoms have resolved.

SPECIAL CONSIDERATIONS
Drug Allergy, Intolerance, and Adverse Reactions

The risk for penicillin cross-reactivity is negligible between all third-generation cephalosporins (e.g., ceftriaxone).

Human Immunodeficiency Virus Infection

Men with HIV infection who have uncomplicated acute epididymitis should receive the same treatment regimen as those who do not have HIV. Other etiologic agents have been implicated in acute epididymitis among men with HIV, including *Cytomegalovirus* (CMV), *Salmonella*, toxoplasmosis, *U. urealyticum*, *Corynebacterium* species, *Mycoplasma* species, and *Mima polymorpha*.[1]

---

[1] "Epididymitis," Centers for Disease Control and Prevention (CDC), July 22, 2021. Available online. URL: www.cdc.gov/std/treatment-guidelines/epididymitis.htm. Accessed May 23, 2023.

Chapter 21 | **Neurosyphilis**

WHAT IS NEUROSYPHILIS?

Neurosyphilis is an infection that affects the coverings of the brain, the brain itself, or the spinal cord. It can occur in people with syphilis, especially if their condition is left untreated. Neurosyphilis is different from syphilis. Syphilis is a sexually transmitted disease (STD) with different signs and symptoms.

The following are the five types of neurosyphilis:

- **Asymptomatic neurosyphilis**. It means that neurosyphilis is present, but the individual reports no symptoms and does not feel sick.
- **Meningeal syphilis**. It can occur between the first few weeks to the first few years of getting syphilis. Individuals with meningeal syphilis can have headache, stiff neck, nausea, and vomiting. Sometimes, there can also be loss of vision or hearing.
- **Meningovascular syphilis**. It causes the same symptoms as meningeal syphilis, but affected individuals also have strokes. This form of neurosyphilis can occur within the first few months to several years after infection.
- **General paresis**. It can occur between 3 and 30 years after getting syphilis. People with general paresis can have personality or mood changes.
- **Tabes dorsalis**. It is characterized by pains in the limbs or abdomen, failure of muscle coordination, and bladder disturbances. Other signs include vision loss, loss of reflexes and loss of sense of vibration, poor gait, and impaired balance. Tabes dorsalis can occur anywhere from 5 to 50 years after the initial syphilis infection.

General paresis and tabes dorsalis are now less common than the other forms of neurosyphilis because of advances made in prevention, screening, and treatment. People with human immunodeficiency virus (HIV)/acquired immunodeficiency syndrome (AIDS) are at higher risk of having neurosyphilis.

Penicillin, an antibiotic, is used to treat syphilis. Some medical professionals recommend another antibiotic called "ceftriaxone" for neurosyphilis treatment. Treatment outcomes are different for every person.

The prognosis can change based on the type of neurosyphilis and how early the disease is diagnosed and treated. Individuals with asymptomatic neurosyphilis or meningeal neurosyphilis usually return to normal health. People with meningovascular syphilis, general paresis, or tabes dorsalis usually do not return to normal health although they may get much better. Individuals who receive treatment many years after they have been infected have a worse prognosis.

HOW TO IMPROVE CARE FOR PEOPLE WITH NEUROSYPHILIS

Consider participating in a clinical trial, so clinicians and scientists can learn more about neurosyphilis and related disorders. Clinical research uses human volunteers to help researchers learn more about a disorder and perhaps find better ways to safely detect, treat, or prevent disease.

All types of volunteers are needed—those who are healthy or may have an illness or disease—of all different ages, sexes, races, and ethnicities to ensure that study results apply to as many people as possible and that treatments will be safe and effective for everyone who will use them.[1]

EVALUATION AND TREATMENT FOR NEUROSYPHILIS

Patients who receive a diagnosis of syphilis and have neurologic, ocular, and/or otologic symptoms should be evaluated for

---

[1] "Neurosyphilis," National Institute of Neurological Disorders and Stroke (NINDS), January 20, 2023. Available online. URL: www.ninds.nih.gov/health-information/disorders/neurosyphilis. Accessed June 1, 2023.

neurosyphilis, ocular syphilis, or otosyphilis according to their clinical presentation.

Patients who have syphilis and symptoms or signs suggestive of neurologic disease (e.g., cranial nerve dysfunction, meningitis, stroke, acute or chronic altered mental status, or motor or sensory deficits) should have an evaluation that includes cerebrospinal fluid (CSF) analysis before treatment. They should receive an HIV test if their status is unknown or previously HIV-negative.[2]

CSF involvement can occur during any stage of syphilis, and CSF laboratory abnormalities are common among persons with early syphilis, even in the absence of clinical neurologic findings. No evidence exists to support variation from recommended diagnosis and treatment for syphilis at any stage for persons without clinical neurologic findings, except tertiary syphilis. If clinical evidence of neurologic involvement is observed (e.g., cognitive dysfunction, motor or sensory deficits, cranial nerve palsies, or symptoms or signs of meningitis or stroke), a CSF examination should be performed before treatment.

Syphilitic uveitis or other ocular syphilis manifestations (e.g., neuroretinitis and optic neuritis) can occur at any stage of syphilis and can be isolated abnormalities or associated with neurosyphilis. All persons with ocular symptoms and reactive syphilis serology need a full ocular examination, including cranial nerve evaluation. If cranial nerve dysfunction is present, a CSF evaluation is needed. Among persons with isolated ocular symptoms (no cranial nerve dysfunction or other neurologic abnormalities), reactive syphilis serology, and confirmed ocular abnormalities on examination, CSF examination is unnecessary before treatment. CSF analysis might be helpful in evaluating persons with ocular symptoms and reactive syphilis serology who do not have ocular findings on examination. If ocular syphilis is suspected, immediate referral to and management in collaboration with an ophthalmologist is crucial. Ocular syphilis should be treated similarly to neurosyphilis, even if a CSF examination is normal.

---

[2] "Neurosyphilis, Ocular Syphilis, and Otosyphilis," Centers for Disease Control and Prevention (CDC), August 24, 2021. Available online. URL: www.cdc.gov/std/syphilis/neuro-ocular-oto.htm. Accessed June 1, 2023.

Hearing loss and other otologic symptoms can occur at any stage of syphilis and can be isolated abnormalities or associated with neurosyphilis, especially of cranial nerve 8. However, among persons with isolated auditory symptoms, normal neurologic examination, and reactive syphilis serology, CSF examination is likely to be normal and is not recommended before treatment. Otosyphilis should be managed in collaboration with an otolaryngologist and treated by using the same regimen as for neurosyphilis.

Recommended Regimen for Neurosyphilis

The following regimen can be used:
- aqueous crystalline penicillin G: 18–24 million units per day, administered as 3–4 million units intravenously (by IV) every four hours or continuous infusion for 10–14 days

Alternative Regimens

If compliance with therapy can be ensured, the following alternative regimens might be considered.
- penicillin G procaine: 2.4 million units intramuscularly (IM) once daily for 10–14 days
- probenecid: 500 mg orally four times/day for 10–14 days

The durations of the recommended and alternative regimens for neurosyphilis are shorter than the duration of the regimen used for latent syphilis. Therefore, benzathine penicillin, 2.4 million units IM once per week for one to three weeks, can be considered after completion of these neurosyphilis treatment regimens to provide a comparable total duration of therapy.[3]

---

[3] "Neurosyphilis, Ocular Syphilis, and Otosyphilis," Centers for Disease Control and Prevention (CDC), July 22, 2021. Available online. URL: www.cdc.gov/std/treatment-guidelines/neurosyphilis.htm. Accessed June 1, 2023.

Chapter 22 | **Pelvic Inflammatory Disease**

WHAT IS PELVIC INFLAMMATORY DISEASE?

Pelvic inflammatory disease (PID) is an infection of a woman's reproductive organs. The reproductive organs include the uterus (womb), fallopian tubes, ovaries, and cervix.

PID can be caused by many different types of bacteria. Usually, PID is caused by bacteria from sexually transmitted infections (STIs). Sometimes, PID is caused by normal bacteria found in the vagina.

WHO GETS PELVIC INFLAMMATORY DISEASE?

Pelvic inflammatory disease affects about 5 percent of women in the United States. Your risk for PID is higher if you:

- have had an STI
- have had PID before
- are younger than 25 and have sex (PID is most common in women aged 15–24.)
- have more than one sex partner or have a partner who has multiple sexual partners
- douche (Douching can push bacteria into the reproductive organs and cause PID. Douching can also hide the signs of PID.)
- recently had an intrauterine device (IUD) inserted (The risk of PID is higher for the first few weeks only after insertion of an IUD, but PID is rare after that. Getting tested for STIs before the IUD is inserted lowers your risk for PID.)

HOW DO YOU GET PELVIC INFLAMMATORY DISEASE?

A woman can get PID if bacteria move up from her vagina or cervix and into her reproductive organs. Many different types of bacteria can cause PID. Most often, PID is caused by infection from two common STIs: gonorrhea and chlamydia. The number of women with PID has dropped in recent years. This may be because more women are getting tested regularly for chlamydia and gonorrhea.

You can also get PID without having an STI. Normal bacteria in the vagina can travel into a woman's reproductive organs and can sometimes cause PID. Sometimes, the bacteria travel up to a woman's reproductive organs because of douching. Do not douche. No doctor or nurse recommends douching.

WHAT ARE THE SIGNS AND SYMPTOMS OF PELVIC INFLAMMATORY DISEASE?

Many women do not know they have PID because they do not have any signs or symptoms. When symptoms do happen, they can be mild or more serious.

Signs and symptoms include:
- pain in the lower abdomen (which is the most common symptom)
- fever (100.4 °F (38 °C) or higher)
- vaginal discharge that may smell foul
- painful sex
- pain when urinating
- irregular menstrual periods
- pain in the upper right abdomen (which is rare)

PID can come on fast, with extreme pain and fever, especially if it is caused by gonorrhea.

HOW IS PELVIC INFLAMMATORY DISEASE DIAGNOSED?

To diagnose PID, doctors usually do a physical exam to check for signs of PID and test for STIs. If you think that you may have PID, see a doctor or nurse as soon as possible.

If you have pain in your lower abdomen, your doctor or nurse will check for:

- unusual discharge from your vagina or cervix
- an abscess (collection of pus) near your ovaries or fallopian tubes
- tenderness or pain in your reproductive organs

Your doctor may do tests to find out whether you have PID or a different problem that looks like PID. These can include:

- tests for STIs, especially gonorrhea and chlamydia as these infections can cause PID
- a test for a urinary tract infection or other conditions that can cause pelvic pain
- ultrasound or another imaging test, so your doctor can look at your internal organs for signs of PID

A Pap test is not used to detect PID.

HOW IS PELVIC INFLAMMATORY DISEASE TREATED?

Your doctor or nurse will give you antibiotics to treat PID. Most of the time, at least two antibiotics are used that work against many different types of bacteria. You must take all of your antibiotics, even if your symptoms go away. This helps make sure the infection is fully cured. See your doctor or nurse again two to three days after starting the antibiotics to make sure they are working.

Your doctor or nurse may suggest going to the hospital to treat your PID if:

- you are very sick
- you are pregnant
- your symptoms do not go away after taking the antibiotics or if you cannot swallow pills (If this is the case, you will need IV antibiotics.)
- you have an abscess in a fallopian tube or ovary

If you still have symptoms or if the abscess does not go away after treatment, you may need surgery. Problems caused by PID, such as chronic pelvic pain and scarring, are often hard to treat. But, sometimes, they get better after surgery.

WHAT CAN HAPPEN IF PELVIC INFLAMMATORY DISEASE IS NOT TREATED?

Without treatment, PID can lead to serious problems such as infertility, ectopic pregnancy, and chronic pelvic pain (pain that does not go away). If you think you may have PID, see a doctor or nurse as soon as possible.

Antibiotics will treat PID, but they will not fix any permanent damage done to your internal organs.

CAN YOU GET PREGNANT IF YOU HAVE HAD PELVIC INFLAMMATORY DISEASE?

Maybe. Your chances of getting pregnant are lower if you have had PID more than once. When you have PID, bacteria can get into the fallopian tubes or cause inflammation of the fallopian tubes. This can cause scarring in the tissue that makes up your fallopian tubes.

Scar tissue can block an egg from your ovary from entering or traveling down the fallopian tube to your uterus (womb). The egg needs to be fertilized by a man's sperm and then attach to your uterus for pregnancy to happen. Even having just a little scar tissue can keep you from getting pregnant without fertility treatment.

Scar tissue from PID can also cause a dangerous ectopic pregnancy (a pregnancy outside of the uterus) instead of a normal pregnancy. Ectopic pregnancies are more than six times more common in women who have had PID compared with women who have not had PID. Most of these pregnancies end in miscarriage.

HOW CAN YOU PREVENT PELVIC INFLAMMATORY DISEASE?

You may not be able to prevent PID. It is not always caused by an STI. Sometimes, normal bacteria in your vagina can travel up to your reproductive organs and cause PID.

But you can lower your risk of PID by not douching. You can also prevent STIs by not having vaginal, oral, or anal sex.

If you do have sex, lower your risk of getting an STI with the following steps:

- **Use condoms**. Condoms are the best way to prevent STIs when you have sex. Because a man does not need to ejaculate (cum) to give or get STIs, make sure to put the condom on before the penis touches the vagina, mouth, or anus. Other methods of birth control, such as birth control pills, shots, implants, or diaphragms, will not protect you from STIs.
- **Get tested**. Be sure you and your partner are tested for STIs. Talk to each other about the test results before you have sex.
- **Be monogamous**. Having sex with just one partner can lower your risk for STIs. After being tested for STIs, be faithful to each other. That means that you have sex only with each other and no one else.
- **Limit your number of sex partners**. Your risk of getting STIs goes up with the number of sex partners you have.
- **Do not douche**. Douching removes some of the normal bacteria in the vagina that protect you from infection. Douching may also raise your risk of PID by helping bacteria travel to other areas, such as your uterus, ovaries, and fallopian tubes.
- **Do not abuse alcohol or drugs**. Drinking too much alcohol or using drugs increases risky behavior and may put you at risk of sexual assault and possible exposure to STIs.

The steps work best when used together. No single step can protect you from every single type of STI.

CAN WOMEN WHO HAVE SEX WITH WOMEN GET PELVIC INFLAMMATORY DISEASE?

Yes. It is possible to get PID or an STI if you are a woman who has sex only with women.

Talk to your partner about her sexual history before having sex and ask your doctor about getting tested if you have signs or symptoms of PID.[1]

---

[1] Office on Women's Health (OWH), "Pelvic Inflammatory Disease," U.S. Department of Health and Human Services (HHS), December 30, 2022. Available online. URL: www.womenshealth.gov/a-z-topics/pelvic-inflammatory-disease. Accessed May 24, 2023.

Chapter 23 | **Pregnancy Complications and Sexually Transmitted Diseases**

If you are pregnant, you can become infected with the same sexually transmitted diseases (STDs) as women who are not pregnant. Pregnant women should ask their doctors about getting tested for STDs since some doctors do not routinely perform these tests.

CAN YOU GET A SEXUALLY TRANSMITTED DISEASE WHILE PREGNANT?

Yes, you can. Women who are pregnant can become infected with the same STDs as women who are not pregnant. Pregnancy does not provide women or their babies any additional protection against STDs. Many STDs are silent or have no symptoms, so you may not know if you are infected. If you are pregnant, you should be tested for STDs, including human immunodeficiency virus (HIV, the virus that causes acquired immunodeficiency syndrome (AIDS)), as a part of your medical care during pregnancy. The results of an STD can be more serious, even life-threatening, for you and your baby if you become infected while pregnant. It is important that you are aware of the harmful effects of STDs and how to protect yourself and your unborn baby against infection. If you are diagnosed with an STD while pregnant, your sex partner(s) should also be tested and treated.[1]

CAN YOU PASS SEXUALLY TRANSMITTED INFECTIONS TO YOUR BABY?

Yes. Some sexually transmitted infections (STIs) can be passed from a pregnant woman to the baby before and during the baby's birth.

- Some STIs, such as syphilis, cross the placenta and infect the baby in the womb.
- Other STIs, such as gonorrhea, chlamydia, hepatitis B, and genital herpes, can pass from the mother to the baby as the baby passes through the birth canal.
- Human immunodeficiency virus (HIV) can cross the placenta during pregnancy and infect the baby during delivery.

WHAT ARE THE HARMFUL EFFECTS OF PASSING A SEXUALLY TRANSMITTED INFECTION TO A BABY?

The harmful effects on babies may include:

- low birth weight (less than five pounds)
- eye infection
- pneumonia
- infection in the baby's blood
- brain damage
- lack of coordination in body movements
- blindness
- deafness
- acute hepatitis
- meningitis
- chronic liver disease (CLD), which can lead to scarring of the liver (cirrhosis)
- stillbirth

---

[1] "STDs during Pregnancy," Centers for Disease Control and Prevention (CDC), April 12, 2022. Available online. URL: www.cdc.gov/std/pregnancy/stdfact-pregnancy.htm. Accessed July 7, 2023.

IF YOU ARE PREGNANT, WHAT CAN YOU DO TO PREVENT PROBLEMS FROM SEXUALLY TRANSMITTED INFECTIONS?

You can prevent some of the health problems caused by STIs and pregnancy with regular prenatal care. Your doctor will test you for STIs early in your pregnancy and again closer to childbirth if needed.

- STIs caused by bacteria, such as chlamydia and gonorrhea, can be cured with antibiotics. Some antibiotics are safe to take during pregnancy. Your doctor can prescribe antibiotics for chlamydia, gonorrhea, syphilis, and trichomoniasis during pregnancy.
- STIs caused by viruses, such as genital herpes and HIV, have no cure.
  - If you have herpes, antiviral medicine may help reduce symptoms. If you have symptoms of herpes or active genital herpes sores at the start of labor, you may need a cesarean section (C-section). This can help lower the risk of passing the infection to your baby.
  - If you have HIV, antiviral medicines can lower the risk of giving HIV to your baby to less than 1 percent. You may also need to have a C-section.

You can also take steps to lower your risk of getting an STI during pregnancy.

CAN YOU BREASTFEED IF YOU HAVE A SEXUALLY TRANSMITTED INFECTION?

Maybe. Some STIs affect breastfeeding, and some do not. The following are some general guidelines, but talk to your doctor, nurse, or lactation consultant about the risk of passing the STI to your baby while breastfeeding:

- If you have HIV, do not breastfeed. You can pass the virus to your baby. In countries, such as the United States, where clean water is available, using a breast milk substitute, such as formula, is recommended.

331

- If you have chlamydia, gonorrhea, or HPV, you can breastfeed your baby.
- If you have trichomoniasis, you can take the antibiotic metronidazole if you are breastfeeding. You may need to wait 12–24 hours after taking the medicine to breastfeed.
- If you have syphilis or herpes, you can breastfeed as long as your baby or pumping equipment does not touch a sore. It is possible to spread syphilis or herpes to any part of your breast, including your nipple and areola. If you have sores on your breast, pump or hand-express your milk until the sores heal. Pumping will help keep up your milk supply and prevent your breast from getting overly full and painful. You can store your milk to give to your baby in a bottle for another feeding. But, if parts of your breast pump also touch the sore(s) while pumping, you should throw the milk away.

ARE SEXUALLY TRANSMITTED INFECTION TREATMENTS SAFE TO USE WHILE BREASTFEEDING?

If you are being treated for an STI, ask your doctor about the possible effects of the medicine on your baby. Most treatments for STIs are safe to take while breastfeeding.[2]

TO PROTECT ALL WOMEN AND INFANTS

The Centers for Disease Control and Prevention (CDC) recommends the following:
- hepatitis B virus (HBV) infection
  - All pregnant women should be tested for hepatitis B surface antigen (HBsAg) during each pregnancy, and those testing positive should be tested for HBV deoxyribonucleic acid (DNA). Women with HBV

---

[2] Office of Research on Women's Health (ORWH), "Sexually Transmitted Infections, Pregnancy, and Breastfeeding," National Institutes of Health (NIH), January 31, 2019. Available online. URL: https://orwh.od.nih.gov/research/maternal-morbidity-and-mortality/information-for-women/sexually-transmitted-infections. Accessed July 7, 2023.

DNA greater than 200,000 IU/mL should receive antiviral therapy to prevent perinatal transmission. If a pregnant woman is infected, HBV transmission to her infant can be prevented by providing hepatitis B immune globulin (HBIG) and hepatitis B vaccine (in separate limbs) to the infant within 12 hours after birth, followed by the completion of the three-dose vaccine series.

- hepatitis C virus (HCV) infection
  - All pregnant women should be tested for hepatitis C during each pregnancy. While there is no treatment available to prevent transmission of HCV infection from mother to child, screening for HCV infection during pregnancy allows health-care providers to identify infected persons who should receive treatment during the postpartum period and infants who should receive testing during a pediatric visit. Identification of HCV infection during pregnancy can also inform pregnancy and delivery management issues that might reduce the risk of HCV transmission to the infant.
- human immunodeficiency virus
  - All pregnant women should be tested for HIV as early as possible, preferably at the first prenatal visit. The earlier HIV is diagnosed and treated, the more effective HIV medicines—called "antiretroviral therapy" (ART)—can be at preventing transmission and improving the health outcomes of both mother and child.
- syphilis
  - All pregnant women should be tested for syphilis at the first prenatal visit, ideally during the first trimester of pregnancy. Among people who may be less likely to receive prenatal care, consider testing at the time of pregnancy testing. The earlier syphilis is diagnosed and treated during pregnancy, the more likely congenital syphilis and its complications (such as stillbirth) can be prevented in the infant.

Penicillin G is effective in preventing maternal transmission to the fetus, as well as treating fetal and maternal infections. Women who live in areas of high syphilis morbidity or who have personal or partner risk for syphilis should be screened again at 28 weeks and at delivery. Any pregnant woman who has a fetal death after 20 weeks of gestation should be tested for syphilis.[3]

[3] "Overview of HIV, Viral Hepatitis, STD, & TB During Pregnancy," Centers for Disease Control and Prevention (CDC), August 11, 2022. Available online. URL: www.cdc.gov/nchhstp/pregnancy/overview.html. Accessed July 7, 2023.

Chapter 24 | Infertility Linked to Sexually Transmitted Diseases/Infections

"Infertility" is a term used to describe the inability of a couple to get pregnant or the inability of a woman to carry a pregnancy to term.

Infertility is defined clinically as not being able to achieve pregnancy after one year of having regular, unprotected intercourse or after six months if the woman is older than 35.

Many different medical conditions and other factors can contribute to fertility problems, and an individual case may have a single cause, several causes, or—in some cases—no identifiable cause.[1]

WHAT IS THE LINK BETWEEN SEXUALLY TRANSMITTED DISEASES/INFECTIONS AND INFERTILITY?

In most cases, sexually transmitted diseases (STDs)/sexually transmitted infections (STIs) are linked to infertility, primarily when they are left untreated.

For instance, chlamydia and gonorrhea are bacterial STIs that can be cured easily with antibiotics. But, if left untreated, 10–20 percent of chlamydial and gonorrheal infections in women

---

[1] "Infertility and Fertility," *Eunice Kennedy Shriver* National Institute of Child Health and Human Development (NICHD), January 31, 2017. Available online. URL: www.nichd.nih.gov/health/topics/infertility. Accessed June 1, 2023.

can result in pelvic inflammatory disease (PID)—a condition that can cause long-term complications, such as chronic pelvic pain, ectopic pregnancy (pregnancy outside of the uterus), and infertility.

Additionally, some infections may not cause symptoms and may go unnoticed. These undiagnosed and untreated infections can lead to severe health consequences, especially in women, causing permanent damage to reproductive organs and infertility.

Infertility from an STI is less common among men, but it does occur. More commonly, untreated chlamydia and gonorrhea infections in men may cause epididymitis, a painful infection in the tissue surrounding the testicles, or urethritis, an infection of the urinary canal in the penis, which causes painful urination and fever.[2]

CHLAMYDIA AND GONORRHEA SCREENING OF SEXUALLY ACTIVE WOMEN YOUNGER THAN 25 YEARS

Chlamydia and gonorrhea are important preventable causes of PID and infertility. Untreated, about 10–15 percent of women with chlamydia will develop PID. Chlamydia can also cause fallopian tube infection without any symptoms. PID and "silent" infection in the upper genital tract may cause permanent damage to the fallopian tubes, uterus, and surrounding tissues, which can lead to infertility.

- In the United States, an estimated 4 million new chlamydia infections and 1.6 million new cases of gonorrhea infections occurred in 2018 alone.*
- Most women infected with chlamydia or gonorrhea have no symptoms.

The Centers for Disease Control and Prevention (CDC) recommends annual chlamydia and gonorrhea screening of all sexually active women younger than 25 years, as well as older women with risk factors such as new or multiple sex partners or a sex partner who has an STI.

Chlamydia and gonorrhea, respectively, are the first and second most commonly reported bacterial STIs in the United States. In 2021,

[2] "Other Sexually Transmitted Diseases (STDs) FAQs," *Eunice Kennedy Shriver* National Institute of Child Health and Human Development (NICHD), January 31, 2017. Available online. URL: www.nichd.nih.gov/health/topics/stds/more_information/other-faqs. Accessed June 1, 2023.

a total of 1,644,614 cases of chlamydia and 710,151 cases of gonor-rhea were reported to the CDC from 50 states and the District of Columbia. The number of reported cases is lower than the estimated total number because infected people are often unaware of, and do not seek treatment for, their infections and because screening for chlamydia is still not routine in many clinical settings.[3]

---

[3] "STDs & Infertility," Centers for Disease Control and Prevention (CDC), April 11, 2023. Available online. URL: www.cdc.gov/std/infertility/default.htm. Accessed June 1, 2023.

Part 4 | Sexually Transmitted Diseases: Testing and Treatment

Chapter 25 | Testing for Sexually Transmitted Diseases

Chapter Contents

Section 25.1 | **Talk. Test. Treat.**

If you are sexually active or thinking of becoming sexually active, it is important that you talk, test, and treat to protect your health. These three small actions can have a big impact on your sexual health!

TALK
Talk openly and honestly to your partner(s) and your health-care provider about sexual health and sexually transmitted infections (STIs).

Talk with your partner(s) before having sex. Not sure how? We have tips to help you start the conversation. Make sure your discussion covers several important ways to make sex safer:
- Talk about when you were last tested and suggest getting tested together.
- If you have any STI, such as herpes or human immunodeficiency virus (HIV), tell your partner.
- Agree to only have sex with each other.
- Use condoms the right way for every act of vaginal, anal, and oral sex throughout the entire sex act (from start to finish).

Talk with your health-care provider about your sex life as it relates to your health. This helps your health-care provider understand what STI tests you should be getting and how often.

Here are a few questions you should expect and be prepared to answer honestly:
- Have you been sexually active in the last year?
- Do you have sex with men, women, or both?
- In the past 12 months, how many sexual partners have you had?
- Do you have anal, oral, or vaginal sex?
- What are you doing to protect yourself from infection?

Not all medical checkups include STI testing, so do not assume that you have been tested unless you discuss it with your provider.

If your provider does not discuss sex or STI testing with you, bring it up.

Ask your health-care provider whether certain vaccines, such as the hepatitis B vaccine or the human papillomavirus (HPV) vaccine, are right for you.

TEST

Get tested. It is the only way to know for sure if you have an STI.

Many STIs do not cause any symptoms, so you could have one and not know. If you are having sex, getting tested is one of the most important things you can do to protect your health.

Even if you are pregnant, you can still get an STI. If you are having sex, you are still at risk.

Find out what STI care options are available near you. In addition to traditional, in-person visits, other options that may be available include:

- video or phone appointments with your health-care provider
- express visits that allow walk-in STI testing and treatment appointments without a full clinical exam
- pharmacies and retail clinics, such as at a grocery store or big-box store, for on-site testing and treatment
- at-home collection, where you collect your own sample and take or mail it to a lab for testing

If you are not comfortable talking with your regular health-care provider about STIs, find a clinic near you that provides confidential testing that is free or low cost.

TREAT

If you test positive for an STI, work with your health-care provider to get the correct treatment.

Some STIs can be cured with the right medicine, and all STIs are treatable. Make sure your treatment works by doing these things:

- Take all of the medication your health-care provider prescribes, even if you start feeling better or your symptoms go away.

- Do not share your medicine with anyone.
- Avoid having sex again until you and your sex partner(s) have all completed treatment.

Your health-care provider can talk with you about which medications are right for you.[1]

Section 25.2 | Sexually Transmitted Disease Testing: Conversation Starters

It might be hard to talk to your partner about getting tested for sexually transmitted diseases (STDs), but it is important. Chances are your partner will be glad you brought it up.

TALK BEFORE YOU HAVE SEX
You can say the following:
- "Let us get tested before we have sex. That way, we can look out for each other."
- "Many people who have an STD do not know it. Why take a chance when we can know for sure?"

There are other things you may want to talk to your partner about. The following are a few examples:
- sexual history, including what type of protection you usually use (e.g., condoms or dental dams) or the last time you got tested for STDs (including human immunodeficiency virus (HIV))
- risk factors, including whether you have had sex without a condom or used drugs with needles

---

[1] "Individuals—#TalkTestTreat," Centers for Disease Control and Prevention (CDC), January 18, 2023. Available online. URL: www.cdc.gov/std/saw/talktesttreat/individuals.htm. Accessed May 29, 2023.

SHARE THE FACTS

You can say the following:

- "Most STDs are easy to treat. And, when they are treated early, STDs are less likely to cause long-term health problems."
- "STD tests are quick, simple, and usually painless. For example, rapid HIV tests can provide results from just a swab inside the mouth in only 20 minutes."
- "If you want to get tested at home, you can get an HIV home test or self-testing kits for other STDs."
- "If you do not feel comfortable talking about STDs with your regular doctor, you can get tested at a clinic instead."

SHOW THAT YOU CARE

You can say the following:

- "I really care about you. I want to make sure we are both healthy."
- "I have been tested for STDs, including HIV. Are you willing to do that, too?"
- "Let us get tested together."

AGREE TO STAY SAFE

You can say the following:

- "If we are going to have sex, using condoms is a good way to protect us from STDs. Let us use condoms every time we have sex."
- "We can enjoy sex more if we know it is safe."[2]

---

[2] Office of Disease Prevention and Health Promotion (ODPHP), "STD Testing: Conversation Starters," U.S. Department of Health and Human Services (HHS), October 20, 2022. Available online. URL: https://health.gov/myhealthfinder/health-conditions/hiv-and-other-stds/std-testing-conversation-starters. Accessed May 29, 2023.

Section 25.3 | **Screening Recommendations**

Parents are a trusted source of health information and can help prepare adolescents for developing healthy relationships and navigating challenges that may lie ahead.

Talking regularly with your adolescent and paying attention to where they are and who they are with can help reduce unhealthy behaviors. Most adolescents report talking about health topics with parents, including sexual and reproductive health.

To prepare for these conversations, parents need to know about options for preventing pregnancy and sexually transmitted diseases (STDs), including human immunodeficiency virus (HIV). In addition, it is important that parents know about key preventive health services.

In addition to unintended pregnancy, young people who choose to be sexually active are at risk of getting an STD.

Getting tested for STDs is important because it is the only way to know if someone has an STD and needs treatment.

The following recommendations are specifically for adolescents, describing which STDs young people should be routinely tested for, who should be tested, and when they should be tested.

Action steps are provided to help parents make sure their adolescent receives the best sexual and reproductive health care possible.

WHY SHOULD ADOLESCENTS BE TESTED FOR SEXUALLY TRANSMITTED DISEASES?

Many STDs do not cause any symptoms, so the only way to know for sure if you have an STD is to get tested. Some curable STDs can be dangerous if they are not treated. For example, if left untreated, chlamydia and gonorrhea can make it difficult—or even impossible—for a woman to get pregnant later in life. The chances of getting HIV if you have an untreated STD also increase. Some STDs, such as HIV, can be fatal if left untreated.

WHAT SEXUALLY TRANSMITTED DISEASE TESTS ARE RECOMMENDED FOR ADOLESCENTS?

A health-care provider can help determine if STD testing is recommended for your adolescent and which STD tests are most appropriate. A health-care provider can also give more information about each type of test.

The following are a few recommendations for STD testing specifically focused on sexually active female adolescents and adults younger than age 25.

Chlamydia Testing

All sexually active women younger than 25 years of age should be tested for chlamydia each year. Sexually active men younger than 25 years of age in areas with a high number of chlamydia cases among males should also be tested each year. Your adolescent's health-care provider should know what is recommended in your area. In addition, all men aged 13 and older who have sex with other men should also be tested each year.

Gonorrhea Testing

All sexually active women younger than 25 years of age should be tested for gonorrhea each year. All men aged 13 and older who have sex with other men should also be tested each year. Typically, anyone testing for chlamydia is tested for gonorrhea at the same time.

Syphilis Testing

Men aged 13 and older who have sex with men should be tested each year.

Human Immunodeficiency Virus Testing

Men aged 13 years and older who have sex with men, people who inject drugs, and people who have a partner with HIV should be tested for HIV at least once a year. Others may also need to be tested if their health-care provider thinks that they may be at higher risk.

Pregnant Women

At their first prenatal visit, pregnant women should be tested for chlamydia, gonorrhea, syphilis, and HIV. For syphilis, retesting early in the third trimester is recommended for women who are at high risk, who live in areas with a high number of syphilis cases, or who tested positive in the first trimester. For HIV, retesting in the third trimester is recommended for women at high risk of acquiring HIV.

WHERE CAN ADOLESCENTS GET TESTED FOR SEXUALLY TRANSMITTED DISEASES?

Sexually transmitted disease testing is typically available from health-care providers and at select outreach events. Your teen's school may also provide testing on-site or resources for where to find testing locations. The STD testing locator available at https://gettested.cdc.gov/ provides nearby testing locations, including those that offer free or low-cost services.

WHAT ARE STEPS PARENTS CAN TAKE TO HELP THEIR ADOLESCENTS?

Support Adolescent Health-Care Seeking and Follow-Up

You play an important role in helping your adolescent regularly access quality health care. The following are a few examples:

- You can help your adolescent find a health-care provider they are comfortable with, schedule appointments, and/or provide or access transportation to the clinic.
- Parents can also help their adolescents fill prescriptions and take medications correctly.

Talk with Your Adolescent

Talking about sex, relationships, and the prevention of HIV, STDs, and pregnancy may not always be comfortable or easy, but you can encourage your teen to ask questions. Be prepared to give fair and honest answers. This will help keep open communication.

- You can tell your teen that the decision to be sexually active comes with the responsibility to keep yourself and your partner safe. Some young people may decide to postpone becoming sexually active until they feel ready to handle this responsibility.
- Explain to your adolescent the range of health services they should discuss or receive when they go to the doctor and why the health services are important. Make sure they are aware of the importance of STD testing.

Prepare for Your Adolescent's Independence

It is important that adolescents have opportunities to seek health care with some independence in order to be prepared to do so as an adult. As a first step, your adolescent should have one-on-one time with their provider routinely, where you step out of the room.

- Let them know early on that as they get older, they will begin to have this one-on-one time so that they will be prepared to ask questions and talk openly and honestly.
- Encourage your adolescent to ask about sexual and reproductive health services when they have one-on-one time with their provider.

As your adolescent gets older, they may go to the doctor and make decisions about services, including STD testing, on their own. Adolescents can consent to STD testing in all 50 states and the District of Columbia, with some variation in the age at which this is allowed. Preparing yourself for these transitions, which are a normal part of adolescent development, can help make them easier for both you and your adolescent.

Stay Informed

Be aware of the quality of the health information your adolescent is receiving from school, friends, online, or other sources. Your adolescent may not be receiving complete or accurate information from these sources. Be available to answer any questions that they may have. The more you know about health topics and services, the easier it will be to talk with your adolescent about them.

Work with Your Adolescent's Health-Care Provider

You and your adolescent's health-care provider can work together as a team with the shared goal of improving your adolescent's health.

- You can let the health-care provider know that you are supportive of your adolescent receiving recommended health services, including those for preventing HIV, other STDs, and unintended pregnancy.
- You can also ask your adolescent's health-care provider to tell you more about newer services or those that you may be less familiar with, such as long-acting reversible contraception (LARC) or HIV pre-exposure prophylaxis (PrEP), which is taking daily medicine to prevent HIV.[3]

WHICH SEXUALLY TRANSMITTED DISEASE TESTS SHOULD ADOLESCENTS GET?

If you are a sexually active adolescent, getting tested for STDs is one of the most important things you can do to protect your health. Make sure you have an open and honest conversation about your sexual history and STD testing with your doctor and ask whether you should be tested for STDs. If you are not comfortable talking with your regular health-care provider about STDs, there are many clinics that provide confidential and free or low-cost testing. The following is a brief overview of STD testing recommendations:

- All adults and adolescents from ages 13–64 should be tested at least once for HIV.
- All sexually active women younger than 25 years should be tested for gonorrhea and chlamydia every year. Women 25 years and older with risk factors such

---

[3] "STD Testing," Centers for Disease Control and Prevention (CDC), June 22, 2020. Available online. URL: www.cdc.gov/healthyyouth/healthservices/infobriefs/std_testing_information.htm. Accessed June 20, 2023.

as new or multiple sex partners or a sex partner who has an STD should also be tested for gonorrhea and chlamydia every year.

- Everyone who is pregnant should be tested for syphilis, HIV, hepatitis B, and hepatitis C starting early in pregnancy. Those at risk for infection should also be tested for chlamydia and gonorrhea starting early in pregnancy. Repeat testing may be needed in some cases.
- All sexually active gay, bisexual, and other men who have sex with men (MSM) should be tested:
    - at least once a year for syphilis, chlamydia, and gonorrhea (Those who have multiple or anonymous partners should be tested more frequently (e.g., every three to six months).)
    - at least once a year for HIV (You may benefit from more frequent HIV testing (e.g., every three to six months).)
    - at least once a year for hepatitis C if living with HIV
- Anyone who engages in sexual behaviors that could place them at risk for infection or shares injection drug equipment should get tested for HIV at least once a year.
- People who have had oral or anal sex should talk with their health-care provider about throat and rectal testing options.[4]

---

[4] "Which STD Tests Should I Get?" Centers for Disease Control and Prevention (CDC), December 14, 2021. Available online. URL: www.cdc.gov/std/prevention/screeningreccs.htm. Accessed June 20, 2023.

Section 25.4 | How Health-Care Providers Diagnose Sexually Transmitted Diseases or Infections

Any person who is sexually active should discuss his or her risk factors for sexually transmitted diseases (STDs)/sexually transmitted infections (STIs) with a health-care provider and ask about getting tested. If you are sexually active, it is important to remember that you may have an STD/STI and not know it because many STDs/STIs do not cause symptoms. You should get tested and have regular checkups with a health-care provider who can help assess and manage your risk, answer your questions, and diagnose and treat an STD/STI if needed.

Starting treatment quickly is important to prevent transmission of infections to other people and to minimize the long-term complications of STDs/STIs. Recent sexual partners should also be treated to prevent reinfection and further transmission.

Some STDs/STIs may be diagnosed during a physical exam or through microscopic examination of a sore or fluid swabbed from the vagina, penis, or anus. This fluid can also be cultured over a few days to see whether infectious bacteria or yeast can be detected. The effects of human papillomavirus (HPV), which causes genital warts and cervical cancer, can be detected in a woman when her health-care provider performs a Pap smear test and takes samples of cells from the cervix to be checked microscopically for abnormal changes. Blood tests are used to detect infections such as hepatitis A, B, and C or human immunodeficiency virus/acquired immunodeficiency syndrome (HIV/AIDS).

Because STDs are passed from person to person and can have serious health consequences, the health department notifies people if they have been exposed to certain STDs/STIs. Not all STDs/STIs are reported, though. If you receive a notice, it is important to see a health-care provider, be tested, and start treatment right away.

Screening is especially important for pregnant women because many STDs/STIs can be passed on to the fetus during pregnancy or delivery. During an early prenatal visit, with the help of her health-care provider, an expectant mother should be screened for these infections, including HIV and syphilis. Some of these STDs/STIs

353

can be cured with drug treatment, but not all of them. However, even if the infection is not curable, a pregnant woman can usually take measures to protect her infant from infection.[5]

Section 25.5 | Sexually Transmitted Disease Testing: An Overview

WHAT ARE SEXUALLY TRANSMITTED DISEASES, AND SHOULD YOU BE TESTED?

The Centers for Disease Control and Prevention (CDC) estimates that there are approximately 19 million new sexually transmitted disease (STD) infections each year—almost half of them among young people aged 15–24. Most infections have no symptoms and often go undiagnosed and untreated, which may lead to severe health consequences, especially for women.

Knowing your STD status is a critical step to stopping STD transmission. If you know you are infected, you can take steps to protect yourself and your partners. Many STDs can be easily diagnosed and treated. If either you or your partner is infected, both of you may need to receive treatment at the same time to avoid getting reinfected.

WHAT IS HUMAN IMMUNODEFICIENCY VIRUS, AND SHOULD YOU BE TESTED?

Human immunodeficiency virus (HIV) is the virus that can lead to acquired immunodeficiency syndrome (AIDS). Unlike some other viruses, the human body cannot get rid of HIV. That means that once you have HIV, you have it for life.

Only certain body fluids, such as blood, semen (cum), preseminal fluid (precum), rectal fluids, vaginal fluids, and breast milk, from a person who has HIV can transmit HIV. These fluids

---

[5] "How Do Health Care Providers Diagnose a Sexually Transmitted Disease (STD) or Sexually Transmitted Infection (STI)?" *Eunice Kennedy Shriver* National Institute of Child Health and Human Development (NICHD), January 31, 2017. Available online. URL: www.nichd.nih.gov/health/topics/stds/conditioninfo/diagnosed. Accessed May 29, 2023.

must come in contact with a mucous membrane or damaged tissue or be directly injected into the bloodstream (from a needle or syringe) for transmission to occur. Mucous membranes are found inside the rectum, vagina, penis, and mouth. Early HIV infection often has no symptoms. The only way to know if you are infected with HIV is to be tested. Currently, there is no effective cure that exists for HIV. However, with proper medical care, HIV can be controlled.

The CDC recommends that everyone between the ages of 13 and 64 get tested at least once as a part of their routine health care. People with higher risk factors, such as more than one sex partner and other STDs, gay and bisexual men, and individuals who inject drugs should be tested at least once a year.

HOW DO YOU KNOW IF YOU ARE AT RISK OF GETTING HUMAN IMMUNODEFICIENCY VIRUS?

Knowing your risk can help you make important decisions to prevent exposure to HIV. The CDC has developed the HIV Risk Reduction Tool (https://hivrisk.cdc.gov/) to help you know risk and better understand how different prevention methods, such as using condoms or taking pre-exposure prophylaxis (PrEP), can reduce your risk. Overall, an American has a 1 in 99 chance of being diagnosed with HIV at some point in his or her lifetime. However, the lifetime risk is much greater among some populations. If current diagnosis rates continue, the lifetime risk of getting HIV is:
- 1 in 6 for gay and bisexual men overall
- 1 in 2 for African American gay and bisexual men
- 1 in 4 for Hispanic gay and bisexual men
- 1 in 11 for White gay and bisexual men
- 1 in 20 for African American men overall
- 1 in 48 for African American women overall
- 1 in 23 for women who inject drugs
- 1 in 36 for men who inject drugs

Your health behaviors also affect your risk. You can get or transmit HIV only through specific activities. HIV is commonly transmitted through anal or vaginal sex without a condom or sharing injection and other drug injection equipment with a person infected with HIV. Substance use can increase the risk of exposure to HIV because alcohol and other drugs can affect your decision to use condoms during sex.

WHAT IS NATIONAL HUMAN IMMUNODEFICIENCY VIRUS TESTING DAY?

National HIV Testing Day (NHTD) is an annual observance to encourage people of all ages to get tested for HIV and to know their status. Too many people do not know they have HIV. At the end of 2014, an estimated 1.1 million persons aged 13 and older were living with HIV infection in the United States, including an estimated 166,000 (15%, or one in seven) persons whose infections had not been diagnosed. Getting tested is the first step to finding out if you have HIV. If you have HIV, getting medical care and taking medicines regularly helps you live a longer, healthier life and also lowers the chances of passing HIV on to others.

Testing is the only way for Americans living with undiagnosed HIV to know their HIV status and get into care. The CDC estimates that more than 90 percent of all new infections could be prevented by proper testing and linking HIV-positive persons to care. HIV testing saves lives! It is one of the most powerful tools in the fight against HIV.

WHAT IS VIRAL HEPATITIS, AND SHOULD YOU BE TESTED?

Viral hepatitis refers to a group of viral infections that affect the liver. The most common types are hepatitis A, B, and C.

Hepatitis A, B, and C are diseases caused by three different viruses. Although each can cause similar symptoms, they have different modes of transmission and can affect the liver differently. Hepatitis A appears only as an acute or newly occurring infection and does not become chronic. People with hepatitis A usually improve without treatment. Hepatitis B and C can also begin as acute infections, but in some people, the virus remains in the body, resulting in chronic disease and long-term liver problems. There are vaccines to prevent hepatitis A and B; however, there is not one for hepatitis C. Recommendations for testing depend on many different factors and on the type of hepatitis.

HOW DO HUMAN IMMUNODEFICIENCY VIRUS, VIRAL HEPATITIS, AND SEXUALLY TRANSMITTED DISEASES RELATE TO EACH OTHER?

Persons who have an STD are at least two to five times more likely than uninfected persons to acquire HIV infection if they are exposed to the virus through sexual contact. In addition, if a person who is HIV-positive also has an STD, that person is more likely to transmit HIV through sexual contact than other HIV-infected persons.

Hepatitis B virus (HBV) and HIV are blood-borne viruses transmitted primarily through sexual contact and injection drug use. Because of these shared modes of transmission, a high proportion of adults at risk for HIV infection are also at risk for HBV infection. HIV-positive persons who become infected with HBV are at increased risk for developing chronic HBV infection and should be tested. In addition, persons who are coinfected with HIV and HBV can have serious medical complications, including an increased risk for liver-related morbidity and mortality.

Hepatitis C virus (HCV) is one of the most common causes of chronic liver disease in the United States. For persons who are HIV-infected, coinfection with HCV can result in a more rapid occurrence of liver damage and may also impact the course and management of HIV infection.[6]

---

[6] "Get Tested—National HIV, STD, and Hepatitis Testing—Frequently Asked Questions," Centers for Disease Control and Prevention (CDC), November 4, 2014. Available online. URL: https://gettested.cdc.gov/faq-page. Accessed May 29, 2023.

Chapter 26 | Talking to Your Health-Care Professional about Sexually Transmitted Diseases

Chapter Contents

Section 26.1 | General Questions to Ask Your Health-Care Professional

ARE YOU AT RISK FOR SEXUALLY TRANSMITTED DISEASES/INFECTIONS?

Sexually transmitted diseases (STDs)/sexually transmitted infections (STIs) affect men and women of all races, backgrounds, sexual orientations, and economic levels. Anyone who is having or has had vaginal, anal, or oral sex has some degree of risk for an STI. In fact, some STIs can be passed through sexual play that does not involve intercourse.

You can analyze your risk for STDs/STIs with the STD Wizard—a free interactive online tool based on the STD Treatment Guidelines of the Centers for Disease Control and Prevention (CDC). The STD Wizard recommends tests and vaccines based on your responses concerning some of your personal characteristics and behaviors. You can use these recommendations to start a discussion with your health-care provider about your STD/STI risk and the tests you may need.

HOW CAN YOU AVOID GETTING A SEXUALLY TRANSMITTED DISEASE/INFECTION?

The most reliable ways to avoid STDs/STIs are to abstain from sexual contact or to be in a long-term monogamous relationship with a partner who has been tested and is uninfected. In addition, the following measures can also help you avoid STIs:

- Know your sexual partners' STI and health history.
- Talk to your health-care provider about your risk and get tested for STIs.
- Get vaccinated against hepatitis A virus, hepatitis B virus, and human papillomavirus (HPV).
- Use latex condoms correctly and for all sexual activities.

Remember, however, that while condoms greatly reduce the chance of getting certain STIs, such as gonorrhea, condoms cannot

361

fully protect against infection because viruses and some bacteria can be passed from person to person by skin-to-skin contact in the genital area not covered by a condom.

WHAT SHOULD YOU DO IF YOU HAVE BEEN DIAGNOSED WITH A SEXUALLY TRANSMITTED DISEASE/INFECTION?

You should see your health-care provider for treatment as soon as possible after receiving a diagnosis of an STD/STI. You should also notify, either yourself or with the help of the local health department, all recent sex partners and advise them to see their health-care providers and be treated. These steps will reduce your risk of becoming reinfected, help avoid spreading the STI to other people, and decrease the risk that your previous sexual partners will develop serious complications from the STI. You and all of your sex partners must avoid sex until treatment is complete and all symptoms have disappeared.

In the case of STIs caused by viruses with no cure (e.g., HIV, genital herpes, or hepatitis), special care and preventive measures can help control the infection, limit symptoms, and help maximize health.

ARE THERE DISORDERS OR CONDITIONS ASSOCIATED WITH SEXUALLY TRANSMITTED DISEASES/INFECTIONS?

Sexually transmitted diseases/infections in women can cause pelvic inflammatory disease (PID), which may result in infertility and chronic pelvic pain.

Men with STIs can also have problems with infertility.

Additionally, a person with an STI other than human immunodeficiency virus (HIV) is two to five times more likely to contract HIV when exposed to an HIV-infected partner than a person without an STI. If a person is already HIV-positive, having another STI increases the chances that he or she will pass the virus on to his or her sexual partner.

Some STIs, such as HPV, viral hepatitis, and HIV, increase the risk of some forms of cancer.

Certain STIs, such as gonorrhea, chlamydia, HIV, and syphilis, can pass from a pregnant woman to the fetus in her womb. The effects can be life-threatening, as is the case with HIV and syphilis.

Other STIs, especially if left untreated, can cause a range of health problems in the infant, including deafness, blindness, and intellectual disability.

CAN A SEXUALLY TRANSMITTED DISEASE/INFECTION LEAD TO CANCER?

Having an STD/STI increases a person's risk for several types of cancer.

Certain high-risk types of HPV can cause cervical cancer in women. In men, HPV infection can lead to the development of penile cancers. HPV can also cause cancers of the mouth, throat, and anus in both sexes.

Acquiring viral hepatitis B or C puts a person at risk for liver cancer, and untreated HIV/acquired immunodeficiency syndrome (AIDS) increases the risk for several types of rare cancers, including lymphomas, sarcomas, and cervical cancer.[1]

Section 26.2 | For Teens: How Do You Discuss Embarrassing Things with Your Doctor?

Talking freely with your doctor can make you feel better and gives your doctor the information he or she needs to give you the best care. You can even discuss personal things about your health with your doctor. Do not be afraid or embarrassed to discuss something that is bothering you.

TIPS FOR TALKING WITH YOUR DOCTOR

- **Stay positive.** Go to your doctor's visits with a good attitude. Remember, your doctor and other caregivers are on your side. Think teamwork! Think positive!

---

[1] "Other Sexually Transmitted Diseases (STDs) FAQs," *Eunice Kennedy Shriver* National Institute of Child Health and Human Development (NICHD), January 31, 2017. Available online. URL: www.nichd.nih.gov/health/topics/stds/more_information/other-faqs. Accessed June 6, 2023.

- **Keep track of how you are feeling**. Before your doctor's visit, keep notes on how you are feeling. This will make it easier for you to answer questions about your symptoms and how medicines make you feel. It also makes it easier for you to bring up anything that you are worried about. Make sure to be honest about how you feel and how long you have felt that way. Also, let your doctor know if you are scared, worried, or sad. Your care will be better if your doctor knows how you are feeling. Your doctor can also tell you about counselors and support groups to help you talk about your feelings.

- **Bring your medical history, including a list of your current medicines**. If you are seeing a doctor for the first time, bring your medical history. Your medical history is a list of your illnesses, dates of operations, treatments (including medicines), names of doctors you have seen, what the doctors told you to do, and anything else you think your doctor should know. If you take medicines that you buy at the pharmacy without a prescription (an order from the doctor), make sure to also include them in your list. That includes things such as vitamins, herbal medicines, and aspirin. Also, if you are allergic to any medicines, such as penicillin, be sure to mention that to your doctor.

- **Ask questions**. Do not be afraid to ask your doctor any questions you have. This will help you understand your own health better. Maybe you have been reading a lot about your health condition, and that has caused you to think of some questions. To remember all the questions you have when you are not in the doctor's office, write them down and bring the list with you to your appointment. Be sure to talk with your parents about the things you want to ask the doctor. This will make getting answers even easier! At your appointment, your doctor may talk about a new treatment that he or she wants you to try. It may involve medicine, surgery, changes in daily habits such as what you eat, or a few of these together. You will get the most out of your treatments if you understand what is involved and why you need them. In case your doctor talks about a new treatment at your next visit, here are some questions you can print or write down to take with you:

- How long will it take?
- What will happen? (Is it a shot, pill, or operation?)
- Will it hurt?
- How many treatments do I have to have?
- Will I be able to go to school?
- Are there things I would not be able to do, such as ride a bike?
- Is this treatment to try to cure my health problem or help take away some of my symptoms?
- Will these treatments make me tired or feel pain? How long will this last?
- What happens if I miss a treatment?
- What will we do if the treatments do not work?
- Is this the best treatment out there for me?
- What will happen to me if I do not have this treatment?

If the treatment you get makes you feel bad, ask if there are others you can try. There may not be others. But you and your doctor can talk about it.

Remember, there is no such thing as a stupid question. If you do not understand the answer to a question, ask the doctor to explain it again until you do understand.

- **Write down what the doctor says**. This will help you remember important information later on. You might even bring a tape recorder and record what the doctor says. But, if you bring a tape recorder, be sure to ask the doctor first if it is okay to use it.

Use a treatment planner to keep track of anything your doctor, counselor, or therapist tells you.

TALKING ABOUT PERSONAL THINGS

It is okay to be nervous about talking to your doctor about things that embarrass you. Who wants to talk to a strange adult about sex, feeling sad, or what you eat? But it is easier than you think. Doctors are there to talk about everything that is going on with your body. They will not think any less of you no matter what you ask or what your problem is. In fact, they are very used to personal issues (and they likely have had to seek help for their own). Telling them everything that is going on with you is very important for your health. By not telling them about a strange smell, rash, pain, or anything else going on with your body, you could be making a health problem worse.

Talking about personal issues with your doctor can be confidential, which means that your doctor has to keep everything you say secret. Doctors might feel they have to tell your parents what you say if they think you are in danger or are not able to make choices on your own. Ask your doctor about the privacy policy before you begin.[2]

[2] girlshealth.gov, "Talking with Your Doctor," Office on Women's Health (OWH), October 31, 2013. Available online. URL: www.girlshealth.gov/disability/medical/talkdr.html. Accessed June 20, 2023.

Chapter 27 | Sexually Transmitted Diseases Reporting and Patient Confidentiality

WILL OTHER PEOPLE KNOW YOUR HUMAN IMMUNODEFICIENCY VIRUS TEST RESULT?

Human immunodeficiency virus (HIV) tests may be anonymous or confidential.

Anonymous testing means only you will know the test result.

- When you take an anonymous HIV test, you get a unique identifier that allows you to get your test results.
- You can also buy an HIV self-test if you want to test anonymously.

Confidential testing means your test result will be part of your medical record.

- Your name and other personal information will be attached to your test results.
- The results will go into your medical record and may be shared with your health-care provider and health insurance company.
- Otherwise, your results are protected by state and federal privacy laws, and they can only be released with your permission.

With confidential testing, if your test result is positive, the result and your name will be reported to the state or local health department to help public health officials estimate HIV rates in the state. The state health department will then remove all personal information about you (name, address, etc.) and share the remaining information with the Centers for Disease Control and Prevention (CDC) and does not share this information with anyone.

SHOULD YOU SHARE YOUR POSITIVE HUMAN IMMUNODEFICIENCY VIRUS TEST RESULT WITH OTHERS?

You should share your HIV status with your sex or needle-sharing partners. Whether you disclose your status to others is your decision.

Partners

You should disclose your HIV status to your sex or needle-sharing partners even if you are uncomfortable talking about it. Communicating your HIV status allows each person to take steps to stay healthy. The more practice you have in disclosing your HIV status, the easier it will become.

Family and Friends

In most cases, your family and friends will only know your test results or HIV status if you tell them. While telling your family that you have HIV may seem hard, disclosure has many benefits. Telling friends and family can provide an important source of support in managing your HIV. Studies show that people who disclose their HIV status respond better to treatment than those who do not.

Employers

In most cases, your employer will only know your HIV status if you tell them. But your employer has the right to ask if you have any health conditions that may affect your ability to do your job or that pose a serious risk to others (e.g., you may have to disclose your health conditions if you are a health-care provider who does procedures where there is a risk of blood or other body fluids being exchanged.)

If you have health insurance through your employer, the insurance company cannot legally tell your employer that you have HIV. But your employer could find out if the insurance company provides detailed information to your employer about the benefits it pays or the cost of insurance.

All people with HIV are covered under the Americans with Disabilities Act (ADA). This means that your employer cannot discriminate against you because of your HIV status if you can do your job.[1]

---

[1] "HIV—Sharing Your Test Result," Centers for Disease Control and Prevention (CDC), June 22, 2022. Available online. URL: www.cdc.gov/hiv/basics/hiv-testing/sharing-test-results.html. Accessed June 12, 2023.

Section 27.2 | At-Home/Mail-Order Sexually Transmitted Disease Tests

WHAT IS THE HOME ACCESS HIV-1 TEST SYSTEM?

The Home Access HIV-1 Test System is a laboratory test sold over the counter (OTC) that uses fingerstick blood mailed to the testing laboratory. The test kit consists of multiple components, including materials for specimen self-collection, prepaid materials for mailing the specimen to a laboratory for testing, testing directions, an information booklet, an anonymous registration system, and a call center to receive your test results and follow-up counseling by telephone.

This approved system uses a finger prick process for home blood collection that results in dried blood spots on special paper. The dried blood spots are mailed to a laboratory with a confidential and anonymous unique personal identification number (PIN) and are analyzed by trained clinicians in a laboratory using the same tests that are used for samples taken in a doctor's office or clinic. Test results are obtained through a toll-free telephone number using the PIN, and posttest counseling is provided by telephone when results are obtained.

WHEN SHOULD YOU TAKE A TEST FOR HUMAN IMMUNODEFICIENCY VIRUS?

If you actively engage in behavior that puts you at risk for human immunodeficiency virus (HIV) infection or your partner engages in such behavior, then you should consider testing on a regular basis. It may take some time for the immune system to produce sufficient antibodies for the test to detect, and this time period can vary from person to person. This time frame is commonly referred to as the "window period" when a person is infected with HIV, but antibodies to the virus cannot be detected; however, the person may be able to infect others. According to the Centers for Disease Control and Prevention (CDC), it can take up to six months to develop antibodies to HIV although most people (97%) will develop detectable antibodies in the first three months following the time of their infection.

HOW RELIABLE IS THE HOME ACCESS HIV-1 TEST SYSTEM?

Clinical studies reported to the U.S. Food and Drug Administration (FDA) showed that the sensitivity (i.e., the percentage of results that will be positive when HIV is present) was estimated to be greater than 99.9 percent. The specificity (i.e., the percentage of results that will be negative when HIV is not present) was also estimated to be greater than 99.9 percent. Results reported as positive have undergone testing using both a screening test and another test to confirm the positive result.

WHAT ABOUT COUNSELING?

The Home Access HIV-1 Test System has a built-in mechanism for pretest and posttest counseling provided by the manufacturer. This counseling is anonymous and confidential. Counseling, which uses both printed material and telephone interaction, provides the user with an interpretation of the test result. Counseling also provides information on how to keep from getting infected if you are negative and how to prevent further transmission of disease if you are infected. Counseling provides you with information about treatment options if you are infected and can even provide referrals to doctors who treat HIV-infected individuals in your area.

IF THE TEST RESULTS ARE POSITIVE, WHAT SHOULD YOU DO?

The counselors can provide you with information about treatment options and referrals to doctors who treat HIV-infected individuals in your area.

DO YOU NEED A CONFIRMATORY TEST?

No, a positive result from the Home Access HIV-1 Test System means that antibodies to the HIV-1 are present in the blood sample submitted to the testing laboratory. The Home Access HIV-1 Test System includes confirmatory testing for HIV-1, and all confirmation testing is completed before the results are released and available to users of the test system.

HOW QUICKLY WILL YOU GET THE RESULTS OF THE HOME ACCESS HIV-1 TEST SYSTEM?

You can anonymously call for the results approximately seven business days (three business days for the Express System) after shipping your specimen to the laboratory by using the unique PIN on the tear-off label included with your test kit. This label includes both the unique PIN and the toll-free number for the counseling center.

HOW ARE UNAPPROVED TEST SYSTEMS DIFFERENT?

The manufacturers of unapproved test systems have not submitted data to the FDA to review to determine whether or not their test systems can reliably detect HIV infection. Therefore, the FDA cannot give the public any assurance that the results obtained using an unapproved test system are accurate.[2]

Section 27.3 | Sexually Transmitted Diseases Diagnoses and Duty to Warn

WHAT IS DUTY TO WARN?

Duty to warn is a legal concept that indicates possible liability for health-care providers if no warning of possible harm is given in certain circumstances.

DOES DUTY TO WARN APPLY TO HEALTH-CARE PROVIDERS AND SEXUALLY TRANSMITTED DISEASE DIAGNOSES?

- A duty to warn exists across various U.S. jurisdictions. Within the health-care field, duty to warn can create an obligation for health-care providers to warn people who

[2] "Information regarding the Home Access HIV-1 Test System," U.S. Food and Drug Administration (FDA), March 7, 2018. Available online. URL: www.fda.gov/vaccines-blood-biologics/approved-blood-products/information-regarding-home-access-hiv-1-test-system. Accessed June 12, 2023.

are not their patients (e.g., third parties) of a serious threat of harm based on conversations with their patients.

- It has been suggested that this duty may extend to infectious diseases, including sexually transmitted diseases (STDs).
- This analysis suggests the following:
  - In a few U.S. jurisdictions, an STD diagnosis may create various physician duties that indirectly extend to people who are not their patients.
  - However, a direct duty to warn third parties that they may need a medical examination because of their potential STD exposure was not found across states despite its existence for other serious medical conditions.

WHAT IS DUTY TO WARN IN HEALTH LAW?

In the area of health law, duty to warn describes a physician's responsibility to warn an identifiable third party of a potential serious threat of harm to their health. It is based on findings from a widely referenced case: Tarasoff v. Regents of the University of California, in which a court found that a psychologist should have warned his patient's girlfriend after his patient told the psychologist of his intention to kill her despite the competing consideration of physician/patient confidentiality.

In the United States, a diagnosed case of certain STDs can trigger:

- reporting by the health-care provider to the state/local government
- investigation by the health department (partner notification, contact tracing, etc.) but not always

Although many health-care providers engaged in STD prevention, diagnosis, and treatment might believe an actual duty to warn law exists in all or most of the states around the country, in reality, very few states have laws or regulations in place specific to common bacterial STDs (e.g., chlamydia, gonorrhea, and syphilis).

The only action that physicians are required to take beyond the diagnosis and treatment of their patient is reporting the case to the state or local health department, per the laws of their state. Physician duties generally do not extend to sex partners of diagnosed patients, and as a result, sex partners are not always notified. Some states may require additional reporting of suspected cases, which can include partners of diagnosed patients.

Many state health departments, however, often use partner notification and contact tracing—two integral components of partner services—to break the chain of STD transmission because these strategies can help pinpoint the window of possible infection. They are most often used when syphilis is the STD in question because of the serious, long-term health risks associated with nontreatment. Limited partner notification services for other STDs (e.g., gonorrhea and chlamydia) may be conducted based on health department resources. Health departments can also encourage patients to notify their partners or provide patients with medication for their partners—a practice known as "expedited partner therapy" (EPT). All patients diagnosed with an STD are covered by patient confidentiality, and specially trained health department staff conduct contact tracing and partner notification while maintaining confidentiality. These activities are widely seen as effective in reducing the STD burden in communities and are supported by the Centers for Disease Control and Prevention (CDC).

WHAT IS THE BOTTOM LINE REGARDING DUTY TO WARN FOR SEXUALLY TRANSMITTED DISEASES IN THE UNITED STATES?

Currently, partner notification and other activities that could be interpreted as "warnings" are limited to health departments, while health-care providers' duties focus on their patients. However, three states do impose legal duties on the health-care provider/patient relationship for third parties, even if these states do not require a warning. These legal duties vary in each of the following three states:

- California
  - "An effort, through the cooperation of the patient," should be made to bring the third party in for examination and treatment.

- If the physician does not have evidence that the third party received treatment within 10 days, the physician must report the suspected case to the health department.
- Nebraska
  - If a patient identifies a third party as someone potentially exposed, this suspected case should be reported to the local or state health department.
  - Physicians should make reasonable efforts to prevent the spread of disease to others, which could include third-party notification depending on the circumstances. However, the state or local health department performs partner notification and referrals, which means the provider's duty is likely limited to health department reporting and actions directed to their patient (i.e., counseling and linkage to care and treatment).
- Indiana
  - If a patient identifies a third party as someone potentially exposed, this suspected case should be reported to the local health officer.

Ultimately, a bacterial STD diagnosis does not automatically trigger a legal requirement for duty to warn because these STDs do not typically represent an imminent danger of serious bodily harm. Currently, the most common bacterial STDs are relatively easily cured with a single or short course of antibiotics. Additionally, practical reasons exist for not routinely performing a duty to warn of STDs, including the following:

- Privacy laws prohibit health-care providers from sharing patient information. Partner notification must ensure partner anonymity. Health departments are trained in the guidelines for partner notification.
- EPT, which is legal in almost every state, is an effective strategy for reaching partners of newly diagnosed patients.

- Partner notification takes time and financial resources, which could make it difficult for a provider to accept this responsibility. This effort is most often handled by health departments as part of their regular practices.

The responsibility for STD reporting and partner notification currently lies in the hands of individual states—there is no universal duty to warn law in place at the present time, although STD diagnoses do sometimes trigger actions beyond the physician's care of their patient and may involve consideration of the care of their patient's sex partner.[3]

Section 27.4 | Sexually Transmitted Diseases Criminalization Laws by State

During the early years of the human immunodeficiency virus (HIV) epidemic, many states implemented HIV-specific criminal exposure laws to discourage actions that might lead to transmission, promote safer sex practices, and, in some cases, receive funds to support HIV prevention activities. These laws were passed at a time when little was known about HIV, including how HIV was transmitted and how best to treat the virus. Many of these state laws, then and now, criminalize actions that cannot transmit HIV—such as biting or spitting—and apply regardless of actual transmission or intent. After more than 40 years of HIV research and significant biomedical advancements to treat and prevent HIV transmission, many state laws are now outdated and do not reflect our current understanding of HIV. In many cases, this same standard is not applied to other infectious, treatable diseases. Furthermore, these

---

[3] "Sexually Transmitted Diseases (STDs)—Duty to Warn," Centers for Disease Control and Prevention (CDC), April 13, 2021. Available online. URL: www.cdc.gov/std/treatment/duty-to-warn.htm. Accessed June 12, 2023.

laws have been shown to increase stigma, exacerbate disparities, and discourage HIV testing.

As of 2022, 35 states have laws that criminalize HIV exposure.

The Centers for Disease Control and Prevention (CDC) researched and analyzed the relevant laws for the 50 states, the District of Columbia, and Puerto Rico and then categorized them into four categories.

- HIV-specific laws that criminalize or control actions that can potentially expose another person to HIV
- sexually transmitted disease (STD), communicable, contagious, infectious disease (STD/communicable/ infectious disease) laws that criminalize or control actions that can potentially expose another person to STDs/communicable/infectious disease, which might include HIV
- sentence enhancement laws specific to HIV, or STDs, that do not criminalize a behavior but increase the sentence length when a person with HIV commits certain crimes
- no specific criminalization laws

General criminal statutes, such as reckless endangerment and attempted murder, can be used to criminalize actions that can potentially expose another to HIV and/or an STD. Many states have laws that fall into more than one of the categories listed above. For this analysis, only HIV-specific laws are captured for states with both HIV-specific laws and STD/communicable/infectious disease laws. Only HIV or STD/communicable/infectious disease laws are captured for states with both HIV and STD/communicable/infectious disease laws and sentence enhancement statutes.

The criminalization of potential HIV exposure is largely a matter of state law, with some federal legislation addressing criminalization in discrete areas, such as blood donation and prostitution (see Figure 27.1). These laws vary as to what actions are criminalized or result in additional penalties. Several states criminalize one or more actions that pose a low or negligible risk for HIV transmission.

Sexually Transmitted Diseases Reporting and Patient Confidentiality

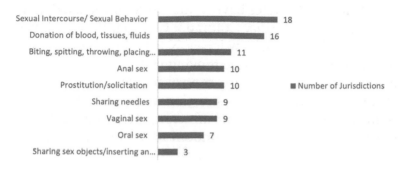

Figure 27.1. Criminalized or Controlled Actions in HIV/STD Criminalization Laws

Centers for Disease Control and Prevention (CDC)
In 35 states that criminalize HIV/STD exposure

In 10 states, laws require people with HIV who are aware of their status to disclose their status to sex partners, and three states require disclosure to needle-sharing partners.

The maximum sentence length for violating an HIV-specific statute is also a matter of state law. Some states have a maximum sentence length of up to life in prison, while others have maximum sentence lengths that are less than 10 years (see Figure 27.2). However, only 10 states have laws that account for HIV prevention measures, such as condom use, antiretroviral therapy (ART), and pre-exposure prophylaxis (PrEP) use.

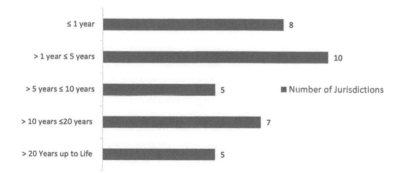

Figure 27.2. Maximum Sentence Length for HIV/STD Criminalization Laws

Centers for Disease Control and Prevention (CDC)
In 35 states, D.C., and Puerto Rico

Since 2014, at least 12 states have modernized or repealed their HIV criminal laws: California, Colorado, Georgia, Illinois, Iowa, Michigan, Missouri, Nevada, New Jersey, North Carolina, Virginia, and Washington. Changes include moving HIV prevention issues from the criminal code to disease control regulations, requiring intent to transmit, actual HIV transmission, or providing defenses for taking measures to prevent transmission, including viral suppression or being noninfectious, condom use, and partner PrEP use.[4]

---

[4] "HIV and STD Criminalization Laws," Centers for Disease Control and Prevention (CDC), March 13, 2023. Available online. URL: www.cdc.gov/hiv/policies/law/states/exposure.html. Accessed June 12, 2023.

Chapter 28 | Understanding Antibiotic Resistance and Sexually Transmitted Disease Treatment

Section 28.1 | About Antibiotic Resistance

Antimicrobial resistance happens when germs, such as bacteria and fungi, develop the ability to defeat the drugs designed to kill them. That means the germs are not killed and continue to grow. Resistant infections can be difficult, and sometimes impossible, to treat.

Antimicrobial resistance is an urgent global public health threat, killing at least 1.27 million people worldwide and associated with nearly 5 million deaths in 2019. In the United States, more than 2.8 million antimicrobial-resistant infections occur each year. More than 35,000 people die as a result, according to the 2019 Antibiotic Resistance (AR) Threats Report of the Centers for Disease Control and Prevention (CDC). When *Clostridioides difficile* —a bacterium that is not typically resistant but can cause deadly diarrhea and is associated with antimicrobial use—is added to these, the U.S. toll of all the threats in the report exceeds 3 million infections and 48,000 deaths.

Antimicrobial resistance has the potential to affect people at any stage of life, as well as the health-care, veterinary, and agriculture industries. This makes it one of the world's most urgent public health problems.

Bacteria and fungi do not have to be resistant to every antibiotic or antifungal to be dangerous. Resistance to even one antibiotic can mean serious problems. The following are a few examples:

- Antimicrobial-resistant infections that require the use of second- and third-line treatments can harm patients by causing serious side effects, such as organ failure, and prolong care and recovery, sometimes for months.
- Many medical advances are dependent on the ability to fight infections using antibiotics, including joint replacements, organ transplants, cancer therapy, and the treatment of chronic diseases such as diabetes, asthma, and rheumatoid arthritis (RA).
- In some cases, these infections have no treatment options.

If antibiotics and antifungals lose their effectiveness, then we lose the ability to treat infections and control these public health threats.

HOW ANTIMICROBIAL RESISTANCE HAPPENS

Antimicrobial resistance is a naturally occurring process. However, increases in antimicrobial resistance are driven by a combination of germs exposed to antibiotics and antifungals and the spread of those germs and their resistance mechanisms.

Definition of Germs and Antimicrobials

Antimicrobial resistance does not mean our body is resistant to antibiotics or antifungals. It means the bacteria or fungi causing the infection are resistant to the antibiotic or antifungal treatment.

Germs are microbes—very small living organisms that include bacteria, fungi, parasites, and viruses.

- Most germs are harmless and even helpful to people, but some can cause infections. Harmful germs are called "pathogens."
- The term "antimicrobials" is used to describe drugs that treat many types of infections by killing or slowing the growth of pathogens causing the infection.
- Bacteria cause infections such as strep throat, foodborne illnesses, and other serious infections. Antibiotics treat bacterial infections.
- Fungi cause infections such as athlete's foot, yeast infections, and other serious infections. Antifungals treat fungal infections.
- People sometimes use "antibiotic" and "antimicrobial" interchangeably.

How Antibiotic and Antifungal Use Affects Resistance

Antibiotics and antifungals save lives, but their use can contribute to the development of resistant germs. Antimicrobial resistance is accelerated when the presence of antibiotics and antifungals pressures bacteria and fungi to adapt.

Antibiotics and antifungals kill some germs that cause infections, but they also kill helpful germs that protect our body from infection. The antimicrobial-resistant germs survive and multiply. These surviving germs have resistance traits in their deoxyribonucleic acid (DNA) that can spread to other germs.

Spread of Germs and Resistance Mechanisms

To survive, germs can develop defense strategies against antibiotics and antifungals called "resistance mechanisms." DNA tells the germ how to make specific proteins, which determine the germ's resistance mechanisms. Bacteria and fungi can carry genes for many types of resistance.

When already hard-to-treat germs have the right combination of resistance mechanisms, it can make all antibiotics or antifungals ineffective, resulting in untreatable infections. Alarmingly, antimicrobial-resistant germs can share their resistance mechanisms with other germs that have not been exposed to antibiotics or antifungals. Table 28.1 gives a few examples of defense strategies used to resist the effects of antibiotics or antifungals.

Table 28.1. Defense Strategies Used to Resist the Effects of Antibiotics or Antifungals[1]

Resistance Mechanisms (Defense Strategies)	Description
Restrict access of the antibiotic	Germs restrict access by changing the entryways or limiting the number of entryways. **Example**: Gram-negative bacteria have an outer layer (membrane) that protects them from their environment. These bacteria can use this membrane to selectively keep antibiotic drugs from entering.

---

[1] "About Antimicrobial Resistance," Centers for Disease Control and Prevention (CDC), October 5, 2022. Available online. URL: www.cdc.gov/drugresistance/about.html. Accessed June 8, 2023.

Table 28.1. Contined

Resistance Mechanisms (Defense Strategies)	Description
Get rid of the antibiotic or antifungal	Germs get rid of antibiotics using pumps in their cell walls to remove antibiotic drugs that enter the cell. **Examples:** • Some *Pseudomonas aeruginosa* bacteria can produce pumps to get rid of several different important antibiotic drugs, including fluoroquinolones, beta-lactams, chloramphenicol, and trimethoprim. • Some *Candida* species produce pumps that get rid of azoles such as fluconazole.
Change or destroy the antibiotic	Germs change or destroy the antibiotics with enzymes, proteins that break down the drug. **Example:** *Klebsiella pneumoniae* bacteria produce enzymes called "carbapenemases," which break down carbapenem drugs and most other beta-lactam drugs.
Change the targets for the antibiotic or antifungal	Many antibiotic drugs are designed to single out and destroy specific parts (or targets) of a bacterium. Germs change the antibiotic's target so the drug can no longer fit and do its job. **Examples:** • *Escherichia coli* bacteria with the *mcr-1* gene can add a compound to the outside of the cell wall so that the drug colistin cannot latch onto it. • *Aspergillus fumigatus* changes the *cyp1A* gene so that triazoles cannot bind to the protein.
Bypass the effects of the antibiotic	Germs develop new cell processes that avoid using the antibiotic's target. **Example:** Some *Staphylococcus aureus* bacteria can bypass the drug effects of trimethoprim.

Section 28.2 | Antimicrobial-Resistant Gonorrhea: A Public Health Threat

WHAT IS GONORRHEA?

People who are sexually active can get gonorrhea, a common sexually transmitted infection (STI) that can affect the genitals, rectum, and throat. It can be treated and cured, but it is highly skilled at outsmarting the antibiotics used to treat it.

WHAT IS DRUG-RESISTANT GONORRHEA?

Drug resistance, also referred to as "antimicrobial resistance," happens when germs such as bacteria and fungi develop the ability to resist, and even defeat, the drugs designed to kill them. That means the germs are not killed and continue to grow. The bacterium that causes gonorrhea has grown resistant to nearly every drug ever used to treat it, and it is only a matter of time until it becomes resistant to the last available cure.

TALK WITH YOUR HEALTH-CARE PROVIDER AND PARTNER(S)

Honest and open conversations, both with your provider and sexual partner(s), are an important part of keeping yourself and your partner(s) safe from infection.[2]

ADDRESSING THE THREAT OF DRUG-RESISTANT GONORRHEA

Antibiotic resistance (AR) is threatening the effectiveness of gonorrhea treatment in the United States. Gonorrhea is one of the most common sexually transmitted diseases (STDs), with more than 1.14 million infections estimated to occur in the United States each year. Left untreated, it can cause serious health problems, particularly for women, including chronic pelvic pain, life-threatening ectopic pregnancy, and even infertility. And, while medication for

---

[2] "Drug-Resistant Gonorrhea: A Public Health Threat," Centers for Disease Control and Prevention (CDC), December 28, 2022. Available online. URL: www.cdc.gov/std/gonorrhea/drug-resistant/public-health-threat/public-health-threat-text-only.htm. Accessed June 8, 2023.

gonorrhea has been available for decades, the bacteria have grown resistant to nearly every drug ever used to treat them.

In response to the ongoing threat of drug resistance, the Centers for Disease Control and Prevention (CDC) has repeatedly revised its gonorrhea treatment guidelines to phase out the use of antibiotics that have become less effective in treating the infection. In the United States, only one recommended treatment option remains for treating gonorrhea—the antibiotic ceftriaxone.

The CDC encourages providers to adhere to the recommended treatment guidelines and urges researchers in the public and private sectors to step up efforts to develop new treatments for this common but potentially serious STD. It is also essential to maintain systems and services across the United States to prevent, diagnose, and treat gonorrhea. Effective diagnosis and treatment are essential to protect individual health and stop the spread of infection, including resistant strains.

GONORRHEA TREATMENT: A SHRINKING ARSENAL

Over the years, gonorrhea has developed resistance to nearly every drug ever used to treat it, including sulfonamides, penicillin, tetracycline, and fluoroquinolones. Due to widespread resistance to each of these antibiotics, by 2007, only cephalosporins—including the oral antibiotic cefixime and the injectable antibiotic ceftriaxone—were left to effectively treat gonorrhea.

The CDC's Gonococcal Isolate Surveillance Project (GISP) closely monitors for early warning signs of resistance to recommended treatments. In 2012, after evidence from the GISP suggested that resistance to cefixime was emerging, the CDC issued new guidelines recommending against its use. Evidence indicates that this change helped slow the emergence of cephalosporin resistance.

While evidence indicates that ceftriaxone continues to be effective for treating gonorrhea, new treatment options are urgently needed.

HISTORICAL TRENDS IN GONORRHEA DRUG RESISTANCE

- **1930s**. Sulfonamide antimicrobials are introduced to treat gonorrhea.

- **1940s.** Due to increasing resistance, sulfonamides are no longer recommended; penicillin has become the treatment of choice for gonorrhea.
- **1980s.** Penicillin and tetracycline are no longer recommended to treat gonorrhea.
- **1990s.** Fluoroquinolones become the predominant treatment for gonorrhea.
- **2007.** Fluoroquinolones are no longer recommended; cephalosporins (including injectable ceftriaxone and oral cefixime) become the backbone of treatment for gonorrhea.
- **2012.** Cefixime is no longer recommended as a first-line regimen for treating gonorrhea.
- **2015.** Ceftriaxone plus azithromycin is the recommended treatment for gonorrhea.
- **2020.** Dual therapy with azithromycin is no longer recommended; ceftriaxone is the only remaining highly effective antibiotic for treating gonorrhea.

MONITORING FOR DRUG RESISTANCE

Since 1986, the GISP has routinely monitored how *Neisseria gonorrhoeae*—the bacterium that causes gonorrhea—responds to antibiotics. The surveillance system annually collects approximately 5–6,000 *N. gonorrhoeae* samples from men with urethral gonorrhea at STD clinics in approximately 25–30 U.S. cities and measures the concentration of various antibiotics needed to stop the bacteria's growth in the laboratory. A "minimum inhibitory concentration" (MIC) is the lowest concentration of drug needed to stop the growth and is an indication of how susceptible the bacterium is to treatment with a given antibiotic. The higher the MIC, the greater the dose of antibiotics required for effective treatment. If MICs become too high, the antibiotic will not work at all.

From 2013 through 2018, the percentage of samples with elevated MICs of azithromycin increased by more than 600 percent (from 0.6% to 4%). Gonorrhea continues to demonstrate resistance to other antibiotics, such as penicillin (13.7% in 2018), tetracycline (25.6% in 2018), and ciprofloxacin (31.2% in 2018). Although increases are seen in other antibiotics, the percentage of samples with elevated MICs to ceftriaxone remains low at 0.2 percent in 2018, making it still an effective treatment option for gonorrhea.

While the currently recommended treatment continues to be effective, there have been reported cases outside the country that required increased drug dosing to cure. Increased action to monitor for and prevent increased resistance is essential.

SEXUALLY TRANSMITTED DISEASE TESTING AND TREATMENT SERVICES ARE VITAL FOR CONTAINING THE THREAT OF ANTIBIOTIC-RESISTANT GONORRHEA

Rates of gonorrhea and several other reportable STDs have been increasing nationwide for years. STD prevention services play a vital role in keeping antibiotic-resistant gonorrhea and other STDs from flourishing in the community by providing critical testing and treatment options. With an estimated more than 20 million new STIs occurring each year, public health agencies cannot provide services to all those who need them.

The public health and health-care systems must work together. The CDC is taking action by collaborating with state and local health departments to extend the reach of existing STD prevention services by providing testing services, medications, and other resources to STD clinics and health departments, improving STD surveillance and electronic health records management, and training disease intervention specialists (DIS) for outbreak response.

IMPROVED SURVEILLANCE AND ACCELERATED DRUG DEVELOPMENT URGENTLY NEEDED

As part of the federal government's broader Combating Antibiotic Resistant Bacteria (CARB) Action Plan, the CDC specifically addresses the threat of antibiotic-resistant gonorrhea by strengthening the timeliness of surveillance systems, working with state and local health departments to enhance their capacity to monitor and test for resistant gonorrhea infections and developing rapid response strategies to effectively contain the spread of resistant gonorrhea, in the event that resistance is detected.

Action from health-care providers, state and local health departments, and public and private partners is urgently needed to prevent untreatable gonorrhea from becoming a reality:

- **Health-care providers**. Physicians and other health-care providers are on the front line in the fight against gonorrhea and play a critical role in our response. The CDC encourages all providers to:
  - take a sexual history (This will help you know which STDs to test your patient for and at which anatomic sites.)
  - adhere to the CDC's recommendations by always treating gonorrhea promptly with injectable ceftriaxone, including posttreatment testing to confirm cure when recommended (www.cdc.gov/std/treatment)
  - follow key CDC screening recommendations, including the following:
    - Screen all sexually active women younger than 25 years, as well as older women with risk factors such as new or multiple sex partners or a sex partner who has an STI.
    - Screen sexually active men who have sex with men (MSM) at anatomic sites of possible exposure at least annually.
  - evaluate and treat all sex partners from the previous 60 days of the patient
  - obtain cultures to test for decreased susceptibility from any patients with suspected or documented gonorrhea treatment failures
  - report any suspected treatment failure to local or state public health officials within 24 hours, helping to ensure that any potential resistance is recognized early
- **Health departments and laboratories**. State and local health departments and other laboratories should enhance or rebuild gonorrhea culture capacity so that AR testing can be performed to ensure resistant infections are quickly detected and reported. If AR

testing cannot be performed locally, facilities should identify and partner with other labs that can perform such testing. Health departments should notify the CDC of treatment failures immediately. Laboratories should also inform local or state public health officials of any isolates with decreased susceptibility to cephalosporins.

- **Researchers and drug developers**. The CDC urges scientists and private sector drug developers to prioritize the identification and study of effective new antibiotic treatments for gonorrhea. With few new drugs in the pipeline, it is important to accelerate research on new drugs or drug combinations now, as it takes years to bring new drugs to market.[3]

Section 28.3 | Can Prophylactic Antibiotics Prevent Sexually Transmitted Diseases?

ANTIBIOTICS CAN HELP PREVENT COMMON SEXUALLY TRANSMITTED INFECTIONS

Sexually transmitted infections (STIs), such as chlamydia, syphilis, and gonorrhea, have been on the rise nationwide. They disproportionally affect men who have sex with men (MSM) and transgender women. Left untreated, they can lead to serious health issues, such as blindness, brain and nerve problems, and infertility in women. Condoms can block many STIs. But condoms are not always used consistently or correctly. So researchers have been exploring other options for preventing STIs, especially among those at elevated risk for repeated infections.

Previous studies found evidence that the antibiotic doxycycline, taken shortly after sex, might reduce the risk of bacterial STIs

---

[3] "Addressing the Threat of Drug-Resistant Gonorrhea," Centers for Disease Control and Prevention (CDC), December 2020. Available online. URL: www.cdc.gov/nchhstp/newsroom/docs/factsheets/drug-resistant-gonorrhea.pdf. Accessed June 8, 2023.

among MSM. This approach is called "doxycycline post-exposure prophylaxis" (doxy-PEP). But some experts have been concerned that the preventive use of antibiotics could lead to antibiotic resistance. This might reduce future options for treating STIs and other bacterial infections.

To learn more, a team led by scientists at the University of California, San Francisco (UCSF), and the University of Washington, Seattle, set out to measure the safety and effectiveness of doxy-PEP. They also looked for evidence of antibiotic resistance. Results were published in the *New England Journal of Medicine* on April 6, 2023.

The study enrolled 501 adults considered at high risk of bacterial STIs, either MSM or transgender women. All had been diagnosed with a bacterial STI in the past year and reported having sex without using a condom in the past year. They were either living with human immunodeficiency virus (HIV) or taking or planning to take medication to prevent HIV infection.

Participants were randomly assigned to receive either doxy-PEP or standard care. Those in the doxy-PEP group were told to take 200 mg of doxycycline tablet as soon as possible, within 72 hours after condomless sex. Participants were tested for STIs every three months and followed for one year.

The researchers found that the doxy-PEP group had a two-thirds lower incidence of syphilis, gonorrhea, and chlamydia compared to the standard care group during each three-month time period. STIs were detected in about 10 percent of the quarterly tests administered to those in the doxy-PEP group, compared to about 30 percent of those in the standard care group.

Gonorrhea was the most often diagnosed STI. The incidence of gonorrhea per quarter in the doxy-PEP group was about 55 percent lower than in the standard care group. Chlamydia and syphilis were each reduced by more than 80 percent per quarter.

The researchers found that the doxy-PEP group had a modestly higher proportion of doxycycline-resistant *Staphylococcus aureus* living in the nose after 12 months. And the incidence of gonorrhea strains resistant to the antibiotic tetracycline, which is in the same antibiotic class as doxycycline, was 38.5 percent in the doxy-PEP group compared to 12.5 percent in the standard care group. This finding suggests doxy-PEP could be less effective in preventing gonorrhea with existing tetracycline resistance; however, the number of available gonorrhea cultures was low.

"It will be important to monitor the impact of doxy-PEP on antimicrobial resistance patterns over time, and weigh this against the demonstrated benefit of reduced STIs and associated decreased antibiotic use for STI treatment in men at elevated risk for recurrent STIs," says Dr. Annie Luetkemeyer of the UCSF, a coleader of the study. "Given its demonstrated efficacy in several trials, doxy-PEP should be considered as part of a sexual health package for MSM and transwomen if they have an increased risk of STIs."[4]

---

[4] News and Events, "Antibiotic Can Help Prevent Common Sexually Transmitted Infections," National Institutes of Health (NIH), April 25, 2023. Available online. URL: www.nih.gov/news-events/nih-research-matters/antibiotic-can-help-prevent-common-sexually-transmitted-infections. Accessed June 8, 2023.

Chapter 29 | Expedited Partner Therapy, an Important Intervention for Disease Control

Chapter Contents

WHAT ARE PARTNER SERVICES?

Partner services provide an array of free services to people diagnosed with human immunodeficiency virus (HIV) or other sexually transmitted diseases (STDs, such as syphilis, gonorrhea, and chlamydia) and their partners. Partner services are functions of local and state health department staff who help identify and locate sexual or drug injection partners to inform them of their risk for HIV and to provide them with testing, counseling, and referrals for other services.

- For those who test negative, partner services can provide them with information on various HIV prevention methods, including pre-exposure prophylaxis (PrEP), condoms, and other sexual and drug-use prevention options.
  - For partners at risk of HIV, consider PrEP. When taken as prescribed, PrEP is highly effective for preventing HIV from sex or injection drug use.
  - Additionally, access to other services, such as risk counseling, may lead to reductions in high-risk sexual and drug-use behaviors.
- For partners who test positive, partner services can provide linkage to treatment and care, risk-reduction counseling, and other services.

HEALTH-CARE PROVIDER ROLE IN INITIATING PARTNER SERVICES

While you are not expected to take on the role of partner notification yourself, it is very helpful for you to educate your patients about partner services and its importance in preventing HIV transmission.

For Patients Being Tested for Human Immunodeficiency Virus/Sexually Transmitted Diseases

- Talk with your patients about partner services and let them know that if they test positive for a reportable disease, they may be contacted by someone from the health department.

- Discuss how partner services can help your patients and their sexual or drug injection partners through early access to testing, treatment, and other services.
- Emphasize the importance of participating in the partner services process as a way to help stop the transmission of HIV/STDs.
- Conduct brief discussions with your patients on how to reduce high-risk sexual and drug-use behaviors.

For People Newly Diagnosed with Human Immunodeficiency Virus

If you are seeing a patient for the first time, speak with them about partner services to determine if partner notification was previously addressed.

FOR PATIENTS WITH HUMAN IMMUNODEFICIENCY VIRUS

- If your patient with HIV presents with an STD, make them aware that they may be contacted by someone from the health department.
- If your patient with HIV informs you of high-risk behavior (e.g., sex without condoms when not virally suppressed or needle sharing during injection drug use), discuss the importance of taking HIV medicine, or antiretroviral therapy, to treat HIV.
  - Viral suppression, or having an undetectable viral load, is the best thing people with HIV can do to stay healthy. Another benefit of reducing the amount of virus in the body is that it helps prevent transmission to others through sex or sharing drug injection equipment and from the mother to the child during pregnancy, birth, and breastfeeding. In fact, a person with HIV who takes HIV medicine as prescribed and gets and stays virally suppressed or undetectable has effectively no risk of sexually transmitting HIV to their HIV-negative partners.

- Refer any of your patients with HIV who present with an STD or need help notifying partners potentially at risk to partner services.

METHODS USED BY HEALTH DEPARTMENTS TO INFORM PARTNERS

Notifying sexual or drug injection partners that they may have been exposed to an infectious disease is formally known as "partner notification." Health departments use one of the following three methods in this process:

- The health department tells the patient's partners ("provider referral"):
  - The patient provides partner contact information to the health department.
  - Partners are located by health department staff and made aware of their potential exposure.
  - Partners are provided, or referred for, counseling, testing, treatment, and other services by the health department.
- The patient tells partners ("self-referral"):
  - The patient takes on the responsibility of letting sexual or drug injection partners know that they have possibly been exposed.
  - The patient provides partners with information about local services, including counseling and testing.
- Both the patient and the health department tell partners ("dual referral"):
  - The patient, with assistance from health department staff, lets partners know of their potential exposure.
  - Health department staff are there to help the patient during the process and provide partners with information and access to counseling, testing, and other resources.

Patients with Human Immunodeficiency Virus Who Present with Gonorrhea or Chlamydia

Due to resource limitations, health departments do not always follow up on cases of gonorrhea or chlamydia. However, if a patient diagnosed with HIV presents with either of these STDs, it is important that you alert health departments of this coinfection with HIV to ensure appropriate follow-up with potentially exposed partners. Certain STDs can increase HIV viral load and genital HIV shedding, which may increase the risk of sexual and perinatal HIV transmission.

FACTS ABOUT PARTNER SERVICES

More than 1 million people in the United States have HIV, and many are unaware of their status. About 40 percent of new HIV infections are transmitted by people undiagnosed and unaware they have HIV.

- The recommendations of the Centers for Disease Control and Prevention (CDC) for partner services for patients diagnosed with HIV and other STDs have created a renewed focus on this public health priority.

Reportable Diseases and Your Patient

Health-care providers and clinical laboratories are required by law to report certain types of infections to their local or state health departments. If your patient tests positive for one of these infections, they will likely be contacted by someone from the health department. Therefore, it is important to let patients know that the health department may contact them if they test positive for one of the reportable infections and that this is a normal procedure.

The list of reportable infections varies from state to state, but it typically includes HIV, syphilis, gonorrhea, and chlamydia. Other infections may also be reportable, and it is important for you as a health-care provider to know which ones are reportable in your area.

GOALS OF PARTNER SERVICES

The goals of partner services include the following:

- providing services to people diagnosed with HIV or other STDs, including risk-reduction counseling and referrals for medical care and other services (e.g., psychosocial support and prevention interventions)

- ensuring that sexual and drug injection partners of people diagnosed with HIV or other STDs are notified of their potential exposure, provided with counseling and testing, treated or linked to medical care if needed, and provided with other appropriate referrals
- reducing future rates of transmission by facilitating early diagnosis

HOW PARTNER SERVICES PROGRAMS HELP YOU

Partner services programs are not intended to have you, the health-care provider, take on more responsibility. In fact, they are designed to ease your workload by offering another free resource to help your patients notify their sexual or drug injection partners of their possible exposure to an infectious disease.

Partner services also do the following:

- Present an opportunity for you to identify behaviors that increase your patient's risk of transmitting HIV or another STD and help you initiate discussions with patients about how to reduce those behaviors.
- Leverage your relationships with patients and maximize the trust they have in you to help prevent the transmission of HIV and other STDs.

HOW PARTNER SERVICES PROGRAMS HELP YOUR PATIENTS

- Ensure that trained professionals contact your patients and inform their partners of their possible exposure without using your patients' names, removing the burden of disclosure from your patients.
- For patients who choose self-referral, ensure that adequate time is spent coaching your patients on how to inform their partners about their potential exposure.
- Increase your patients' knowledge about how to protect themselves and maintain their own health.
- Present another free resource for your patients to access education and counseling about how to live well with HIV.
- Help partners get tested quickly and facilitate timely treatment or linkage to care.

RESOURCES FOR PARTNER SERVICES

- To obtain additional free partner services materials for health-care providers or patients, go to cdc.gov/hiv/clinicians/screening/partnernotification-services.html or call 800-CDC-INFO (800-232-4636).
- For more information about HIV screening, prevention, treatment, and care, visit cdc.gov/HIVNexus.
- Visit the American Academy of HIV Medicine's website (aahivm.org) for health-care provider resources, such as the robust Referral Link database.[1]

Section 29.2 | What Is Expedited Partner Therapy?

Expedited partner therapy (EPT) is the clinical practice of treating the sex partners of patients diagnosed with chlamydia or gonorrhea by providing prescriptions or medications to the patient to take to his/her partner without the health-care provider first examining the partner.

Effective clinical management of patients with treatable sexually transmitted diseases (STDs) requires treatment of the patients' current sex partners to prevent reinfection and curtail further transmission. The standard approach to partner treatment has included clinical evaluation in a health-care setting, with partner notification accomplished by the index patient, by the provider or an agent of the provider, or a combination of these methods. Provider-assisted referral is considered the optimal strategy for partner treatment but is not available to most patients with gonorrhea or chlamydial infection because of resource limitations. The usual alternative is to advise patients to refer their partners for treatment.

The Centers for Disease Control and Prevention (CDC) has concluded that EPT is a useful option to facilitate partner management, particularly for the treatment of male partners of women with chlamydial infection or gonorrhea. Although ongoing evaluation

---

[1] "Partner Services for HIV and STDs," Centers for Disease Control and Prevention (CDC), March 2021. Available online. URL: www.cdc.gov/stophivtogether/library/topics/treatment/brochures/cdc-hiv-lsht-treatment-brochure-partner-services-provider.pdf. Accessed June 8, 2023.

will be needed to define when and how EPT can be best utilized, the evidence indicates that EPT should be available to clinicians as an option for partner treatment. EPT represents an additional strategy for partner management that does not replace other strategies, such as provider-assisted referral, when available.[2]

EVIDENCE SUPPORTING EXPEDITED PARTNER THERAPY FOR CHLAMYDIA AND GONORRHEA

Expedited partner therapy is a harm-reduction strategy and the clinical practice of treating the sex partners of persons with diagnosed chlamydia or gonorrhea, who are unable or unlikely to seek timely treatment, by providing medications or prescriptions to the patient as allowable by law. Patients then provide partners with these therapies without the health-care provider having examined the partner (www.cdc.gov/std/ept). Unless prohibited by law or other regulations, medical providers should routinely offer EPT to patients with chlamydia when the provider cannot ensure that all of a patient's sex partners from the previous 60 days will seek timely treatment. If the patient has not had sex during the 60 days before diagnosis, providers should offer EPT for the patient's most recent sex partner. Because EPT must be an oral regimen and current gonorrhea treatment involves an injection, EPT for gonorrhea should be offered to partners unlikely to access timely evaluation after linkage is explored. EPT is legal in the majority of states but varies by chlamydial or gonococcal infection. Providers should visit www.cdc.gov/std/ept to obtain updated information for their state. Providing patients with packaged oral medication is the preferred approach because the efficacy of EPT using prescriptions has not been evaluated, obstacles to EPT can exist at the pharmacy level, and many persons (especially adolescents) do not fill the prescriptions provided to them by a sex partner. Medication or prescriptions provided for EPT should be accompanied by educational materials for the partner, including treatment instructions, warnings about taking medications (e.g., if the partner is pregnant or has an allergy to the medication), general health counseling,

---

[2] "Expedited Partner Therapy," Centers for Disease Control and Prevention (CDC), April 19, 2021. Available online. URL: www.cdc.gov/std/ept/default.htm. Accessed June 8, 2023.

and a statement advising that partners seek medical evaluation as soon as possible for HIV infection and any symptoms of STIs, particularly pelvic inflammatory disease (PID).

Evidence supporting EPT is based on three U.S. clinical trials involving heterosexual men and women with chlamydia or gonorrhea. All three trials reported that more partners were treated when patients were offered EPT. Two reported statistically significant decreases in the rate of reinfection, and one observed a lower risk for persistent or recurrent infection that was statistically nonsignificant. A fourth trial in the United Kingdom did not demonstrate a difference in the risk of reinfection or in the number of partners treated between persons offered EPT and those advised to notify their sex partners. U.S. trials and a meta-analysis of EPT revealed that the magnitude of reduction in reinfection of index patients, compared with patient referral, differed according to the STI and the sex of the index patient. However, across trials, reductions in chlamydia prevalence at follow-up were approximately 20 percent, and reductions in gonorrhea were approximately 50 percent at follow-up.

DATA ON USE OF EXPEDITED PARTNER THERAPY FOR SEXUALLY TRANSMITTED INFECTIONS AMONG MEN WHO HAVE SEX WITH MEN

Existing data indicate that EPT might also have a role in partner management for trichomoniasis; however, no partner management intervention has been reported to be more effective than any other in reducing trichomoniasis reinfection rates. No data support use of EPT in the routine management of patients with syphilis.

Data are limited regarding the use of EPT for gonococcal or chlamydial infections among men who have sex with men (MSM), compared with heterosexuals. Published studies, including recent data regarding extragenital testing, indicated that male partners of MSM with diagnosed gonorrhea or chlamydia might have other bacterial STIs (gonorrhea or syphilis) or HIV. Studies have reported that 5 percent of MSM have a new diagnosis of HIV when evaluated as partners of men with gonococcal or chlamydial infections; however, more recent data indicate that in certain settings, the frequency of HIV infection is much lower. Considering limited data and the potential for other bacterial STIs among MSM partners, shared clinical decision-making regarding EPT is recommended.

Expedited Partner Therapy, an Important Intervention for Disease Control

All persons who receive bacterial STI diagnoses and their sex partners, particularly MSM, should be tested for HIV, and those at risk for HIV infection should be offered HIV PrEP (www.cdc.gov/hiv/pdf/risk/prep/cdc-hiv-prep-guidelines-2017.pdf).[3]

Section 29.3 | Legal Status of Expedited Partner Therapy

Assuring treatment of the sex partners of persons with sexually transmitted diseases (STDs) has been a central component of the prevention and control of bacterial STDs in the United States for decades. Traditional practices to inform, evaluate, and treat sex partners of persons infected with STDs have relied upon patients or health-care providers to notify partners of infected persons of their exposure to an STD. Initially developed to help control syphilis, partner management became widely recommended for gonorrhea, chlamydial, and, most recently, human immunodeficiency virus (HIV) infection. However, for STDs other than syphilis, partner management based on provider referral is rarely assured, while patient referral has had only modest success in assuring partner treatment.

An alternative approach to assuring the treatment of partners is expedited partner therapy (EPT). EPT is the delivery of medications or prescriptions by persons infected with an STD to their sex partners without clinical assessment of the partners. Clinicians (e.g., physicians, nurse practitioners, physician assistants, pharmacists, and public health workers) provide patients with sufficient medications directly or via prescription for the patients and their partners. After evaluating multiple studies involving EPT, the Centers for Disease Control and Prevention (CDC) concluded that EPT is a "useful option" to further partner treatment, particularly for male partners of women with chlamydia or gonorrhea. In August 2006, the CDC recommended the practice of EPT for certain populations and specific conditions, and the CDC continues to recommend it in Sexually Transmitted Diseases Treatment Guidelines, 2010.

---

[3] "Expedited Partner Therapy," Centers for Disease Control and Prevention (CDC), July 22, 2021. Available online. URL: www.cdc.gov/std/treatment-guidelines/clinical-EPT.htm. Accessed June 8, 2023.

Throughout discussions of EPT, the legal status of the practice remained an area of uncertainty. To assist state and local STD programs in their efforts to implement EPT as an additional partner services tool, the CDC collaborated with the Center for Law and the Public's Health at Georgetown and Johns Hopkins Universities to assess the legal framework concerning EPT across all 50 states and other jurisdictions (the District of Columbia and Puerto Rico; Figure 29.1). The primary research objective was to conceptualize, frame, and identify legal provisions that implicate a clinician's ability to provide a prescription for a patient's sex partner, without prior evaluation of that partner, for purposes of treating an STD (specifically chlamydia or gonorrhea).

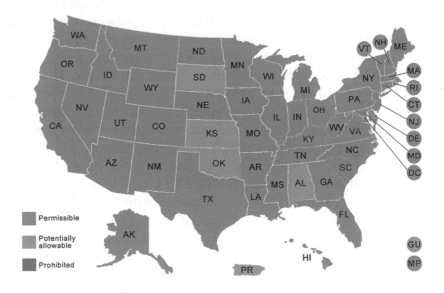

Figure 29.1. Legal Status of Expedited Partner Therapy in the United States

Centers for Disease Control and Prevention (CDC)

LIMITATIONS

The information presented here is not legal advice, nor is it a comprehensive analysis of all the legal provisions that could implicate the legality of EPT in a given jurisdiction. Rather, it provides a comparative snapshot of legal provisions that may highlight legislative, regulatory, and judicial laws and policies concerning EPT based on currently available information. This snapshot is subject to change. Measuring the legal weight of nonbinding legal sources, such as policy guidance documents or administrative decisions, must be done locally within the context of applicable statutes and regulations. The data and assessment are intended to be used as a tool to assist state and local health departments as they determine locally appropriate ways to control STDs. The data and assessment are not intended to be used for research purposes; dates are provided for the most recent legal change regardless of whether it resulted in a changed status. Assessment of local statutes was not undertaken, with the exception of the District of Columbia. Assessment of tribal laws for sovereign nations was also not undertaken.[4]

---

[4] "Legal Status of Expedited Partner Therapy (EPT)," Centers for Disease Control and Prevention (CDC), April 19, 2021. Available online. URL: www.cdc.gov/std/ept/legal/default.htm. Accessed June 8, 2023.

Chapter 30 |
Complementary and Alternative Therapies for Sexually Transmitted Diseases

Many people use complementary and integrative therapies and activities in addition to traditional medical care. With most complementary therapies, your health is looked at from a holistic (or "whole picture") point of view. Think of your body as working as one big system. From a holistic viewpoint, everything you do, from what you eat to what you drink to how stressed you are, affects your health and well-being.

DO THESE THERAPIES WORK?
Healthy people use these kinds of therapies to try to make their immune systems stronger and to make themselves feel better in general. People who have diseases or illnesses, such as human immunodeficiency virus (HIV), use these therapies for the same reasons. They can also use these therapies to help deal with symptoms of the disease or side effects from the medicines that treat the disease.

If you want to try complementary treatments to help you cope with HIV, remember the following things:

- Always talk to your health-care provider before you start any kind of treatment, even if you think it is safe.
- Just because something is "natural" (e.g., a herb) does not mean that it is safe to take. Sometimes, these products can interact with your HIV medications or cause side effects on their own. St. John's wort, for example, decreases levels of some HIV medications in your blood.
- The federal government does not require that herbal remedies and dietary supplements be tested in the same way that standard medicines are tested before they are sold. Many of the treatments out there have not been studied as much as the HIV drugs you are taking. It is always a risk to take something or try something that has not been fully studied or researched.
- Be careful of treatments that claim to be "miracle cures"—ones that claim to cure HIV/acquired immunodeficiency syndrome (AIDS). There are people out there who may try to trick you into buying an expensive product that does not work. Always do your research and ask your provider for help.
- Complementary therapies are not substitutes for the treatment and medicines you receive from your provider. Never stop taking your HIV medications just because you have started a complementary therapy.
- The federal government is funding studies of how well some complementary therapies work to treat disease, so look for news about these studies.[1]

COMPLEMENTARY AND INTEGRATED MEDICINE FOR HEPATITIS C

The use of complementary and alternative medicine (CAM) is widespread, with approximately 40 percent of Americans using

---

[1] "Complementary and Integrative Therapies for HIV," U.S. Department of Veterans Affairs (VA), February 24, 2022. Available online. URL: www.hiv.va.gov/patient/daily/alternative-therapies/index.asp. Accessed June 9, 2023.

some form of this therapy. Although most utilize this therapy as a supplement to conventional medicine, some have substituted alternative treatments for scientifically accepted treatment modalities. Some of the reasons why patients are turning to alternative therapies may include:

- a perception that traditional therapies are not successful
- a desire to have more autonomy in choosing their treatments
- a perception that alternative therapies are safer or more natural
- a concern over the cost and side effects of conventional medicine
- a sense that they will be able to spend more time with practitioners than in a conventional medical setting

Many clinicians have limited knowledge or understanding of the possible benefits and risks of alternative therapies. The primary criticism of alternative therapies is that claims of efficacy are often based solely on anecdotal or personal experience. In addition, there is a lack of standardization in the preparation and formulation of these products whose use is not regulated by the U.S. Food and Drug Administration (FDA). Many patients with hepatitis C virus (HCV) infection are turning to alternative approaches for treatment and management of their infection. In particular, the use of herbs has become increasingly popular in patients who are nonresponders to conventional HCV treatments. The following is a discussion of alternative treatments used by patients with chronic hepatitis C, including four of the most popular herbs that patients are taking for chronic HCV infection.

Note: The following four alternative therapies described were selected because they are cited the most in the literature on alternative treatments for hepatitis C. By no means should they be advocated for use until randomized, double-blinded, and placebo-controlled studies with large numbers of patients are completed. Until these therapies are better evaluated, there is always the potential for harmful effects and drug interactions.

Acupuncture

Acupuncture is the art and science of manipulating the flow of qi and other essential substances through the organ channels of the body. Approximately 1 million Americans utilize acupuncture annually, primarily for the relief of chronic pain. One popular theory explaining how acupuncture modulates pain is the neurohumoral hypothesis, which states that the pain-relieving properties of acupuncture are, in part, mediated by a cascade of endorphins and monoamines that are activated by stimulating "De qi," a sensation of numbness and fullness. "De qi" is associated with the stimulation of A-delta afferents, which set the cascade in motion. Acupuncture has been tried in the treatment of pain associated with chronic pancreatitis. Yet no studies addressing acupuncture in the treatment of pain associated with cirrhosis or fibrosis from chronic hepatitis C have been published to date. Ironically, the potential for acupuncture to transmit hepatitis C infection is well recognized. As such, providers should caution patients about this mode of treatment.

Yoga

Yoga advocates controlled breathing, concentration of mind, mastery over senses, and intense meditation. In addition, certain postures or exercises for psychosomatic harmony are involved. Although yoga has been recommended by clinicians for those with chronic hepatitis C, no studies to date have been published demonstrating any effect of yoga on HCV ribonucleic acid (RNA) levels. Consequently, yoga cannot be recommended as a conclusive treatment for chronic hepatitis C.

Qigong

Qigong is the traditional Chinese discipline that focuses on breathing and movement of qi to increase physical harmony and strength and establish spiritual and emotional peace. Some studies indicate that patients with symptoms or complications associated with HCV, such as excessive fatigue, portal hypertension, cirrhosis, or fluid retention, should avoid stressful activities. The energy-conserving, qi-channeling practice of qigong is perfectly designed to keep an individual in shape without causing stress and exhaustion. However, again no studies to date have been published demonstrating an effect of qigong on HCV RNA levels.

Milk Thistle (Silymarin)

This herbal compound, extracted with 95 percent ethanol, is prepared from the leaves of the plant *Silybum marianum*, a member of the aster family, which encompasses daisies, thistles, and artichokes. The name "milk thistle" derives from its characteristic spiked leaves with white veins.

Milk thistle has three active flavonoid components: silybin, silydianin, and silychristin. Silybin has the greatest degree of biologic activity, and standard silymarin extracts contain 70 percent silybin.

PUTATIVE HEPATOPROTECTIVE PROPERTIES

- It acts as an antioxidant and scavenges free radicals (superoxide anion radical and nitric oxide) produced by activated Kupffer cells to protect against genomic injury—in vitro concentrations were quite high (higher than the dose given therapeutically).
- It inhibits lipid peroxidation and stabilizes the phospholipid composition of the hepatocyte plasma membrane.
- It protects against glutathione depletion.
- It selectively inhibits leukotriene formation and inhibits the 5-lipooxygenase pathway at in vivo doses to protect against genomic injury.
- It has anti-inflammatory effects and stabilizes mast cells and inhibits neutrophil migration.

Stronger Neo-Minophagen C

The usual formulation contains 200 mg of glycyrrhizin (a major component of the licorice root), 100 mg of cysteine, and 2,000 mg of glycine in 100 cc of saline. Most studies have used daily intravenous injections of stronger neo-minophagen C (SNMC); however, more recent studies suggest that an oral form may have equivalent efficacy.

The reported beneficial effects of glycyrrhizin on liver tissue include:

- stabilization of hepatic cellular membranes
- inhibition of the production of prostaglandin E2 (PGE2)
- augmentation of the effects of interferon

Cathy Herbal Tablet

Cathy herbal tablet (CH100) is a compound that contains 19 different Chinese herbs used to treat chronic liver disease. This compound's mechanism of action is unknown.

Thymus Extracts

Oral thymus preparations include components such as bovine thymopoietin and thymic humoral factor. The supposed immunological properties of thymus extracts include the following:

- stimulation of interferon production
- enhancement of T-cell-dependent antibody production
- enhancement of helper T-cell activity
- increased production of suppressor cells and natural killer cell activity

CONCLUSION

- All studies to date have been hampered by the small sample size, the different forms of thymus extract used (oral versus parenteral), and the different doses and regimens.
- If a standardized formulation of thymus extract is developed and shown to have some effect in chronic hepatitis C, either by itself or in combination with interferon, further investigation with large controlled trials would be warranted.[2]

---

[2] "Complementary and Integrated Medicine for Hepatitis C," U.S. Department of Veterans Affairs (VA), October 23, 2018. Available online. URL: www.hepatitis.va.gov/hcv/treatment/alternative-therapies.asp. Accessed June 9, 2023.

Chapter 31 | **Health Insurance Coverage**

SEXUALLY TRANSMITTED INFECTION SCREENINGS AND COUNSELING

Medicare Part B (Medical Insurance) covers sexually transmitted infection (STI) screenings for chlamydia, gonorrhea, syphilis, and/or hepatitis B if you are pregnant or at increased risk for an STI.

Medicare also covers up to two face-to-face, high-intensity behavioral counseling sessions if you are a sexually active adult at increased risk for these infections. Each session can be 20–30 minutes long.

Medicare covers STI screenings once every 12 months or at certain times during pregnancy. Medicare covers up to two behavioral counseling sessions each year.

Your Costs in Original Medicare

You pay nothing for the screenings and counseling if your primary care doctor or other health-care provider accepts assignment.

Note: Your doctor or other health-care provider may recommend you get services more often than Medicare covers. Or they may recommend services that Medicare does not cover. If this happens, you may have to pay some or all of the costs. Ask questions, so you understand why your doctor is recommending certain services and if, or how much, Medicare will pay for them.

Things to Know

Your primary care provider must order the screening or refer you for behavioral counseling. Medicare will only cover counseling

415

sessions with a Medicare-eligible primary care provider in a primary care setting (such as a doctor's office). Medicare would not cover counseling as a preventive service in an inpatient setting (such as a skilled nursing facility).[1]

HUMAN IMMUNODEFICIENCY VIRUS SCREENINGS
Medicare Part B (Medical Insurance) covers a human immunodeficiency virus (HIV) screening once per year if you meet one of the following conditions:
- You are aged 15–65.
- You are younger than 15 or older than 65 and are at an increased risk for HIV.

If you are pregnant, you can get the screening up to three times during your pregnancy.

Your Costs in Original Medicare
You pay nothing for the test if your doctor or other health-care provider accepts assignment.[2]

SEXUALLY TRANSMITTED DISEASE PREVENTIVE SERVICES COVERAGE
Provisions and Application to Plan Types
NON-GRANDFATHERED PRIVATE HEALTH INSURANCE PLANS
Section 2713 of the Public Health Service (PHS) Act, as added by the Affordable Care Act (ACA) and incorporated into the Employee Retirement Income Security Act of 1974 (ERISA) and the Code, requires that non-grandfathered group health plans and health insurance issuers offering non-grandfathered group or individual health insurance coverage provide coverage of certain specified

---

[1] "Sexually Transmitted Infection Screenings & Counseling," Centers for Medicare & Medicaid Services (CMS), January 21, 2021. Available online. URL: www.medicare.gov/coverage/sexually-transmitted-infection-screenings-counseling. Accessed June 9, 2023.
[2] "HIV Screenings," Centers for Medicare & Medicaid Services (CMS), February 21, 2013. Available online. URL: www.medicare.gov/coverage/hiv-screenings. Accessed June 9, 2023.

preventive services without cost-sharing. These preventive services include:

- evidence-based items or services that have an "A" or "B" recommendation rating from the United States Preventive Services Task Force (USPSTF)
- immunizations recommended for routine use in children, adolescents, and adults by the Advisory Committee on Immunization Practices (ACIP)
- evidence-informed recommendations to improve the health and well-being of infants, children, and adolescents that are included in the Bright Futures Project of the Health Resources and Services Administration (HRSA)
- recommended services included in the HRSA-supported Women's Preventive Services Guidelines, including all contraceptives approved by the U.S. Food and Drug Administration (FDA), sterilization procedures, and patient education and counseling for women with reproductive capacity, as prescribed by a health-care provider

MEDICARE

Under the ACA, USPSTF services with a Grade "A" or "B" must be covered without cost-sharing if the secretary determines they are reasonable and necessary for the prevention or early detection of an illness or disability appropriate for individuals entitled to benefits under part A or enrolled under part B preventive care recommendations.

MEDICAID EXPANSION PLANS

Medicaid expansion plans offered by states that extend Medicaid eligibility to nonelderly individuals with annual incomes at or below 133 percent of the federal poverty level ($16,611 for an individual or $34,247 for a family of four in 2019) are required to cover the full range of preventive services required in the essential health benefits (EHB) final rule. This encompasses coverage without cost sharing for all services outlined in Section 2713 of the PHS Act.

TRADITIONAL MEDICAID PLANS

Section 4106 provides that states who elect to cover all USPSTF Grade "A" or "B" recommended preventive services, as well as ACIP-recommended vaccines and their administration, without cost-sharing shall receive a one-percentage-point increase in the federal medical assistance percentage (FMAP) for those services.

In addition to these services, private and public plans may cover other preventive services without cost-sharing.

Chlamydia Testing

Preventive services coverage for chlamydia testing is shown in Table 31.1.

Table 31.1. Preventive Services Coverage for Chlamydia Testing

Recommending Authority	Eligible Populations and Service Specifics	Plans That Cover without Cost-Sharing
USPSTF (Grade "B"; September 2014)	Screen the following groups for chlamydia: • sexually active women (including pregnant women) aged 24 and younger • sexually active older women (including pregnant women) who are at increased risk for chlamydia infection	• non-grandfathered private health insurance plans • Medicare • Medicaid expansion plans • traditional Medicaid plans*
Bright Futures/AAP recommendations for pediatric preventive health care (March 2020)	Screen all adolescents between the ages of 11 and 21 according to recommendations in the current edition of the AAP *Red Book: Report of the Committee on Infectious Diseases.* These include at least annual screening for: • all sexually active girls and young women • sexually active boys and young men who are at increased risk for infection (e.g., men who have sex with men)	• non-grandfathered private health insurance plans • Medicaid expansion plans • traditional Medicaid plans

*Optional for adults, depending on state policy; however, preventive services for children are often covered as part of the Early and Periodic Screening, Diagnostic, and Treatment (EPSDT) benefit for children.

Syphilis Testing

Preventive services coverage for syphilis testing is shown in Table 31.2.

Table 31.2. Preventive Services Coverage for Syphilis Testing

Recommending Authority	Eligible Populations and Service Specifics	Plans That Cover without Cost-Sharing
USPSTF (Grade "A"; June 2016)	Screen nonpregnant adults and adolescents at increased risk for syphilis infection.	• non-grandfathered private health insurance plans • Medicare • Medicaid expansion plans • traditional Medicaid plans*
USPSTF (Grade "A"; September 2018)	Screen all pregnant women for syphilis infection.	• non-grandfathered private health insurance plans • Medicare • Medicaid expansion plans • traditional Medicaid plans*
Bright Futures/AAP recommendations for pediatric preventive health care (March 2020)	Screen sexually active adolescents between the ages of 11 and 21 who are at increased risk for infection in accordance with recommendations in the current edition of the AAP *Red Book: Report of the Committee on Infectious Diseases.*	• non-grandfathered private health insurance plans • Medicaid expansion plans • traditional Medicaid plans

Optional for adults, depending on state policy; however, preventive services for children are often covered as part of the EPSDT benefit for children.

Gonorrhea Testing

Preventive services coverage for gonorrhea testing is shown in Table 31.3.

Table 31.3. Preventive Services Coverage for Gonorrhea Testing

Recommending Authority	Eligible Populations and Service Specifics	Plans That Cover without Cost-Sharing
USPSTF (Grade "B"; September 2014)	Screen the following groups for gonorrhea: • sexually active women (including pregnant women) aged 24 and younger • sexually active older women (including pregnant women) who are at increased risk for chlamydia infection	• non-grandfathered private health insurance plans • Medicare • Medicaid expansion plans • traditional Medicaid plans*

Table 31.3. Continued

Recommending Authority	Eligible Populations and Service Specifics	Plans That Cover without Cost-Sharing
Bright Futures/AAP recommendations for pediatric preventive health care (March 2020)	Screen all adolescents between the ages of 11 and 21 according to recommendations in the current edition of the AAP *Red Book: Report of the Committee on Infectious Diseases.* These include at least annual screening for: • all sexually active girls and young women • sexually active boys and young men who are at increased risk for infection (e.g., men who have sex with men)	• non-grandfathered private health insurance plans • Medicaid expansion plans • traditional Medicaid plans

* Optional for adults, depending on state policy; however, preventive services for children are often covered as part of the EPSDT benefit for children.

Ocular Prophylaxis for Gonococcal Ophthalmia Neonatorum

Preventive services coverage for gonococcal ophthalmia neonatorum testing is shown in Table 31.4.

Table 31.4. Preventive Services Coverage for Gonococcal Ophthalmia Neonatorum Testing

Recommending Authority	Eligible Populations and Service Specifics	Plans That Cover without Cost-Sharing
USPSTF (Grade "A"; January 2019)	Provide prophylactic ocular topical medication to all newborns for the prevention of gonococcal ophthalmia neonatorum.	• non-grandfathered private health insurance plans • Medicaid expansion plans • traditional Medicaid plans*

* Optional for adults, depending on state policy; however, preventive services for children are often covered as part of the EPSDT benefit for children.

Human Papillomavirus: Testing

Preventive services coverage for human papillomavirus (HPV) testing is shown in Table 31.5.

420

Table 31.5. Preventive Services Coverage for Human Papillomavirus Testing

Recommending Authority	Eligible Populations and Service Specifics	Plans That Cover without Cost-Sharing
Women's Preventive Services Guidelines (December 2016)	Screen average-risk women aged 21–65 for cervical cancer. • For women aged 21–29, cervical cytology (Pap test) should be used every three years. • Women aged 30–65 years should be screened with cytology and human papillomavirus testing every five years or cytology alone every three years.	• non-grandfathered private health insurance plans • Medicaid expansion plans
USPSTF (Grade "A"; August 2018)	Screen women aged 21–65 for cervical cancer. Ages 21–29: • every three years with cervical cytology testing Ages 30–65: • every three years with cervical cytology testing • every five years with high-risk human papillomavirus testing (hrHPV) • every five years with hrHPV testing in combination with cytology testing (co-testing)	• non-grandfathered private health insurance plans • Medicare • Medicaid expansion plans • traditional Medicaid plans*

Optional for adults, depending on state policy; however, preventive services for children are often covered as part of the EPSDT benefit for children.

Human Papillomavirus: Vaccination

Preventive services coverage for HPV vaccination is shown in Table 31.6.

Table 31.6. Preventive Services Coverage for Human Papillomavirus Vaccination

Recommending Authority	Eligible Populations and Service Specifics	Plans That Cover without Cost-Sharing
Advisory Committee on Immunization Practices (August 2019)	Vaccination against human papillomavirus (HPV) is routinely recommended at age 11 or 12. • For persons initiating vaccination before their 15th birthday, the recommended immunization schedule is two doses of the HPV vaccine. • For persons initiating vaccination on or after their 15th birthday or for persons with certain immunocompromising conditions, the recommended immunization schedule is three doses of the HPV vaccine.	• non-grandfathered private health insurance plans • Medicaid expansion plans • traditional Medicaid plans*

Optional for adults, depending on state policy; however, preventive services for children are often covered as part of the EPSDT benefit for children.

Sexually Transmitted Infection and Human Immunodeficiency Virus Prevention Counseling

Preventive services coverage for HIV prevention counseling is shown in Table 31.7.

Table 31.7. Preventive Services Coverage for Sexually Transmitted Infection and Human Immunodeficiency Virus Prevention Counseling[3]

Recommending Authority	Eligible Populations and Service Specifics	Plans That Cover without Cost-Sharing
USPSTF (Grade "B"; September 2014)	Provide intensive behavioral counseling to prevent STIs for all sexually active adolescents and adults at increased risk for STIs.	• non-grandfathered private health insurance plans • Medicare • Medicaid expansion plans • traditional Medicaid plans*
Women's Preventive Services Guidelines (December 2016)	Provide counseling on STIs, including HIV, for all sexually active women.	• non-grandfathered private health insurance plans • Medicaid expansion plans

Optional for adults, depending on state policy; however, preventive services for children are often covered as part of the EPSDT benefit for children.

[3] "Sexually Transmitted Disease Preventive Services Coverage," Centers for Disease Control and Prevention (CDC), August 18, 2020. Available online. URL: www.cdc.gov/nchhstp/highqualitycare/preventiveservices/std. html. Accessed June 9, 2023.

Part 5 | Sexually Transmitted Diseases: Risks and Prevention

Chapter 32 | High-Risk Sexual Behavior and Sexually Transmitted Infections

Chapter Contents

Section 32.1 | An Overview of Risky Sexual Behaviors

YOUTH ENGAGE IN SEXUAL RISK BEHAVIORS
Many young people engage in health-risk behaviors and experiences that can result in unintended health outcomes. The Youth Risk Behaviour Survey data of the Centers for Disease Control and Prevention (CDC; www.cdc.gov/healthyyouth/data/yrbs/pdf/YRBS_Data-Summary-Trends_Report2023_508.pdf) show protective sexual behaviors (i.e., condom use, sexually transmitted disease (STD) testing, and human immunodeficiency virus (HIV) testing), experiences of violence, mental health, and suicidal thoughts and behaviors worsened from 2011 to 2021.

FAST FACTS ON NATIONAL YOUTH RISK BEHAVIOR SURVEY
Among U.S. high school students surveyed in 2021:
- 30 percent had ever had sexual intercourse
- 48 percent did not use a condom the last time they had sex
- 8 percent had been physically forced to have sexual intercourse when they did not want to
- 9 percent of all students have ever been tested for HIV
- 5 percent of all students have been tested for STDs during the past year

HUMAN IMMUNODEFICIENCY VIRUS, SEXUALLY TRANSMITTED DISEASES, AND TEEN PREGNANCY ARE HEALTH CONSEQUENCES
Sexual risk behaviors place youth at risk for HIV infection, other STDs, and unintended pregnancy:
- HIV infection:
  - About 20 percent of all new HIV diagnoses were among young people (aged 13–24) in 2020.
- other STDs:
  - More than half of the nearly 20 million new STDs reported in 2020 were among young people (aged 15–24).

- teen pregnancy:
  - More than 145,000 infants were born to adolescent females in 2021.

SCHOOLS AND YOUTH SERVING ORGANIZATIONS CAN HELP

School health programs can help young people adopt lifelong attitudes and behaviors that support their health and well-being—including behaviors that can reduce their risk for HIV and other STDs.

HIV, STD, and teen pregnancy prevention programs in schools should do the following:

- Provide health information that is basic, accurate, and directly contributes to health-promoting decisions and behaviors.
- Address the needs of youth who are not having sex as well as youth who are currently sexually active.
- Ensure that all youth are provided with effective education and skills to protect themselves and others from HIV infection, other STDs, and unintended pregnancy.
- Be developed with the active involvement of students and parents.
- Be locally determined and consistent with community values and relevant policies.[1]

Section 32.2 | Having Multiple Sexual Partners

The term "people who exchange sex for money or nonmonetary items" (hereinafter referred to as "people who exchange sex") includes a broad range of persons who trade sex for income or other items, including food, drugs, medicine, and shelter. Persons who exchange sex are at increased risk of getting or transmitting human immunodeficiency virus (HIV) and other sexually transmitted diseases (STDs) because they are more likely to engage in

[1] "Sexual Risk Behaviors," Centers for Disease Control and Prevention (CDC), March 16, 2023. Available online. URL: www.cdc.gov/healthyyouth/sexualbehaviors/index.htm. Accessed June 27, 2023.

risky sexual behaviors (e.g., sex without a condom, sex with multiple partners) and substance use. Those who exchange sex more regularly as a source of ongoing income are at higher risk for HIV than those who do so infrequently. Persons who engage in such activities include escorts; people who work in massage parlors, brothels, and the adult film industry; exotic dancers; state-regulated prostitutes (in Nevada); and men, women, and transgender persons who participate in survival sex, that is, trading sex to meet basic needs of daily life. For any of the above, sex can be consensual or nonconsensual.

It is important for people who exchange sex to get tested for HIV regularly and know their status. Knowing one's status helps determine the best prevention or care options:

- Condoms are highly effective in preventing a person from getting or transmitting HIV infection if used the right way every time during sex.
- For persons who are HIV-negative, prevention options such as pre-exposure prophylaxis (PrEP), taking HIV medicines as prescribed to prevent getting HIV, may be beneficial.
- For people who are living with HIV, taking medicines to treat HIV (called "antiretroviral therapy" (ART)) the right way every day can help keep them healthy and greatly reduce their chance of transmitting HIV to others.

PREVENTION CHALLENGES
Lack of Data

There is a lack of population-based studies on persons who exchange sex although some studies have been done in singular settings such as prisons and exotic dance clubs. However, the illegal—and often criminalized—nature of the exchange of sex makes it difficult to gather population-level data on HIV risk among this population. This lack of data creates significant barriers to developing targeted HIV prevention efforts.

Socioeconomic Factors

Many persons who exchange sex face stigma, poverty, and lack of access to health care and other social services—all of which pose challenges to HIV prevention efforts. Existing research shows the following:

- Many persons who exchange sex may have a history of homelessness, unemployment, incarceration, mental health issues, violence, emotional/physical/sexual abuse, and drug use.
- Some transgender persons may turn to exchange sex because of discrimination and lack of economic opportunities. They may exchange sex to generate income for rent, drugs, medicines, hormones, and gender-related surgeries.

Sexual Risk Factors

Persons who exchange sex may not use condoms consistently. Several factors may contribute to this behavior, including the following:

- **Economics**. Persons who exchange sex may receive more money for sex without a condom.
- **Partner type**. Persons who exchange sex may use condoms less often with regular clients than with one-time clients and even less frequently with intimate partners.
- **Power dynamics**. Unequal power in a relationship with clients may make it difficult for persons who exchange sex to negotiate condom use.

Other risk factors for this population include the following:

- multiple high-risk sex partners, for example, partners who do not know they are living with HIV or other STDs
- more money for sex with partners known to be HIV-positive

Drug and Alcohol Use

There is a strong link between the exchange of sex and drug and alcohol use. Under the influence of drugs or alcohol, persons who exchange sex may have impaired judgment; engage in riskier forms of sex, such as anal sex; and have difficulty negotiating safer sex (e.g., condom use) with their customers. People who trade sex for drugs tend to have more clients, use condoms less often, and are more likely to share needles and other drug works.

Knowledge of Human Immunodeficiency Virus Status

Many persons who exchange sex may not know their HIV status because they:

- do not know where to access available services
- are uncomfortable sharing information about sexual and substance use histories as part of HIV testing protocol

Some persons who know their HIV status may be reluctant to seek or stay in care because of:

- mistrust of the health-care system
- concern that they may lose income if identified as being HIV-positive
- financial circumstances and other barriers (e.g., health insurance) that affect health-care access[2]

Section 32.3 | Oral Sex and Risk of Sexually Transmitted Diseases

WHAT IS ORAL SEX?

Oral sex involves using the mouth to stimulate the genitals or genital area of a sex partner. Types of oral sex include the penis (fellatio), vagina (cunnilingus), and anus (anilingus).

Oral sex is commonly practiced by sexually active adults. More than 85 percent of sexually active adults aged 18–44 years reported having oral sex at least once with a partner of the opposite sex. A separate survey conducted during 2011–2015 found that 41 percent

---

[2] "HIV Risk among Persons Who Exchange Sex for Money or Nonmonetary Items," Centers for Disease Control and Prevention (CDC), March 16, 2022. Available online. URL: www.cdc.gov/hiv/group/sexworkers.html. Accessed June 1, 2023.

of teenagers aged 15–19 years reported having oral sex with a partner of the opposite sex.

CAN SEXUALLY TRANSMITTED DISEASES SPREAD DURING ORAL SEX?

Yes. Many sexually transmitted diseases (STDs) and other infections are spread through oral sex. Anyone exposed to an infected partner can get an STD in the mouth, throat, genitals, or rectum. The risk of getting an STD or spreading an STD to others through oral sex depends on several things, including the particular STD, type of sex, and number of sex acts performed.

- It is possible to get some STDs in the mouth or throat after giving oral sex to a partner who has a genital or anal/rectal STD.
- It is possible to get certain STDs on the genitals and genital areas after receiving oral sex from a partner with a mouth or throat infection.
- It is possible to have an STD in more than one area at the same time. For example, you can have an STD in the throat and the genitals.
- Several STDs (i.e., syphilis, gonorrhea, and intestinal infections) that are transmitted by oral sex can spread in the body.
- Oral sex involving the anus (or anilingus) can transmit hepatitis A and B. It can also transmit intestinal parasites, such as *Giardia*, and bacteria, such as *Escherichia coli* (*E. coli*) and *Shigella*.
- If you have an STD, you might not know it because many STDs are symptomless. It is possible to spread STDs even when you do not have any signs or symptoms.

WHICH SEXUALLY TRANSMITTED DISEASES CAN BE PASSED ON FROM ORAL SEX?

Chlamydia

RISK OF INFECTION FROM ORAL SEX

- Giving oral sex to a partner with an infected penis can cause chlamydia in the throat.

- Giving oral sex to a partner with an infected vagina or urinary tract may cause chlamydia in the throat.*
- Giving oral sex to a partner with an infected rectum might cause chlamydia in the throat.*
- Getting oral sex on the penis from a partner with chlamydia in the throat can cause chlamydia of the penis.
- Getting oral sex on the vagina from a partner with chlamydia in the throat might cause chlamydia of the vagina or urinary tract.*
- Getting oral sex on the anus from a partner with chlamydia in the throat might cause chlamydia in the rectum.*

Needs more research.

AREAS OF INITIAL INFECTION
- throat
- genitals
- urinary tract
- rectum

Gonorrhea
RISK OF INFECTION FROM ORAL SEX
- Giving oral sex to a partner with an infected penis can cause gonorrhea in the throat.
- Giving oral sex to a partner with an infected vagina or urinary tract might cause gonorrhea in the throat.*
- Giving oral sex to a partner with an infected rectum might cause gonorrhea in the throat.*
- Receiving oral sex on the penis from a partner with gonorrhea in the throat may cause gonorrhea of the penis.
- Receiving oral sex on the vagina from a partner with gonorrhea in the throat might cause gonorrhea of the vagina or urinary tract.*
- Receiving oral sex on the anus from a partner with gonorrhea in the throat might cause gonorrhea in the rectum.*

Needs more research.

AREAS OF INITIAL INFECTION

- throat
- genitals
- urinary tract
- rectum

Syphilis
RISK OF INFECTION FROM ORAL SEX

- Giving oral sex to a partner with a syphilis sore or rash on the genitals or anus can cause syphilis.
- Receiving oral sex from a partner with a syphilis sore or rash on the lips or mouth or in the throat can cause syphilis.
- Another important factor that affects risk of spreading syphilis is how long your partner had syphilis.

AREAS OF INITIAL INFECTION

- lips
- mouth
- throat
- genitals
- anus
- rectum

Herpes (Herpes Simplex Virus Types 1 and 2)
RISK OF INFECTION FROM ORAL SEX

- Giving oral sex to a partner with herpes on the genital area, anus, or buttocks or in the rectum may cause oral herpes.
- Receiving oral sex from a partner with herpes on the lips or mouth or in the throat can cause herpes on the genital area, anus, or buttocks or in the rectum.

AREAS OF INFECTION

- lips
- mouth

- throat
- genital area
- anus
- rectum
- buttocks

Human Papillomavirus
RISK OF INFECTION FROM ORAL SEX
- Giving oral sex to a partner who has a penis or genital area infected with human papillomavirus (HPV) can cause HPV in the throat.
- Giving oral sex to a partner with an HPV-infected vagina or genital area can cause HPV in the throat.
- Giving oral sex to a partner with HPV on the anus or in the rectum may cause HPV in the throat.*
- Receiving oral sex from a partner with HPV in the throat might cause HPV in the genital area, anus, or rectum.*

Needs more research.

AREAS OF INFECTION
- mouth
- throat
- genital area
- vagina
- cervix
- anus
- rectum

Human Immunodeficiency Virus
RISK OF INFECTION FROM ORAL SEX
- Giving oral sex on the penis of a partner with human immunodeficiency virus (HIV) can cause HIV. The risk of infection is lower than the risks from vaginal or anal sex.
- Giving oral sex on the vagina of a partner with HIV may cause HIV. The risk of infection is thought to be very low.

- Giving oral sex on the anus of a partner with HIV may cause HIV. There are few reports of transmission from this type of oral sex.
- Receiving oral sex on the penis from a partner with HIV may cause HIV. This risk is thought to be very low and has not been well studied.
- Receiving oral sex on the vagina from a partner with HIV might cause HIV. This risk is thought to be extremely low and has not been well studied.
- Receiving oral sex on the anus from a partner with HIV might cause HIV. There are few reports of transmission from this type of oral sex.
- The virus level (or viral load) in an infected partner's blood and other body fluids during a sexual encounter. An undetectable HIV viral load eliminates the risk of spreading HIV from oral sex.

AREAS OF INFECTION
- infection of the immune system throughout the body

Trichomoniasis
RISK OF INFECTION FROM ORAL SEX
- Giving oral sex to a partner with an infection in their genitals might cause trichomoniasis of the throat. There are few reports of potential spread from oral sex.
- Spread of trichomoniasis by other oral sex practices has not been reported.

AREAS OF INITIAL INFECTION
- vagina
- penis
- mouth/throat (possibly)

IS ORAL SEX SAFER THAN VAGINAL OR ANAL SEX?
- It is difficult to compare the risks of getting specific STDs from specific types of sexual activities.

- Most people who have oral sex also have vaginal or anal sex.
- Few studies look at the risks of getting STDs, other than HIV, from giving oral sex on the vagina or anus, compared to the penis.
- Studies show the risk of getting HIV from oral sex (giving or receiving) with a partner who has the infection is much lower than the risk of getting HIV from anal or vaginal sex. This may not be true for other STDs.
  - In a study of gay men with syphilis, one out of five reported having only oral sex.
  - Getting HIV from oral sex may be extremely low, but it is hard to know the exact risk. If you are having oral sex, you should protect yourself.
- It is possible that getting certain STDs in the throat, such as chlamydia or gonorrhea, may not be as harmful as getting an STD in the genital area or rectum. Having these infections in the throat might increase the risk of getting HIV. Having gonorrhea in the throat may also lead to the spread of disease throughout the body.
  - Having infections of chlamydia and gonorrhea in the throat may make it easier to spread these infections to others through oral sex. This is especially important for gonorrhea since throat infections can be harder to treat.
  - Infections from certain STDs, such as syphilis and HIV, spread throughout the body. Therefore, infections acquired in the throat may lead to the same health problems as infections acquired in the genitals or rectum.
  - Mouth and throat infections by certain types of HPV may develop into oral or neck cancer.

WHAT MAY INCREASE THE CHANCES OF GIVING OR GETTING A SEXUALLY TRANSMITTED DISEASE THROUGH ORAL SEX?

Certain factors may increase a person's chances of getting HIV or other STDs during oral sex if exposed to an infected partner. Factors include:

- poor oral health, which can include tooth decay, gum disease or bleeding gums, and oral cancer

- sores in the mouth or on the genitals
- exposure to the "pre-cum" or "cum" (also known as "pre-ejaculate" or "ejaculate")

However, there are no scientific studies that show whether these factors increase the risk of getting HIV or STDs from oral sex.

WHAT CAN YOU DO TO PREVENT SEXUALLY TRANSMITTED DISEASE TRANSMISSION DURING ORAL SEX?

You can lower your chances of giving or getting STDs during oral sex. Use a condom, dental dam, or other barrier methods every time you have oral sex.

- For oral sex on the penis, do the following:
  - Cover the penis with a nonlubricated latex condom.
  - Use plastic (polyurethane) condoms if you or your partner is allergic to latex.
- For oral sex on the vagina or anus, do the following:
  - Use a dental dam.
  - Cut open a condom to make a square and put it between your mouth and your partner's vagina or anus.

The only way to avoid STDs is not to have vaginal, anal, or oral sex.

If you are having sex, you can lower your chances of getting an STD by:

- being in a long-term mutually monogamous relationship with a partner who does not have an STD (e.g., a partner with negative STD test results)
- using latex condoms the right way every time you have sex

It is important to remember that many people with an STD may be unaware of their infection. STDs often have no symptoms and are unrecognized.[3]

---

[3] "STD Risk and Oral Sex," Centers for Disease Control and Prevention (CDC), December 31, 2021. Available online. URL: www.cdc.gov/std/healthcomm/stdfact-stdriskandoralsex.htm. Accessed July 13, 2023.

Chapter 33 | Nonsexual Factors That Raise Risk of Sexually Transmitted Diseases

Chapter Contents

WHAT IS A HUMAN IMMUNODEFICIENCY VIRUS VIRAL LOAD?

A human immunodeficiency virus (HIV) viral load is a blood test that measures the amount of HIV in a sample of your blood. The test looks for genetic material from the virus in your blood. These tests are called "molecular tests" or "nucleic acid amplification tests" (NAATs or NATs). There are several types of NAATs. A polymerase chain reaction (PCR) test is one type of NAAT that may be used to find HIV.

HIV is a virus that damages immune system cells. These cells protect your body against diseases from germs, such as viruses, bacteria, and fungi. If you lose too many immune cells, your body will have trouble fighting off infections and other diseases.

You can get HIV from contact with the blood of a person who has an HIV infection. This usually happens through sex or sharing needles or other equipment used to inject drugs.

This virus is the cause of acquired immunodeficiency syndrome (AIDS). AIDS is the final, most serious stage of an HIV infection. Without treatment, the amount of HIV in your body can increase. It can gradually destroy your immune system and become AIDS. With AIDS, your body has trouble fighting off infections from germs that usually do not cause problems in healthy people. These are called "opportunistic infections," and they can become life-threatening. AIDS increases your risk of developing certain cancers, too.

Most people with HIV do not have AIDS. If you have HIV, you can take HIV medicines that protect your immune system and help prevent you from getting AIDS. Medicines that treat HIV are called "antiretroviral therapy" (ART). ART cannot get rid of HIV completely, so you will need to take medicines for the rest of your life. But ART can control HIV and help you live a longer, healthier life.

Having regular HIV viral load tests is an important part of making sure your HIV medicines are keeping your viral load low, so you stay healthy.

Other names are nucleic acid testing, NAT, NAAT, HIV PCR, ribonucleic acid test (RNA test), and HIV quantification.

441

WHAT IS IT USED FOR?

An HIV viral load test is mainly used after you are diagnosed with HIV to:

- guide decisions about your treatment
- check how well your HIV medicines are working
- watch for any changes in your HIV infection

HIV viral load testing is also used to test newborn babies when they are born to a person who has HIV. That is because HIV can be passed to a baby during pregnancy, during childbirth, and through breast milk.

In certain cases, an HIV viral load test may be used to diagnose HIV. Usually, HIV screening tests are used first. That is because HIV viral load tests are expensive. But viral load tests can find HIV sooner after infection than screening tests. So your health-care provider may order this test if your risk of having HIV is very high.

WHY DO YOU NEED A HUMAN IMMUNODEFICIENCY VIRUS VIRAL LOAD TEST?

A viral load test is needed to guide treatment decisions. If you have HIV, you will probably start taking HIV medicines soon after your diagnosis. But, first, you will need a viral load test to find out how much virus is in your blood. This information helps your provider choose the right medicines for you. Your first test result will be compared with later test results to see if the medicines are working.

A viral load test is needed to see how well treatment is working and to monitor your HIV infection. The goal of HIV treatment is to reduce the amount of virus in your blood until there is too little to show up on a test. You will need to have regular viral load tests to see whether your viral load is dropping enough. HIV viral load tests are usually done:

- before you start taking medicine
- about two to eight weeks after starting or changing HIV medicines
- every three to six months to monitor your infection when your treatment is working well

Your provider may order an HIV viral load test to diagnose HIV if:

- you recently had a high-risk exposure to HIV that include:
  - having vaginal or anal sex with someone who has HIV or whose HIV status you do not know
  - sharing needles, syringes, or other items used to inject drugs with other people
  - exchanging sex for money or drugs
  - having a sexually transmitted disease (STD), such as syphilis
  - having sex with anyone who has done anything listed above
- you had recent possible exposure to HIV and you have early symptoms of HIV infection that may include (the early stage of HIV does not always cause symptoms):
  - flu-like symptoms, such as fever, chills, aches
  - extreme fatigue
  - swollen lymph nodes (in your neck, groin, or armpit)
  - rash
  - sores in your mouth

If you think you were exposed to HIV, talk with your provider right away about getting tested. You may also be able to have emergency treatment to prevent HIV infection within the first three days after a possible exposure.

WHAT HAPPENS DURING A HUMAN IMMUNODEFICIENCY VIRUS VIRAL LOAD TEST?

A health-care professional will take a blood sample from a vein in your arm using a small needle. After the needle is inserted, a small amount of blood will be collected into a test tube or vial. You may feel a little sting when the needle goes in or out. This usually takes less than five minutes.

WILL YOU NEED TO DO ANYTHING TO PREPARE FOR THE TEST?

You do not need any special preparations for an HIV viral load test. But, if you are getting this test to find out if you are infected with

HIV, you should talk with a counselor before or after your test, so you can better understand the results and your treatment options.

ARE THERE ANY RISKS IN THE TEST?

There is very little risk in having a blood test. You may have slight pain or bruising at the spot where the needle was put in, but most symptoms go away quickly.[1]

WHAT CAN INCREASE THE RISK OF GETTING OR TRANSMITTING HUMAN IMMUNODEFICIENCY VIRUS?

Viral Load

The higher someone's viral load, the more likely that person is to transmit HIV.

- Viral load is the amount of HIV in the blood of someone who has HIV.
- Viral load is highest during the acute phase of HIV and without HIV treatment.
- Taking HIV medicine can make the viral load very low— so low that a test cannot detect it (called an "undetectable viral load").
- People with HIV who keep an undetectable viral load (or stay virally suppressed) can live long, healthy lives. Having an undetectable viral load also helps prevent transmitting the virus to others through sex or sharing needles, syringes, or other injection equipment and from the mother to the child during pregnancy, birth, and breastfeeding.

Other Sexually Transmitted Diseases

If you have another STD, you may be more likely to get or transmit HIV.

- Getting tested and treated for STDs can lower your chances of getting or transmitting HIV and other STDs.

---

[1] MedlinePlus, "HIV Viral Load," National Institutes of Health (NIH), August 29, 2022. Available online. URL: https://medlineplus.gov/lab-tests/hiv-viral-load/. Accessed June 6, 2023.

- If you have HIV and get and keep an undetectable viral load, getting an STD does not appear to increase the risk of transmitting HIV. But STDs can cause other problems.
- Using condoms can reduce your chances of getting or transmitting STDs that can be transmitted through genital fluids, such as gonorrhea, chlamydia, and HIV.
- Condoms are less effective at preventing STDs that can be transmitted through sores or cuts on the skin, such as human papillomavirus (HPV), genital herpes, and syphilis.

If you are sexually active, you and your partners should get tested for STDs, even if you do not have symptoms. To get tested for HIV or other STDs, find a testing site near you.

Alcohol and Drug Use

When you are drunk or high, you are more likely to engage in risky sexual behaviors, such as having sex without protection (such as condoms or medicine to prevent or treat HIV).

- Being drunk or high affects your ability to make safe choices.
- Drinking alcohol, particularly binge drinking, and using "club drugs" can alter your judgment, lower your inhibitions, and impair your decisions about sex or drug use.
- You may be more likely to have unplanned sex, have a harder time using a condom the right way every time you have sex, have more sexual partners, or use other drugs.

If you are going to a party or another place where you know you will be drinking or using drugs, you can bring a condom so that you can reduce your risk of getting or transmitting HIV if you have vaginal or anal sex.

Counseling, medicines, and other methods are available to help you stop or cut down on drinking or using drugs. Talk with a counselor, doctor, or other health-care provider about options that might be right for you.[2]

WHAT DO THE RESULTS MEAN?

If you have an HIV viral load test because you have HIV, the following would be the results:

- A negative or undetectable viral load means that you have so little HIV in your blood that the test cannot find it. This means that your HIV medicines are working well to protect your immune system, and you are unlikely to spread HIV through sex. It does not mean you are cured. You must continue to take your medicines as prescribed to keep your HIV in control.
- A low viral load means your medicine is stopping the virus from growing, and your infection is unlikely to get worse.
- A high viral load means the virus is growing, and your treatment is not working well. The higher the viral load, the more risk you have for infections and diseases related to a weak immune system. It may also mean you have a higher risk of developing AIDS. If your results show a high viral load, your provider will probably change your medicines.

If you had an HIV viral load test to diagnose whether you have HIV, the following would be the results:

- A normal or negative result means that no HIV was found in your blood, and you are probably not infected with HIV.
- A result that shows any amount of virus in your blood means you have an HIV infection. Your provider will likely order other tests, including a CD4 count, to see how much HIV has damaged your immune system.

If you have questions about your results, talk with your provider.

---

[2] "Factors That Increase HIV Risk," Centers for Disease Control and Prevention (CDC), April 21, 2021. Available online. URL: www.cdc.gov/hiv/basics/hiv-transmission/increase-hiv-risk.html. Accessed June 6, 2023.

IS THERE ANYTHING ELSE YOU NEED TO KNOW ABOUT A HUMAN IMMUNODEFICIENCY VIRUS VIRAL LOAD?

If you are living with HIV, you will have regular viral load tests to monitor your infection and treatment. It is best to have the same type of test done at the same lab if possible. That is because labs have different ways of measuring HIV viral load. Your provider needs to compare your test results over time to see if your viral load is going up or down, and different tests from different labs can be difficult to compare.[3]

Section 33.2 | Substance Use and Sexual Risk Behaviors

According to the Surgeon General's Report Facing Addiction in America, the misuse of substances such as alcohol and drugs is a growing problem in the United States. Although substance misuse can occur at any age, the teenage and young adult years are particularly critical at-risk periods. Research shows that the majority of adults who meet the criteria for having a substance use disorder started using substances during their teen and young adult years. Teen substance use is also associated with sexual risk behaviors that put young people at risk of human immunodeficiency virus (HIV), sexually transmitted diseases (STDs), and pregnancy. To address these issues, more needs to be done to lessen risks and increase protective factors for teens.

WHAT WE KNOW ABOUT SUBSTANCE USE AND SEXUAL RISK BEHAVIORS

Studies conducted among teens have identified an association between substance use and sexual risk behaviors such as ever having sex, having multiple sex partners, not using a condom, and pregnancy before the age of 15.

---

[3] See footnote [1].

Researchers have found that as the frequency of substance use increases, the likelihood of sex and the number of sex partners also increases. In addition, studies show that sexual risk behaviors increase in teens who use alcohol and are highest among students who use marijuana, cocaine, prescription drugs (such as sedatives, opioids, and stimulants), and other illicit drugs. Teens who reported no substance use are the least likely to engage in sexual risk-taking.

According to the 2017 National Youth Risk Behavior Survey (YRBS), 40 percent of high school students have ever had intercourse, and 29 percent of high school students are currently sexually active. Of the students who are currently sexually active, 19 percent drank alcohol or used drugs before their last sexual intercourse.

RISK FACTORS AND PREVENTION ACTIVITIES

Substance use and sexual risk behaviors share some common underlying factors that may predispose teens to these behaviors. Because substance use clusters with other risk behaviors, it is important to learn whether precursors can be determined early to help identify youth who are most at risk.

Primary prevention approaches that are most effective are those that address common risk factors. Prevention programs for substance use and sexual risk behaviors should include a focus on individuals, peers, families, schools, and communities. When students' school environments are supportive and their parents are engaged in their lives, they are less likely to use alcohol and drugs and engage in sexual behaviors that put them at risk for HIV, STDs, or pregnancy.

Common risk factors for substance use and sexual risk behaviors include:

- extreme economic deprivation (poverty and overcrowding)
- family history of the problem behavior, family conflict, and family management problems
- favorable parental attitudes toward the problem behavior and/or parental involvement in the problem behavior

- lack of positive parent engagement
- association with substance-using peers
- alienation and rebelliousness
- lack of school connectedness

For primary prevention activities targeting substance use and sexual risk behaviors to be effective, they should include:
- school-based programs that promote social and emotional competence
- peer-led drug and alcohol resistance programs
- parenting skills training
- parent engagement
- family support programs[4]

HOW CAN ALCOHOL PUT YOU AT RISK OF GETTING OR TRANSMITTING HUMAN IMMUNODEFICIENCY VIRUS?

Drinking alcohol, particularly binge drinking, affects your brain, making it hard to think clearly. When you are drunk, you may be more likely to make poor decisions that put you at risk of getting or transmitting HIV, such as having sex without medicine to prevent or treat HIV or without a condom.

You may also be more likely to have a harder time using a condom the right way, have more sexual partners, or use other drugs. Those behaviors can increase your risk of exposure to HIV and other STDs. Or, if you have HIV, they can also increase your risk of transmitting HIV to others.

What Can You Do?

If you drink alcohol, do the following:
- **Drink in moderation**. Moderate drinking is up to one drink per day for women and up to two drinks per day for men. One drink is a 12-ounce bottle of beer, a 5-ounce glass of wine, or a shot of liquor.

---

[4] "Substance Use and Sexual Risk Behaviors among Youth," Centers for Disease Control and Prevention (CDC), March 29, 2019. Available online. URL: www.cdc.gov/healthyyouth/factsheets/substance_use_fact_sheet-basic. htm. Accessed June 9, 2023.

- **Visit Rethinking Drinking (www.rethinkingdrinking. niaaa.nih.gov)**. This is a website of the National Institute on Alcohol Abuse and Alcoholism (NIAAA) of the National Institutes of Health (NIH). This website can help you evaluate your drinking habits and consider how alcohol may be affecting your health.
- **Do not have sex if you are drunk or high from other drugs**. Sex under the influence of drugs or alcohol is associated with high-risk sexual behavior that will eventually lead to exposure to HIV and other STDs.
- **If you are HIV-negative, talk to your health-care provider about pre-exposure prophylaxis (PrEP)**. PrEP is medicine people at risk for HIV take to prevent getting HIV from sex or injection drug use. PrEP can stop HIV from taking hold and spreading throughout your body. PrEP must be taken as prescribed, and alcohol use can make it hard to stick to an HIV regimen. Be open and honest about your alcohol use, so you and your doctor can develop a plan for you to stick to your HIV medicine.
- **If you are not taking PrEP as prescribed, condom use is also important to help prevent HIV**. And, since PrEP only protects against HIV, condom use is still important for the protection against other sexually transmitted infections (STIs).
- **If you have HIV, take HIV medicine (called "antiretroviral therapy" (ART)) as prescribed**. People with HIV who take HIV medication as prescribed and get and keep an undetectable viral load can live long and healthy lives and will not transmit HIV to their HIV-negative partners through sex.

Need Help?
- If you feel you are drinking too much, too fast, or too often, therapy and other methods are available to help you stop or cut down on your alcohol use (if you have a problem). Talk with a counselor, doctor, or other

health-care providers about options that might be right for you.

- The NIAAA offers an Alcohol Treatment Navigator (https://alcoholtreatment.niaaa.nih.gov/). This online tool helps you find the right treatment for you—and near you. It guides you through a step-by-step process to finding a highly qualified professional treatment provider.
- You can also use the Substance Abuse and Mental Health Services Administration (SAMHSA) Behavioral Health Treatment Locator (https://findtreatment.gov/) or call 800-662-HELP (4357). Open 24/7.

Staying Healthy

If you have HIV, alcohol use can be harmful to your brain and body and affect your ability to stick to your HIV treatment. Learn about the health effects of alcohol and other drug use and how to access alcohol treatment programs if you need them at www.hiv.gov/hiv-basics/staying-in-hiv-care/other-related-health-issues/alcohol-and-drug-use/.[5]

Section 33.3 | Injection Drug Use

Sharing needles, syringes, or other equipment (works) to inject drugs puts people at high risk of getting or transmitting human immunodeficiency virus (HIV) and other infections. People who inject drugs (PWIDs) account for about 1 in 10 HIV diagnoses in the United States. Syringe services programs (SSPs) can play a role in preventing HIV and other health problems among PWIDs, by providing access to sterile syringes. These programs can also provide comprehensive services such as help with stopping substance

[5] HIV.gov, "Alcohol and HIV Risk," U.S. Department of Health and Human Services (HHS), June 28, 2022. Available online. URL: www.hiv.gov/hiv-basics/hiv-prevention/reducing-risk-from-alcohol-and-drug-use/alcohol-and-hiv-risk/. Accessed June 9, 2023.

misuse; testing and linkage to treatment for HIV, hepatitis B, and hepatitis C; education on what to do for an overdose; and other prevention services.[6]

CAN YOU GET HUMAN IMMUNODEFICIENCY VIRUS FROM INJECTING DRUGS?

Yes, if you share needles, syringes, or other injection equipment with someone who has HIV. Sharing can transfer blood from person to person, and blood can carry HIV.

Also, when you use drugs, you may be more likely to take risks with sex, which can increase your chances of getting HIV.

HOW CAN YOU PREVENT GETTING HUMAN IMMUNODEFICIENCY VIRUS?

The best way is to stop injecting drugs. To find a treatment program to help you quit, visit findtreatment.samhsa.gov or call 800-662-HELP (4357).

If you continue to inject drugs, here are some ways to lower your risk of HIV:

- Use new, clean needles and syringes every time you inject and never share injection equipment.
- If you do share needles and syringes, always clean used needles and syringes with bleach.
- Cleaning your needles and syringes can greatly reduce your risk of HIV and viral hepatitis.
- Bleach cannot be used to clean water or cotton. Use new, clean water and cotton each time.
- Take pre-exposure prophylaxis (PrEP) to prevent getting HIV. When taken as prescribed, PrEP is highly effective for preventing HIV.
- Take post-exposure prophylaxis (PEP) if you think you have been exposed to HIV in the past 72 hours and are not on PrEP.

---

[6] "Injection Drug Use," Centers for Disease Control and Prevention (CDC), March 16, 2022. Available online. URL: www.cdc.gov/hiv/risk/drugs/index.html. Accessed June 9, 2023.

- Use condoms the right way every time you have anal or vaginal sex or choose less risky activities, such as oral sex. Abstinence (not having sex) is always an option.

WHERE CAN YOU GET NEW, CLEAN NEEDLES AND SYRINGES?

- Many communities have SSPs that give out new, clean needles, syringes, bleach kits, and other supplies. To find one near you, visit nasen.org/map.
- Some pharmacies sell new, clean needles and syringes.
- In some places, health-care providers can write prescriptions for new, clean needles and syringes.[7]

RISK OF HUMAN IMMUNODEFICIENCY VIRUS FROM INJECTING DRUGS

The risk of getting or transmitting HIV is very high if an HIV-negative person uses injection equipment that someone with HIV has used. This is because the needles, syringes, or other injection equipment may have blood in them, and blood can carry HIV. HIV can survive in a used syringe for up to 42 days, depending on temperature and other factors.

Substance use disorder can also increase the risk of getting HIV through sex. When people are under the influence of substances, they are more likely to engage in risky sexual behaviors, such as having anal or vaginal sex without protection (such as a condom or medicine to prevent or treat HIV), having sex with multiple partners, or trading sex for money or drugs.

RISK OF OTHER INFECTIONS AND OVERDOSE

Sharing needles, syringes, or other injection equipment also puts people at risk for getting HIV and viral hepatitis. PWIDs should talk to a health-care provider about getting a blood test for hepatitis B and C and getting vaccinated for hepatitis A and B.

---

[7] "HIV and Injecting Drugs 101," Centers for Disease Control and Prevention (CDC), October 2022. Available online. URL: www.cdc.gov/hiv/pdf/library/consumer-info-sheets/cdc-hiv-consumer-info-sheet-injecting-drugs-101. pdf. Accessed June 9, 2023.

In addition to being at risk of HIV and viral hepatitis, PWIDs can have other serious health problems, such as skin infections and heart infections. People can also overdose and get very sick or even die from having too many drugs or too much of one drug in their body or from products that may be mixed with the drugs without their knowledge (e.g., fentanyl).[8]

Section 33.4 | Vaginal Douching: Helpful or Harmful?

WHAT IS DOUCHING?

The word "douche" means to wash or soak. Douching is washing or cleaning out the inside of the vagina with water or other mixtures of fluids. Most douches are sold in stores as prepackaged mixes of water and vinegar, baking soda, or iodine. The mixtures usually come in a bottle or bag. You squirt the douche upward through a tube or nozzle into your vagina. The water mixture then comes back out through your vagina.

Douching is different from washing the outside of your vagina during a bath or shower. Rinsing the outside of your vagina with warm water will not harm your vagina. But douching can lead to many different health problems.

Most doctors recommend that women do not douche.

HOW COMMON IS DOUCHING?

In the United States, almost one in five women aged 15–44 douche.

More African American and Hispanic women douche than White women. Douching is also common in teens of all races and ethnicities.

Studies have not found any health benefit to douching. But studies have found that douching is linked to many health problems.

---

[8] "HIV and Injection Drug Use," Centers for Disease Control and Prevention (CDC), April 21, 2021. Available online. URL: www.cdc.gov/hiv/basics/hiv-transmission/injection-drug-use.html. Accessed June 9, 2023.

WHY SHOULD WOMEN NOT DOUCHE?

Most doctors recommend that women do not douche. Douching can change the necessary balance of vaginal flora (bacteria that live in the vagina) and natural acidity in a healthy vagina.

A healthy vagina has good and harmful bacteria. The balance of bacteria helps maintain an acidic environment. The acidic environment protects the vagina from infections or irritation.

Douching can cause an overgrowth of harmful bacteria. This can lead to a yeast infection or bacterial vaginosis (BV). If you already have a vaginal infection, douching can push the bacteria causing the infection up into the uterus, fallopian tubes, and ovaries. This can lead to pelvic inflammatory disease (PID), a serious health problem.

Douching is also linked to other health problems.

WHAT HEALTH PROBLEMS ARE LINKED TO DOUCHING?

Health problems linked to douching include:
- BV, which is an infection in the vagina (Women who douche often (once a week) are five times more likely to develop BV than women who do not douche.)
- PID, an infection in the reproductive organs that is often caused by a sexually transmitted infection (STI)
- problems during pregnancy, including preterm birth and ectopic pregnancy
- STIs, including human immunodeficiency virus (HIV)
- vaginal irritation or dryness

Researchers are studying whether douching causes these problems or whether women at higher risk for these health problems are more likely to douche.

SHOULD YOU DOUCHE TO GET RID OF VAGINAL ODOR OR OTHER PROBLEMS?

No. You should not douche to try to get rid of vaginal odor or other vaginal problems such as discharge, pain, itching, or burning.

Douching will only cover up the odor for a short time and will make other problems worse. Call your doctor or nurse if you have:
- vaginal discharge that smells bad
- vaginal itching and thick, white, or yellowish-green discharge with or without an odor
- burning, redness, and swelling in or around the vagina
- pain when urinating
- pain or discomfort during sex

These may be signs of a vaginal infection or an STI. Do not douche before seeing your doctor or nurse. This can make it hard for the doctor or nurse to find out what may be wrong.

SHOULD YOU DOUCHE TO CLEAN INSIDE YOUR VAGINA?

No. Doctors recommend that women do not douche. You do not need to douche to clean your vagina. Your body naturally flushes out and cleans your vagina. Any strong odor or irritation usually means something is wrong.

Douching can also raise your chances of a vaginal infection or an STI. If you have questions or concerns, talk to your doctor.

WHAT IS THE BEST WAY TO CLEAN YOUR VAGINA?

It is best to let your vagina clean itself. The vagina cleans itself naturally by making mucous. The mucous washes away blood, semen, and vaginal discharge.

If you are worried about vaginal odor, talk to your doctor or nurse. But you should know that even healthy, clean vaginas have a mild odor that changes throughout the day. Physical activity can also give your vagina a stronger, muskier scent, but this is still normal.

Keep your vagina clean and healthy by doing the following:
- **Washing the outside of your vagina with warm water when you bathe**. Some women also use mild soaps. But, if you have sensitive skin or any current vaginal infections, even mild soaps can cause dryness and irritation.

- **Avoiding scented tampons, pads, powders, and sprays**. These products may increase your chances of getting a vaginal infection.

CAN DOUCHING BEFORE OR AFTER SEX PREVENT SEXUALLY TRANSMITTED INFECTIONS?

No. Douching before or after sex does not prevent STIs. In fact, douching removes some of the normal bacteria in the vagina that protect you from infection. This can actually increase your risk of getting STIs, including HIV, the virus that causes acquired immunodeficiency syndrome (AIDS).[9]

Know That Washing the Vagina or Douching after Sex Will Not Prevent STIs

- The American Congress of Obstetricians and Gynecologists (ACOG) recommends that women do not douche.
- Douching can change the balance of germs and acidity in a healthy vagina.
- Any changes in that balance can cause an overgrowth of bad bacteria. This can lead to a yeast infection or bacterial vaginosis.
- If you have a vaginal infection, douching can push infection-causing bacteria up into the uterus, fallopian tubes, and ovaries. This can cause more serious problems.[10]

SHOULD YOU DOUCHE IF YOU HAD SEX WITHOUT USING PROTECTION OR IF THE CONDOM BROKE?

No. Douching removes some of the normal bacteria in the vagina that protect you from infection. This can increase your risk of getting STIs, including HIV. Douching does not also protect against pregnancy.

---

[9] Office on Women's Health (OWH), "Douching," U.S. Department of Health and Human Services (HHS), December 29, 2022. Available online. URL: www.womenshealth.gov/a-z-topics/douching. Accessed July 24, 2023.
[10] "Sexually Transmitted Diseases - Women's Health Guide," U.S. Department of Veterans Affairs (VA), June 3, 2015. Available online. URL: www.publichealth.va.gov/infectiondontpassiton/womens-health-guide/stds/index.asp. Accessed July 24, 2023.

If you had sex without using protection or if the condom broke during sex, see a doctor right away. You can get medicine to help prevent HIV and unwanted pregnancy.

SHOULD YOU DOUCHE IF YOU WERE SEXUALLY ASSAULTED?

No, you should not douche, bathe, or shower. As hard as it may be to not wash up, you may wash away important evidence if you do. Douching may also increase your risk of getting STIs, including HIV. Go to the nearest hospital emergency room as soon as possible. The National Sexual Assault Hotline at 800-656-HOPE (4673) can help you find a hospital able to collect evidence of sexual assault. Your doctor or nurse can help you get medicine to prevent HIV and unwanted pregnancy.

CAN DOUCHING AFTER SEX PREVENT PREGNANCY?

No. Douching does not prevent pregnancy. It should never be used for birth control. If you had sex without using birth control or if your birth control method did not work correctly (failed), you can use emergency contraception to keep from getting pregnant.

If you need birth control, talk to your doctor or nurse about which type of birth control method is best for you.

HOW DOES DOUCHING AFFECT PREGNANCY?

Douching can make it harder to get pregnant and can cause problems during pregnancy:

- **Trouble getting pregnant**. Women who douched at least once a month had a harder time getting pregnant than those women who did not douche.
- **Higher risk of ectopic pregnancy**. Douching may increase a woman's chance of damaged fallopian tubes and ectopic pregnancy. Ectopic pregnancy is when the fertilized egg attaches to the inside of the fallopian tube instead of the uterus. If left untreated, ectopic pregnancy can be life-threatening. It can also make it hard for a woman to get pregnant in the future.

- **Higher risk of early childbirth**. Douching raises your risk for premature birth. One study found that women who douched during pregnancy were more likely to deliver their babies early. This raises the risk of health problems for you and your baby.[11]

---

[11] See footnote [9].

Chapter 34 | Prevention of Sexually Transmitted Diseases

Chapter Contents

Section 34.1 | The Lowdown on How to Prevent Sexually Transmitted Diseases

The Centers for Disease Control and Prevention (CDC) estimates that there are millions of new sexually transmitted diseases (STDs) in the United States each year.

Anyone who is sexually active can get an STD. The following are a few groups who are more affected by STDs:

- adolescents and young adults
- gay, bisexual, and other men who have sex with men (MSM)
- pregnant women and infants
- racial and ethnic minorities

The good news is that STDs are preventable. There are steps you can take to keep yourself and your partner(s) healthy. Here is how you can avoid giving or getting an STD.

PRACTICE ABSTINENCE

The surest way to avoid STDs is not to have sex. This means not having vaginal, oral, or anal sex.

USE CONDOMS

Using a condom correctly every time you have sex can help you avoid STDs. Condoms lessen the risk of infection for all STDs. You can still get certain STDs, such as herpes or human papillomavirus (HPV), from contact with your partner's skin, even when using a condom.

Most people say they used a condom the first time they ever had sex, but when asked about the last four weeks, less than a quarter said they used a condom every time.

HAVE FEWER PARTNERS

Agree to only have sex with one person who agrees to only have sex with you. Make sure you both get tested to know for sure that neither of you has an STD. This is one of the most reliable ways to avoid STDs.

GET VACCINATED

The most common STD can be prevented by a vaccine. The HPV vaccine is safe and effective and can help you avoid HPV-related health problems, such as genital warts and some cancers.

Who Should Get the Human Papillomavirus Vaccine?

- All boys and girls aged 11–12 should get the vaccine, but the vaccine can start at age 9.
- Everyone through age 26 should get the vaccine if not vaccinated already.

TALK WITH YOUR PARTNER

Talk with your sex partner(s) about STDs and staying safe before having sex. It might be uncomfortable to start the conversation, but protecting your health is your responsibility.

GET TESTED

Many STDs do not have symptoms, but they can still cause health problems.

- Talk with your health-care provider.
- Search for CDC-recommended tests.
- Find a location to get tested for STDs.

The only way to know for sure if you have an STD is to get tested.

IF YOU TEST POSITIVE

Getting an STD is not the end. Many STDs are curable, and all are treatable. If either you or your partner is infected with an STD that can be cured, both of you need to start treatment immediately to avoid getting reinfected.[1]

---

[1] Sexually Transmitted Diseases (STDs)—Prevention," Centers for Disease Control and Prevention (CDC), January 21, 2021. Available online. URL: www.cdc.gov/std/prevention/lowdown/lowdown-text-only.htm. Accessed June 12, 2023.

Section 34.2 | Impact of Fewer Sex Partners and Male Circumcision on Disease Risk

ABSTINENCE

Abstinence means not having oral, vaginal, or anal sex. An abstinent person is someone who has never had sex or someone who has had sex but has decided not to continue having sex for some period of time.

What We Know about Abstinence

Abstinence is a 100 percent effective way to prevent human immunodeficiency virus (HIV), other sexually transmitted diseases (STDs), and pregnancy. The longer you wait to start having oral, vaginal, or anal sex, the fewer sex partners you are likely to have in your lifetime. Having fewer partners lowers your chances of having sex with someone who has HIV or another STD.

What You Can Do

Choose to be abstinent and talk to your partner about that decision. Not having sex is a 100 percent effective way to prevent getting or transmitting HIV.

CHOOSING LESS RISKY SEXUAL ACTIVITIES

Some sexual activities are riskier for HIV transmission than others. By choosing less risky sexual activities, you can reduce your risk of getting or transmitting HIV.

What We Know about Choosing Less Risky Sexual Activities

HIV is mainly spread by having anal or vaginal sex without using a condom or without taking medicine to prevent or treat HIV. Anal sex is the riskiest type of sex for transmitting HIV. It is possible for either partner—the partner inserting the penis in the anus or the partner receiving the penis—to get HIV, but it is much riskier for an HIV-negative partner to be the receptive partner.

Vaginal sex is less risky than anal sex, and oral sex and touching are much less risky than anal or vaginal sex for getting or transmitting HIV. There is extremely low-to-no risk of getting or transmitting HIV through oral sex or touching.

What You Can Do

Choosing activities with little-to-no risk, such as oral sex, instead of higher-risk activities, such as anal or vaginal sex, can lower your chances of getting or transmitting HIV. If you have anal sex, it is riskier for the HIV-negative partner to be the receptive partner. You can do other things to reduce your risk, including taking medicine to prevent or treat HIV and using condoms the right way every time you have sex. If the partner with HIV takes HIV medicine (called "antiretroviral therapy" (ART)) as prescribed and keeps an undetectable viral load, they will not transmit HIV through sex.

REDUCING THE NUMBER OF PARTNERS

Reducing the number of partners refers to choosing to limit how many sex partners you have in your lifetime.

What We Know about Reducing the Number of Partners

The more sex partners you have in your lifetime, the more likely you are to have a sex partner who does not know their status, is not taking medicine to treat HIV, and/or does not have an undetectable viral load. Having more sex partners also increases your chances of having a partner with another STD.

What You Can Do

Not having sex is a 100 percent effective way to prevent getting or transmitting HIV. If you are sexually active, you can choose to have fewer partners. You can also choose sexual activities that are lower risk for HIV than anal or vaginal sex.

Limiting the number of partners you have can lower your risk of getting or transmitting HIV. You can decrease your risk even more by taking other actions, including using a condom the right way every time you have sex and taking medicine to prevent or treat HIV.

Talking openly and frequently with your partner about sex can help you make decisions that may decrease your risk of getting or transmitting HIV.

MALE CIRCUMCISION

Male circumcision is removing some or all the foreskin (the fold of skin that covers the head, or glans, of the penis) from the penis is called "male circumcision." This procedure is done for hygiene and health reasons or as part of religious or cultural traditions.

What We Know about Male Circumcision

When men are circumcised, they are less likely than uncircumcised men to get HIV from a female partner who has HIV. There are biological reasons why, for some men, male circumcision may decrease the risk of getting HIV during vaginal sex with a female partner who has HIV. Male circumcision also reduces the risk of a man getting herpes and human papillomavirus (HPV) from a woman who has those infections. However, there is no evidence that circumcision decreases the risk of HIV-negative receptive partners getting HIV from a circumcised partner with HIV.

The evidence about the benefits of circumcision among gay and bisexual men is inconclusive. More studies are underway.

What You Can Do

Male circumcision decreases the risk that an HIV-negative heterosexual man will get HIV from a woman with HIV. But there is no evidence that circumcision decreases any other person's risk of getting HIV. Also, circumcised men and their partners can still get other STDs. Take other actions to prevent getting or transmitting HIV, such as using condoms the right way every time you have sex or taking medicine to prevent or treat HIV to further reduce your chance of getting HIV.

If you are a parent, talk to your health-care provider about the risks and benefits of male circumcision for your newborn.[2]

MALE CIRCUMCISION FOR HUMAN IMMUNODEFICIENCY VIRUS PREVENTION

- **Heterosexually active adolescent and adult males (including bisexual males)**. Health-care providers should inform all uncircumcised adolescent and adult males that male circumcision reduces, but does not eliminate, the chance of acquiring HIV and other sexually transmitted infections (STIs) during heterosexual contact. Additionally, the patients should be informed of the potential risks associated with the procedure. Health-care providers should assess the sexual risk behaviors of their male patients, and the patients who engage in activities that may increase their chances of acquiring HIV should be counseled about voluntary male circumcision as another potential strategy. Those patients who choose to be circumcised should be offered medically performed circumcision services and information on HIV prevention. Heterosexual males who engage in behaviors that increase the chances of getting HIV include:
  - males who are in sexual relationships with HIV-infected female partners
  - males with multiple female partners
  - males in relationships with females who engage in behaviors that may increase their chances of getting HIV or are part of communities overrepresented in the HIV epidemic (e.g., commercial sex workers, females who inject drugs, and females in defined populations with HIV prevalence of 1 percent or higher)
- **Gay and bisexual males**. Providers should inform uncircumcised gay and bisexual males that data from several observational studies indicate that male

---

[2] "What Can Decrease HIV Risk?" Centers for Disease Control and Prevention (CDC), May 26, 2020. Available online. URL: https://hivrisk.cdc.gov/can-decrease-hiv-risk/. Accessed June 13, 2023.

circumcision provides partial protection from HIV acquisition for gay and bisexual males who practice mainly or exclusively insertive anal sex (top). However, no clinical trials have included large enough numbers of gay and bisexual males to make a definitive conclusion regarding the usefulness of male circumcision in reducing the chances of acquiring HIV in this community. Additionally, there is no evidence that male circumcision reduces the chances of acquiring HIV through receptive anal sex (bottom).

- **Parents and guardians of male newborns, children, and adolescents**. Parents should be informed of the medical benefits—including a lower chance of getting HIV—and the risks of male circumcision and should make decisions in consultation with a health-care provider. When providing information to parents about male circumcision for an adolescent minor, the adolescent should be included in the decision-making process.

CONSIDERATIONS

The following key issues should be considered during the decision-making process:

- **Health benefits**: Male circumcision can reduce a male's chances of acquiring HIV by 50–60 percent during heterosexual contact with female partners with HIV, according to data from three clinical trials. Circumcised men, compared with uncircumcised men, have also been shown in clinical trials to be less likely to acquire new infections with syphilis (by 42%), genital ulcer disease (by 48%), genital herpes (by 28–45%), and high-risk strains of human papillomavirus associated with cancer (by 24–47%). While male circumcision has not been shown to reduce the chances of HIV transmission to female partners, it does reduce the chance that a female partner will acquire a new syphilis infection by 59 percent. In observational studies, circumcision has been shown

469

to lower the risk of penile cancer, cervical cancer in female sexual partners, and infant urinary tract infections in male infants.

- **Health risks**. The overall risk of adverse events associated with male circumcision is low, with minor bleeding and inflammation cited as the most common complications. The Centers for Disease Control and Prevention (CDC) analysis found that the rate of adverse events for medically attended male circumcision is 0.4 percent for infants under one year, about 9 percent for children aged one to nine years, and about 5 percent for males 10 years and older. More severe complications can occur but are exceedingly rare. Adult men who undergo circumcision generally report minimal or no change in sexual satisfaction or function.

- **Stage of life**. Circumcision is simpler, safer, and less expensive for newborns and infants than for adult males. Delaying circumcision until adolescence or adulthood enables the male to participate in—or make—the decision but could diminish the potential benefits related to sexual health and increases the risks.

- **Informed choice**. Male circumcision is a voluntary procedure. The decision regarding circumcision should be made in consultation with a health-care provider and consider personal, cultural, religious, and ethical beliefs.

IMPLICATIONS FOR HUMAN IMMUNODEFICIENCY VIRUS PREVENTION IN THE UNITED STATES

Given the urgency of ending the HIV epidemic in the United States, the CDC believes it is essential to maximize the impact of all available prevention options and is working to provide clinicians with the best possible information on the full range of proven approaches. Male circumcision is one strategy that may help reduce the continued spread of HIV in the United States. Ultimately, the degree to which male circumcision affects overall HIV transmission in the United States in the future will depend on a number of factors whose impact is not yet known. Those factors include the future contribution of heterosexual contact to the number of HIV infections that occur each year, future rates of infant male circumcision, the percentage of males who engage in heterosexual contact as well as behaviors that increase their chances of getting HIV who elect to be circumcised, and whether the approach can be effectively integrated with other proven HIV prevention strategies. Data on the cost-effectiveness of male circumcision to prevent HIV in the United States are limited but suggest that newborn circumcision would offer long-term cost savings by reducing their lifetime risk of HIV infection.

At an individual level, male circumcision may help reduce the risk of acquiring HIV among males and may be combined with other proven risk-reduction strategies to provide even greater protection. While the benefits of circumcision can be high for males without HIV who engage in behaviors that may increase their chances of getting HIV, the overall public health benefit for the entire U.S. population may be limited due to the lack of definitively proven benefits among HIV transmission categories at a national level, including male-to-male sexual contact and heterosexual contact. The greatest benefit will be among uncircumcised males who engage in heterosexual contact living in geographic areas with a high prevalence of HIV.[3]

Section 34.3 | Human Immunodeficiency Virus Treatment as Prevention

People with human immunodeficiency virus (HIV) should take medicine to treat HIV as soon as possible. HIV medicine is called "antiretroviral therapy" (ART). If taken as prescribed, HIV

---

[3] "Male Circumcision for HIV Prevention Fact Sheet," Centers for Disease Control and Prevention (CDC), July 12, 2022. Available online. URL: www.cdc.gov/nchhstp/newsroom/fact-sheets/hiv/male-circumcision-HIV-prevention-factsheet.html. Accessed June 13, 2023.

medicine reduces the amount of HIV in the body (viral load) to a very low level, which keeps the immune system working and prevents illness. This is called "viral suppression"—defined as having less than 200 copies of HIV per milliliter of blood. HIV medicine can even make the viral load so low that a test cannot detect it. This is called an "undetectable viral load."

Getting and keeping an undetectable viral load is the best thing people with HIV can do to stay healthy. Another benefit of reducing the amount of virus in the body is that it prevents transmission to others through sex or syringe sharing and from the mother to the child during pregnancy, birth, and breastfeeding. This is sometimes referred to as "treatment as prevention." There is strong evidence about treatment as prevention for some of the ways HIV can be transmitted, but more research is needed for other ways.

RISK OF HUMAN IMMUNODEFICIENCY VIRUS TRANSMISSION WITH UNDETECTABLE VIRAL LOAD BY TRANSMISSION CATEGORY

Risk of HIV transmission with undetectable viral load by transmission category is shown in Table 34.1.

Table 34.1. Undetectable Viral Load by Transmission Category and Who Are at Risk[4]

Transmission Category	Risk for People Who Keep an Undetectable Viral Load
Sex (oral, anal, or vaginal)	No risk of transmission, according to studies
Pregnancy, labor, and delivery	1 percent or less†
Sharing syringes or other drug injection equipment	Unknown but likely reduced risk
Breastfeeding	Substantially reducing but not eliminating risk

†*The risk of transmitting HIV to the baby can be 1 percent or less if the pregnant person takes HIV medicine daily as prescribed throughout pregnancy, labor, and delivery and gives HIV medicine to their baby for four to six weeks after giving birth.*

---

[4] "HIV Treatment as Prevention," Centers for Disease Control and Prevention (CDC), July 21, 2022. Available online. URL: www.cdc.gov/hiv/risk/art/index.html. Accessed June 13, 2023.

WHAT IS TREATMENT AS PREVENTION?

Treatment as prevention (TasP) refers to taking HIV medicine to prevent the sexual transmission of HIV. It is one of the most highly effective options for preventing HIV transmission.

People with HIV who take HIV medicine (called "antiretroviral therapy" (ART)) as prescribed and get and keep an undetectable viral load—a very low level of HIV in the blood—can live long and healthy lives and will not transmit HIV to their HIV-negative partners through sex. This is sometimes called "undetectable=un-transmittable" (U=U).

TasP works when a person with HIV takes HIV medicine exactly as prescribed and has regular follow-up care, including routine viral load tests to ensure their viral load stays undetectable.

TAKING HUMAN IMMUNODEFICIENCY VIRUS MEDICINE TO STAY HEALTHY AND PREVENT TRANSMISSION

Human immunodeficiency virus treatment involves taking highly effective medicine that reduces the amount of HIV in your body. HIV medicine is recommended for everyone with HIV, and people with HIV should start HIV medicine as soon as possible after diagnosis, even on that same day.

People on HIV treatment take a combination of HIV medicines (called an "HIV treatment regimen"). A person's initial HIV treatment regimen generally includes three HIV medicines from at least two different HIV drug classes that must be taken every day. Many people with HIV take two or more different HIV medicines combined in one pill. Long-acting injections of HIV medicine, given every two months, are also available if your health-care provider determines that you meet certain requirements.

If taken as prescribed, HIV medicine reduces the amount of HIV in your blood (also called your "viral load") to a very low level, which keeps your immune system working and prevents illness. This is called "viral suppression," defined as 200 copies of HIV per milliliter of blood.

HIV medicine can also make your viral load so low that a standard lab test cannot detect it. This is called having an "undetectable viral load." Almost everyone who takes HIV medicine as

473

prescribed can achieve an undetectable viral load, usually within one to six months after starting treatment. Many will bring their viral load to an undetectable level very quickly, but it could take more time for a small portion of people just starting HIV medicine.

There are important health benefits to getting the viral load as low as possible. People with HIV who know their status, take HIV medicine as prescribed, and get and keep an undetectable viral load can live long and healthy lives.

There is also a major prevention benefit. People with HIV who take HIV medicine as prescribed and get and keep an undetectable viral load will not transmit HIV to their HIV-negative partners through sex.

KEEP YOUR VIRAL LOAD UNDETECTABLE

Stay undetectable. Make HIV care and treatment a part of your daily routine. Keep your medical appointments and take your medications as directed.

HIV treatment is not a cure, and HIV is still in your body, even when your viral load is undetectable, so you need to keep taking your HIV medicine as prescribed. If you skip doses of your HIV medicine, even now and then, you give HIV the chance to multiply rapidly. This could weaken your immune system, and you could become sick.

If you have stopped taking your HIV medicine or are having trouble taking all the doses as prescribed, talk to your health-care provider as soon as possible. Your provider can help you get back on track and discuss the best strategies to prevent transmitting HIV to your sexual partners until your viral load is confirmed to be undetectable again.

Get tips on taking HIV medicine as prescribed.

HOW DO WE KNOW TREATMENT AS PREVENTION WORKS?

Large research studies with newer HIV medicines have shown that treatment is prevention. Over several years, these studies monitored thousands of male-female and male-male couples in which one partner has HIV and the other does not. No HIV transmissions were observed when the partner with HIV was virally suppressed. This means that if you keep your viral load undetectable, you will not transmit HIV to someone you have vaginal, anal, or oral sex with.

In addition to preventing sexual transmission of HIV, studies have shown that there are other prevention benefits of taking HIV medicine to get and keep an undetectable viral load:

- It reduces the risk of HIV transmission to the child during pregnancy, labor, and delivery. If a pregnant person takes HIV medicine daily as prescribed throughout pregnancy, labor, and delivery and gives HIV medicine to the infant for two to six weeks after giving birth, the risk of transmitting HIV to the baby can be 1 percent or less.
- It substantially decreases the risk of transmitting HIV to your baby through breastfeeding to less than 1 percent. However, the risk is not zero. If you are pregnant or thinking of becoming pregnant, talk to your health-care provider as early as possible about what infant feeding choice is right for you.
- It may reduce HIV transmission risk for people who inject drugs. Scientists do not have enough data to know whether having a suppressed or undetectable viral load prevents HIV transmission through sharing needles, syringes, or other injection drug equipment (e.g., cookers). It very likely reduces risk, but it is unknown by how much. Even if you are taking HIV medicine and have an undetectable viral load, use new equipment each time you inject and do not share needles and syringes with other people.

TALK WITH YOUR HEALTH-CARE PROVIDER ABOUT GETTING TO UNDETECTABLE

Talk with your health-care provider about the benefits of HIV treatment and which HIV medicine is right for you. Discuss how frequently you should get your viral load tested to make sure you get and keep an undetectable viral load. If your lab results show that the virus is detectable or if you are having trouble taking every dose of your medicine, you can still protect your HIV-negative partner by using other methods of preventing sexual transmission of HIV such as condoms, safer sex practices, and/or pre-exposure prophylaxis (PrEP) for an HIV-negative partner until your viral load is undetectable again. Talk to your partner about post-exposure prophylaxis (PEP) if you think they may have had a possible exposure to HIV (e.g., if the condom breaks during sex and you do not have an undetectable viral load).

Taking HIV medicine to maintain an undetectable viral load does not protect you or your partner from getting other sexually transmitted infections (STIs), so talk to your provider about ways to prevent other STIs.

TALK TO YOUR PARTNER

Treatment as prevention can be used alone or in conjunction with other prevention strategies. Talk about your HIV status with your sexual partners and decide together which prevention methods to use. Some states have laws that require you to tell your sexual partner that you have HIV in certain circumstances.[5]

---

[5] HIV.gov, "HIV Treatment as Prevention," U.S. Department of Health and Human Services (HHS), February 1, 2023. Available online. URL: www.hiv.gov/tasp/. Accessed June 13, 2023.

Chapter 35 | Pre-exposure Vaccination for Sexually Transmitted Diseases

Chapter Contents

Section 35.1 | Hepatitis A Vaccine Can Prevent Hepatitis A

WHY GET VACCINATED?

Hepatitis A vaccine can prevent hepatitis A.

Hepatitis A is a serious liver disease. It is usually spread through close, personal contact with an infected person or when a person unknowingly ingests the virus from objects, food, or drinks that are contaminated by small amounts of stool (poop) from an infected person.

Most adults with hepatitis A have symptoms, including fatigue, low appetite, stomach pain, nausea, and jaundice (yellow skin or eyes, dark urine, light-colored bowel movements). Most children less than six years of age do not have symptoms.

A person infected with hepatitis A can transmit the disease to other people even if he or she does not have any symptoms of the disease.

Most people who get hepatitis A feel sick for several weeks, but they usually recover completely and do not have lasting liver damage. In rare cases, hepatitis A can cause liver failure and death; this is more common in people older than 50 years and people with other liver diseases.

The hepatitis A vaccine has made this disease much less common in the United States. However, outbreaks of hepatitis A among unvaccinated people still happen.

DOSAGE OF THE HEPATITIS A VACCINE

Children need two doses of the hepatitis A vaccine:

- first dose: 12–23 months of age
- second dose: at least six months after the first dose

Infants aged 6–11 months traveling outside the United States when protection against hepatitis A is recommended should receive one dose of the hepatitis A vaccine. These children should still get two additional doses at the recommended ages for long-lasting protection.

Older children and adolescents aged 2–18 who were not vaccinated previously should be vaccinated.

Adults who were not vaccinated previously and want to be protected against hepatitis A can also get the vaccine.

The hepatitis A vaccine is also recommended for the following people:

- international travelers
- men who have sexual contact with other men
- people who use injection or non-injection drugs
- people who have occupational risk for infection
- people who anticipate close contact with an international adoptee
- people experiencing homelessness
- people with human immunodeficiency virus (HIV)
- people with chronic liver disease

In addition, a person who has not previously received the hepatitis A vaccine and who has direct contact with someone with hepatitis A should get the hepatitis A vaccine as soon as possible and within two weeks after exposure.

The hepatitis A vaccine may be given at the same time as other vaccines.

TALK WITH YOUR HEALTH-CARE PROVIDER

Tell your vaccination provider if the person getting the vaccine has had an allergic reaction after a previous dose of the hepatitis A vaccine or has any severe, life-threatening allergies.

In some cases, your health-care provider may decide to postpone hepatitis A vaccination until a future visit.

Pregnant or breastfeeding people should be vaccinated if they are at risk for getting hepatitis A. Pregnancy or breastfeeding are not reasons to avoid hepatitis A vaccination.

People with minor illnesses, such as a cold, may be vaccinated. People who are moderately or severely ill should usually wait until they recover before getting the hepatitis A vaccine.

Your health-care provider can give you more information.

RISKS OF A VACCINE REACTION

Soreness or redness where the shot is given, fever, headache, tiredness, or loss of appetite can happen after hepatitis A vaccination.

People sometimes faint after medical procedures, including vaccination. Tell your provider if you feel dizzy or have vision changes or ringing in the ears.

As with any medicine, there is a very remote chance of a vaccine causing a severe allergic reaction, other serious injury, or death.

WHAT IF THERE IS A SERIOUS PROBLEM?

An allergic reaction could occur after the vaccinated person leaves the clinic. If you see signs of a severe allergic reaction (hives, swelling of the face and throat, difficulty breathing, a fast heartbeat, dizziness, or weakness), call 911 and get the person to the nearest hospital.

For other signs that concern you, call your health-care provider.

Adverse reactions should be reported to the Vaccine Adverse Event Reporting System (VAERS). Your health-care provider will usually file this report, or you can do it yourself. Visit the VAERS website (https://vaers.hhs.gov/) or call 800-822-7967. VAERS is only for reporting reactions, and VAERS staff members do not give medical advice.

THE NATIONAL VACCINE INJURY COMPENSATION PROGRAM

The National Vaccine Injury Compensation Program (VICP) is a federal program that was created to compensate people who may have been injured by certain vaccines. Claims regarding alleged injury or death due to vaccination have a time limit for filing, which may be as short as two years. Visit the VICP website (www.hrsa.gov/vaccine-compensation) or call 800-338-2382 to learn about the program and about filing a claim.[1]

---

[1] "Hepatitis A VIS," Centers for Disease Control and Prevention (CDC), October 15, 2021. Available online. URL: www.cdc.gov/vaccines/hcp/vis/vis-statements/hep-a.html. Accessed June 2, 2023.

Section 35.2 | **Hepatitis B Vaccination for All Age Groups**

WHY GET VACCINATED?

Hepatitis B vaccine can prevent hepatitis B. Hepatitis B is a liver disease that can cause mild illness lasting a few weeks, or it can lead to a serious, lifelong illness.

- **Acute hepatitis B**. It is a short-term illness that can lead to fever, fatigue, loss of appetite, nausea, vomiting, jaundice (yellow skin or eyes, dark urine, clay-colored bowel movements), and pain in the muscles, joints, and stomach.
- **Chronic hepatitis B**. It is a long-term illness that occurs when the hepatitis B virus remains in a person's body. Most people who go on to develop chronic hepatitis B do not have symptoms, but it is still very serious and can lead to liver damage (cirrhosis), liver cancer, and death. Chronically infected people can spread hepatitis B virus to others, even if they do not feel or look sick themselves.

Hepatitis B is spread when blood, semen, or other body fluid infected with the hepatitis B virus enters the body of a person who is not infected. People can become infected through:

- birth (If a pregnant person has hepatitis B, their baby can become infected.)
- sharing items such as razors or toothbrushes with an infected person
- contact with the blood or open sores of an infected person
- sex with an infected partner
- sharing needles, syringes, or other drug-injection equipment
- exposure to blood from needlesticks or other sharp instruments

Most people who are vaccinated with hepatitis B vaccine are immune for life.

HEPATITIS B VACCINE

- Hepatitis B vaccine is usually given as 2, 3, or 4 shots.
- Infants should get their first dose of the hepatitis B vaccine at birth and will usually complete the series at 6–18 months of age. The birth dose of the hepatitis B vaccine is an important part of preventing long-term illness in infants and the spread of hepatitis B in the United States.
- Anyone aged 59 or younger who has not yet gotten the vaccine should be vaccinated.
- Hepatitis B vaccination is recommended for adults aged 60 or older at increased risk of exposure to hepatitis B who were not vaccinated previously. Adults aged 60 or older who are not at increased risk and were not vaccinated in the past may also be vaccinated.
- The hepatitis B vaccine may be given as a stand-alone vaccine or as part of a combination vaccine (a type of vaccine that combines more than one vaccine together into one shot).
- The hepatitis B vaccine may be given at the same time as other vaccines.

TALK WITH YOUR HEALTH-CARE PROVIDER

Tell your vaccination provider if the person getting the vaccine has had an allergic reaction after a previous dose of the hepatitis B vaccine or has any severe, life-threatening allergies.

In some cases, your health-care provider may decide to postpone hepatitis B vaccination until a future visit.

Pregnant or breastfeeding people who were not vaccinated previously should be vaccinated. Pregnancy or breastfeeding are not reasons to avoid hepatitis B vaccination.

People with minor illnesses, such as a cold, may be vaccinated. People who are moderately or severely ill should usually wait until they recover before getting the hepatitis B vaccine.

Your health-care provider can give you more information.[2]

---

[2] "Hepatitis B VIS (Interim)," Centers for Disease Control and Prevention (CDC), May 12, 2023. Available online. URL: www.cdc.gov/vaccines/hcp/vis/vis-statements/hep-b.html. Accessed June 2, 2023.

ADULTS ARE RECOMMENDED TO RECEIVE THE HEPATITIS B VACCINE

The Advisory Committee on Immunization Practices (ACIP) recommends that the following people should receive hepatitis B vaccination:

- all infants
- unvaccinated children younger than 19 years of age
- adults aged 19–59
- adults aged 60 and older with risk factors for hepatitis B

The following group may receive hepatitis B vaccination:

- adults aged 60 and older without known risk factors for hepatitis B

Risk factors for hepatitis B are as follows:

- persons at risk of infection by sexual exposure
- sex partners of persons who test positive for hepatitis B surface antigen (HBsAg)
- sexually active persons who are not in a long-term, mutually monogamous relationship (e.g., persons with more than one sex partner during the previous six months)
- persons seeking evaluation or treatment for a sexually transmitted infection (STI)
- men who have sex with men (MSM)
- persons at risk of infection by percutaneous or mucosal exposure to blood
- persons with current or recent injection use
- household contacts of persons who test positive for HBsAg
- residents and staff of facilities for persons with developmental disabilities
- health-care and public safety personnel with reasonably anticipated risk for exposure to blood or blood-contaminated body fluids
- persons on maintenance dialysis, including in-center or home hemodialysis and peritoneal dialysis, and persons who are on predialysis

- persons with diabetes at the discretion of the treating clinician

Other factors for hepatitis B are as follows:
- international travelers to countries with high or intermediate levels of endemic hepatitis B virus (HBV) infection (HBsAg prevalence of 2% or more)
- persons with hepatitis C virus (HCV) infection
- persons with chronic liver disease (including, but not limited to, persons with cirrhosis, fatty liver disease, alcoholic liver disease, autoimmune hepatitis, or an alanine aminotransferase (ALT) or aspartate aminotransferase (AST) level more than twice the upper limit of normal)
- persons with HIV infection
- incarcerated persons

IMPLEMENTATION GUIDELINES

To ensure vaccination of persons at risk of HBV infection, health-care providers should do the following:
- Offer hepatitis B vaccination to all adults aged 19–59 who have not previously completed vaccination, as well as adults aged 60 and older with risk factors for hepatitis B or without identified risk factors but seeking protection.
- Implement standing orders to administer the hepatitis B vaccine as part of routine services to adults who have not completed the vaccine series.
- Offer hepatitis B vaccination, when feasible, in outreach and other settings in which services are provided to persons at risk for HBV infection (e.g., syringe services programs, HIV testing sites, HIV prevention programs, and homeless shelters).[3]

---

[3] "Hepatitis B Vaccination of Adults," Centers for Disease Control and Prevention (CDC), March 28, 2022. Available online. URL: www.cdc.gov/hepatitis/hbv/vaccadults.htm. Accessed June 2, 2023.

Section 35.3 | **Human Papillomavirus Vaccination**

WHY IS THE HUMAN PAPILLOMAVIRUS VACCINE IMPORTANT?

Genital human papillomavirus (HPV) is a common virus that is passed from one person to another through direct skin-to-skin contact during sexual activity. Most sexually active people will get HPV at some time in their lives though most will never even know it. HPV infection is most common in people in their late teens and early 20s. There are about 40 types of HPV that can infect the genital areas of men and women. Most HPV types cause no symptoms and go away on their own. But some types can cause cervical cancer in women and other less common cancers—such as cancers of the anus, penis, vagina, vulva, and oropharynx. Other types of HPV can cause warts in the genital areas of men and women, called "genital warts." Genital warts are not life-threatening. But they can cause emotional stress, and their treatment can be very uncomfortable. Every year, about 12,000 women are diagnosed with cervical cancer, and 4,000 women die from this disease in the United States. About 1 percent of sexually active adults in the United States have visible genital warts at any point in time.

WHICH GIRLS/WOMEN SHOULD RECEIVE HUMAN PAPILLOMAVIRUS VACCINATION?

Human papillomavirus vaccination is recommended for 11- and 12-year-old girls. It is also recommended for girls and women aged 13–26 who have not yet been vaccinated or completed the vaccine series. The HPV vaccine can also be given to girls beginning at age 9. The Centers for Disease Control and Prevention (CDC) recommends 11- and 12-year-olds get two doses of HPV vaccine to protect against cancers caused by HPV.

WILL SEXUALLY ACTIVE FEMALES BENEFIT FROM THE VACCINE?

Ideally, females should get the vaccine before they become sexually active and exposed to HPV. Females who are sexually active may also benefit from vaccination, but they may get less benefit. This is because they may have already been exposed to one or more of the HPV types targeted by the vaccines. However, few sexually active young women are infected with all HPV types prevented by the vaccines, so most young women could still get protection by getting vaccinated.

CAN PREGNANT WOMEN GET THE VACCINE?

The vaccine is not recommended for pregnant women. Studies show that the HPV vaccine does not cause problems for babies born to women who were vaccinated while pregnant, but more research is still needed. A pregnant woman should not get any doses of the HPV vaccine until her pregnancy is completed.

Getting the HPV vaccine when pregnant is not a reason to consider ending a pregnancy. If a woman realizes that she got one or more shots of an HPV vaccine while pregnant, she should do the following two things:

- Wait until after her pregnancy to finish any remaining HPV vaccine doses.
- Call the pregnancy registry (800-986-8999 for Gardasil® and Gardasil® 9 or 888-825-5249 for Cervarix).

SHOULD GIRLS AND WOMEN BE SCREENED FOR CERVICAL CANCER BEFORE GETTING VACCINATED?

Girls and women do not need to get an HPV test or Pap test to find out if they should get the vaccine. However, it is important that women continue to be screened for cervical cancer, even after getting all recommended shots of the HPV vaccine. This is because the vaccine does not protect against all types of cervical cancer.

HOW EFFECTIVE IS THE HUMAN PAPILLOMAVIRUS VACCINE?

The HPV vaccine targets the HPV types that most commonly cause cervical cancer and can cause some cancers of the vulva, vagina, anus, and oropharynx. It also protects against the HPV types that cause most genital warts. The HPV vaccine is highly effective in preventing the targeted HPV types, as well as the most common health problems caused by them.

The vaccine is less effective in preventing HPV-related disease in young women who have already been exposed to one or more HPV types. That is because the vaccine prevents HPV before a person is exposed to it. The HPV vaccine does not treat existing HPV infections or HPV-associated diseases.

HOW LONG DOES VACCINE PROTECTION LAST?

Research suggests that vaccine protection is long-lasting. Current studies have followed vaccinated individuals for 10 years and show that there is no evidence of weakened protection over time.

WHAT DOES THE VACCINE NOT PROTECT AGAINST?

The vaccine does not protect against all HPV types—so it will not prevent all cases of cervical cancer. Since some cervical cancers will not be prevented by the vaccine, it will be important for women to continue getting screened for cervical cancer. Also, the vaccine does not prevent other sexually transmitted infections (STIs). So it will still be important for sexually active persons to lower their risk for other STIs.

HOW SAFE IS THE HUMAN PAPILLOMAVIRUS VACCINE?

The HPV vaccine has been licensed by the U.S. Food and Drug Administration (FDA). The CDC has approved this vaccine as safe and effective. The vaccine was studied in thousands of people around the world, and these studies showed no serious safety concerns. Side effects reported in these studies were mild, including pain where the shot was given, fever, dizziness, and nausea. Vaccine safety continues to be monitored by the CDC and the FDA. More than 60 million doses of HPV vaccine have been distributed in the United States as of March 2014.

Fainting, which can occur after any medical procedure, has also been noted after HPV vaccination. Fainting after any vaccination is more common in adolescents. Because fainting can cause falls and injuries, adolescents and adults should be seated or lying down during HPV vaccination. Sitting or lying down for about 15 minutes after a vaccination can help prevent fainting and injuries.

WHY IS HUMAN PAPILLOMAVIRUS VACCINATION ONLY RECOMMENDED FOR WOMEN THROUGH AGE 26?

Human papillomavirus vaccination is not currently recommended for women over 26 years of age. Clinical trials showed that overall, HPV vaccination offered women limited or no protection against HPV-related diseases. For women over 26 years of age, the best way to prevent cervical cancer is to get routine cervical cancer screening, as recommended.

WHAT ABOUT VACCINATING BOYS AND MEN?

The HPV vaccine is licensed for use in boys and men. It has been found to be safe and effective for males 9 26 years. The Advisory Committee on Immunization Practices (ACIP) recommends routine vaccination of boys aged 11 or 12 with a series of doses. The vaccination series can be started beginning at age nine. Vaccination is recommended for males aged 13–21 who have not already been vaccinated or who have not received all recommended doses. The vaccine is most effective when given at younger ages; males aged 22–26 may be vaccinated. The CDC recommends 11- and 12-year-olds get two doses of the HPV vaccine to protect against cancers caused by HPV.

IS HUMAN PAPILLOMAVIRUS VACCINE COVERED BY INSURANCE PLANS?

Health insurance plans cover the cost of HPV vaccines. If you do not have insurance, the Vaccines for Children (VFC) program may be able to help.

HOW CAN YOU GET HELP TO PAY FOR HUMAN PAPILLOMAVIRUS VACCINE?

The Vaccines for Children (VFC) program helps families of eligible children who might not otherwise have access to vaccines. The program provides vaccines at no cost to doctors who serve eligible children. Children younger than 19 years of age are eligible for VFC vaccines if they are Medicaid-eligible, American Indian, or Alaska Native or have no health insurance. "Underinsured" children who have health insurance that does not cover vaccination can receive VFC vaccines through Federally Qualified Health Centers (FQHCs) or Rural Health Centers (RHCs). Parents of uninsured or underinsured children who receive vaccines at no cost through the VFC program should check with their health-care providers about possible administration fees that might apply. These fees help providers cover the costs that result from important services such as storing the vaccines and paying staff members to give vaccines to patients. However, VFC vaccines cannot be denied to an eligible child if a family cannot afford the fee.

WHAT VACCINATED GIRLS/WOMEN NEED TO KNOW: WILL GIRLS/WOMEN WHO HAVE BEEN VACCINATED STILL NEED CERVICAL CANCER SCREENING?

Yes, vaccinated women will still need regular cervical cancer screening because the vaccine protects against most but not all HPV types that cause cervical cancer. Also, women who got the vaccine after becoming sexually active may not get the full benefit of the vaccine if they have already been exposed to HPV.

ARE THERE OTHER WAYS TO PREVENT CERVICAL CANCER?

Regular cervical cancer screening (Pap and HPV tests) and follow-up can prevent most cases of cervical cancer. The Pap test can detect cell changes in the cervix before they turn into cancer. The HPV test looks for the virus that can cause these cell changes. Screening can detect most, but not all, cervical cancers at an early, treatable stage. Most women diagnosed with cervical cancer in the United States have either never been screened or have not been screened in the past five years.

ARE THERE OTHER WAYS TO PREVENT HUMAN PAPILLOMAVIRUS?

For those who are sexually active, condoms may lower the chances of getting HPV if used with every sex act from start to finish. Condoms may also lower the risk of developing HPV-related diseases (genital warts and cervical cancer). But HPV can infect areas that are not covered by a condom—so condoms may not fully protect against HPV.

People can also lower their chances of getting HPV by being in a faithful relationship with one partner, limiting their number of sex partners, and choosing a partner who has had no or few prior sex partners. But even people with only one lifetime sex partner can get HPV. And it may not be possible to determine if a partner who has been sexually active in the past is currently infected. That is why the only sure way to prevent HPV is to avoid all sexual activities.[4]

Section 35.4 | How Close Are We to an Effective Human Immunodeficiency Virus Vaccine?

PROGRESS TOWARD A HUMAN IMMUNODEFICIENCY VIRUS VACCINE

The development of a safe, effective, preventive human immunodeficiency virus (HIV) vaccine remains key to realizing a durable end to the HIV/acquired immunodeficiency syndrome (AIDS) pandemic. The National Institute of Allergy and Infectious Diseases (NIAID) and its global partners are pursuing numerous research strategies to develop next-generation vaccine candidates.

Developing a Human Immunodeficiency Virus Vaccine Is Challenging

HIV mutates rapidly and has unique ways of evading the immune system. Most vaccines do the following:

- **Mimic the immune responses of recovered patients.** There are no documented cases of a person living with HIV developing an immune response that clears

---

[4] "HPV Vaccine Information for Young Women," Centers for Disease Control and Prevention (CDC), April 18, 2022. Available online. URL: www.cdc.gov/std/hpv/stdfact-hpv-vaccine-young-women.htm. Accessed June 5, 2023.

the infection. Researchers are working to define and understand the responses that may protect against HIV.

- **Are inactivated or weakened viruses**. Inactivated HIV was not effective at eliciting immune responses in clinical trials. A live form of HIV is too dangerous to use.
- **Are effective against pathogens that are rarely encountered**. People in high-risk groups might be exposed to HIV daily.

WE HAVE MADE PROGRESS

Results from the landmark RV144 clinical trial in Thailand, reported in 2009, provided the first signal of the HIV vaccine efficacy, a 31 percent reduction in HIV infection among vaccinees. RV144 evaluated the safety and efficacy of a prime-boost combination of two vaccine components given in sequence: one using a harmless virus as a vector—or carrier—to deliver HIV genes and a second containing a protein found on the HIV surface.

Broadly neutralizing antibodies (bNAbs) can stop many HIV strains from infecting human cells in the laboratory. A minority of people living with HIV naturally produce bNAbs but usually too late after infection to overcome the virus. Researchers have isolated bNAbs from the blood of people living with HIV and are studying them in detail in an effort to design novel vaccine candidates.

WE ARE WORKING TO DO MORE

To build on this progress, the NIAID is pursuing two general approaches, each of which has many components. Numerous investigational vaccines are at different stages of development.

- basic and preclinical research
- manufacture of vaccines for human testing
- clinical trials to test for safety and efficacy in humans

Scientists are developing novel prime-boost regimens that elicit strong, long-lasting protective immune responses.

- The Pox-Protein Public-Private Partnership, or P5, comprises organizations, including the NIAID, working to build on the modest success of RV144 and increase understanding of the immune responses linked to protection against an HIV infection.
- Scientists are developing improved vectors that deliver HIV genes to host cells, resulting in the production of HIV proteins, and trigger anti-HIV immune responses. In the Imbokodo vaccine efficacy trial, researchers are evaluating a prime-boost regimen that includes mosaic antigens created from genes from many HIV variants.
- Researchers are working to determine how adjuvants—vaccine components that enhance antigen-specific immune responses—affect the potency, durability, and other aspects of vaccine-induced immunity.
- Scientists are working to harness the potential of bNAbs to protect HIV negative people from acquiring HIV.
  - Scientists are studying the design and delivery of antigens—vaccine components that stimulate specific immune responses—to develop vaccine candidates that may induce HIV-negative people's immune systems to make bNAbs.
  - Passive immunization involves giving injections or intravenous infusions of bNAbs as an HIV prevention strategy. The ongoing antibody-mediated prevention (AMP) studies aim to determine whether giving HIV-negative people bNAb infusions is safe, tolerable, and effective at preventing HIV infection.
  - Researchers are also investigating vectored immunoprophylaxis, which involves injecting a vector containing bNAb genes to produce antibodies that may prevent HIV infection.[5]

---

[5] "Progress towards an HIV Vaccine," National Institute of Allergy and Infectious Diseases (NIAID), June 22, 2018. Available online. URL: www.niaid.nih.gov/sites/default/files/hivvaccineinfographic.pdf. Accessed June 5, 2023.

A THEORETICAL APPROACH TO HUMAN IMMUNODEFICIENCY VIRUS VACCINE DEVELOPMENT

This approach to developing an HIV vaccine is based on theory and involves establishing an understanding of the immune response to HIV infection and finding ways to generate and enhance that response through vaccination. Some strategies aim to prevent HIV infection via antibodies, while others strive to generate a protective cellular response.

DESIGNING AN ANTIBODY-BASED HUMAN IMMUNODEFICIENCY VIRUS VACCINE

No one with HIV has ever developed an immune response that cleared the infection, so scientists do not yet know what constitutes an effective immune response to the virus. However, researchers have observed that some people living with HIV naturally develop bNAbs against the virus after months or years of infection. These bNAbs have been shown in the laboratory to stop most HIV strains from infecting human cells. They do not eradicate the virus from people living with HIV, however, because by the time a bNAb appears in a mature form, HIV has proliferated and mutated to escape neutralization by that antibody. But, if a vaccine could generate bNAbs in healthy people before exposure to HIV, the antibodies potentially could fight the virus off completely.

Numerous studies by NIAID scientists, grantees, and others have provided evidence that a vaccine eliciting bNAbs might protect people from HIV. First, researchers have shown that infusing bNAbs into monkeys protects them from infection by a human-monkey hybrid virus similar to HIV. Second, clinical studies have demonstrated that infusing bNAbs into people living with HIV reduces the amount of virus circulating in their blood. Third, laboratory studies have shown that bNAbs markedly suppress HIV production from infected immune cells where the virus hides in the body.

To directly test the hypothesis that bNAbs can prevent HIV infection, a pair of large, multinational, NIAID-funded clinical trials launched in the spring of 2016, called the AMP studies, are giving intravenous infusions of bNAbs to healthy adults at high risk for HIV to see if that protects them from the virus.

One of the first potent bNAbs to be discovered, VRC01, was identified and isolated by scientists at the NIAID Vaccine Research Center (VRC) in 2010. Since that time, researchers have isolated hundreds of other bNAbs, and many scientists have embarked on projects to reverse-engineer an HIV vaccine that elicits one of these antibodies. The basic process involves identifying the site where a bNAb binds to the virus, characterizing the molecular structure of that site in detail, designing a protein replica of the binding site, and testing the replica, called an "immunogen," in animals and people to see if it elicits the desired bNAb.

In 2018, VRC scientists reported that a vaccine based on the fusion peptide—a vulnerable site on HIV that helps the virus fuse with a cell to infect it—elicited neutralizing antibodies in mice, guinea pigs, and monkeys. VRC scientists first identified the fusion peptide target in 2016 and considered it particularly promising for use as a vaccine because its sequence is the same across most strains of HIV, it is exposed on the spike on HIV's surface, it lacks the sugars that obscure the immune system's view of other sites on the virus's outer shell, and the immune system makes a strong response to it. The experimental vaccine includes a portion of the fusion peptide bonded to a carrier that evokes a strong immune response. This immunogen is paired with a replica of the spike on HIV's surface. The scientists are working to optimize the vaccine and ultimately aim to manufacture a version of it suitable for safety testing in human volunteers in a carefully designed and monitored clinical trial.

One of the signature characteristics of powerful HIV bNAbs is that they mutate dozens of times before achieving their mature HIV-fighting form. This means eliciting such antibodies through vaccination likely would involve an initial vaccine to kick-start bNAb development followed by a series of vaccinations to coax the bNAb along the desired developmental pathway. A 2011 VRC-led study of antibody genetics enabled scientists to deduce the step-by-step evolution of VRC01 and related antibodies. Moreover, studies by VRC scientists and NIAID grantees have revealed how bNAbs and HIV stimulate each other to evolve, shedding light on the necessary structures of the initial and intermediate immunogens of an HIV vaccine regimen that would generate a nascent bNAb and coax it to mature. A 2015 trio of animal studies by NIAID grantees provided evidence that such a strategy could generate the desired antibody response.

A related approach to creating an HIV vaccine is to elicit a variety of HIV antibodies, each of which neutralizes only a modest variety of HIV strains but together neutralize a wide range. This strategy is attractive because some modestly neutralizing antibodies have a much shorter developmental pathway than bNAbs, thus requiring far fewer immunogens.

UNDERSTANDING HUMAN IMMUNODEFICIENCY VIRUS STRUCTURE

Broadly neutralizing antibodies bind mainly to five unchanging sites located on spikes on HIV's surface. These spikes are known as the "envelope glycoprotein" (Env). Each spike is composed of three identical pairs of proteins, collectively called the "trimer." Many attempts to immunize against HIV used just one segment of the trimer, yielding suboptimal results. Eventually, it became clear that the whole trimer would be a more effective immunogen. However, Env is extremely difficult to stabilize as a stand-alone molecule separate from HIV. So it was a major advance when, in 2013, NIAID grantees engineered a more stable form of Env and obtained an atomic-level image of it.

The following year, a study co-led by National Institutes of Health (NIH) scientists discovered that an HIV vaccine that teaches the immune system to neutralize the virus should be based on the configuration Env takes before it fuses with a cell. VRC researchers produced a high-resolution structural model of this pre-fusion viral spike, a valuable tool for HIV immunogen design. Furthermore, studies by NIAID grantees have demonstrated that it is possible to immunize animals with HIV trimer proteins and to modify Env immunogens, so they stimulate the production of the earliest precursors of particular bNAbs. Such experimental structure-based vaccines are currently being evaluated in early-stage clinical trials at the NIAID and elsewhere.

Structural studies by VRC scientists led to the 2016 discovery of the fusion peptide as a vaccine target. The scientists characterized in atomic-level detail how a bNAb isolated from the blood of a person living with HIV binds to the fusion peptide and stops the virus from infecting a cell. These insights led to the development of a fusion peptide-based vaccine that can elicit neutralizing antibodies in animal models.

DESIGNING A CELL-BASED HUMAN IMMUNODEFICIENCY VIRUS VACCINE

An alternative theoretical approach to HIV vaccine design aims to elicit a potent cell-based immune response rather than an antibody response. Some NIAID grantees pursuing this strategy aim to elicit cellular immune responses to the most static regions of HIV's proteins by creating vaccine components focused solely on these regions. In contrast, other grantees strive to elicit cellular immune responses using so-called mosaic antigens, which are computationally derived proteins created by stitching together genetic sequences from across the whole HIV genome.

Taking a different tack, another NIAID grantee pursuing a cell-based response to HIV created an immunogen by placing selected HIV genes into an unrelated virus called "cytomegalovirus" (CMV). Most people naturally acquire CMV, which usually does not cause any symptoms in healthy adults and which persists in the body at very low levels yet garners a large immune response as T-cells armed to fight the virus circulate in high numbers in the blood. In a preliminary test of this approach, monkeys infected with simian immunodeficiency virus (SIV), the simian form of HIV, were vaccinated with a monkey version of the CMV immunogen. More than half of the vaccinated animals completely controlled SIV and ultimately eliminated it from their bodies within a year or two, marking the first time an immune response cleared an AIDS-causing virus. Scientists are still investigating how this vaccine works at the cellular and molecular levels, and clinical trials are awaiting the selection and manufacture of a final vaccine candidate.[6]

---

[6] "A Theoretical Approach to HIV Vaccine Development," National Institute of Allergy and Infectious Diseases (NIAID), May 15, 2019. Available online. URL: www.niaid.nih.gov/diseases-conditions/theoretical-approach. Accessed June 5, 2023.

Chapter 36 |
Preventing Perinatal Transmission of Human Immunodeficiency Virus

WHAT IS PERINATAL TRANSMISSION OF HUMAN IMMUNODEFICIENCY VIRUS?

Perinatal transmission of human immunodeficiency virus (HIV) is when HIV is passed from a woman with HIV to her child during pregnancy, childbirth (also called "labor and delivery"), or breastfeeding (through breast milk). Perinatal transmission of HIV is also called "mother-to-child transmission of HIV."

The use of HIV medicines and other strategies have helped lower the rate of perinatal transmission of HIV to 1 percent or less in the United States and Europe. (HIV medicines are called "antiretrovirals.")[1]

CAN A PREGNANT PERSON TRANSMIT HUMAN IMMUNODEFICIENCY VIRUS TO THEIR BABY?

Yes, however, treatment with a combination of HIV medicines (called "antiretroviral therapy" (ART)) can prevent transmission of HIV to your baby and protect your health.

[1] HIVinfo, "Preventing Perinatal Transmission of HIV," U.S. Department of Health and Human Services (HHS), January 31, 2023. Available online. URL: https://hivinfo.nih.gov/understanding-hiv/fact-sheets/preventing-perinatal-transmission-hiv. Accessed June 14, 2023.

HOW CAN YOU PREVENT TRANSMITTING HUMAN IMMUNODEFICIENCY VIRUS TO YOUR BABY?

If you have HIV, the following are a few steps you can take to reduce your risk of transmitting HIV to your baby.

Get Tested for Human Immunodeficiency Virus as Soon as Possible to Know Your Status

- If you are pregnant or planning to get pregnant, get tested for HIV as early as possible during each pregnancy. Knowing your HIV status gives you powerful information.
- If you learn you have HIV, the sooner you start treatment, the better—for your health and your baby's health and to prevent transmitting HIV to your partner.
- If you learn you do not have HIV but are at increased risk of acquiring it, get tested again in your third trimester.
- Know your HIV status. Encourage your partner to get tested for HIV.

Human Immunodeficiency Virus–Negative but at Risk? Take Medicine to Prevent Human Immunodeficiency Virus

- If you have a partner with HIV and you are considering getting pregnant, talk to your health-care provider about pre-exposure prophylaxis (PrEP).
- PrEP is medicine people at risk for HIV take to prevent getting HIV from sex or injection drug use. PrEP can stop HIV from taking hold and spreading throughout your body.
- PrEP may be an option to help protect you and your baby from getting HIV while you try to get pregnant, during pregnancy, or while breastfeeding. Find out if PrEP is right for you.
- If your partner has HIV, also encourage them to get and stay on HIV medicine. This will keep them healthy and help prevent them from transmitting HIV to you.

Human Immunodeficiency Virus–Positive? Take Medicine to Treat Human Immunodeficiency Virus

- Taking HIV medicine reduces the amount of HIV in your body (your viral load) to a very low level, called "viral suppression." If your viral load is so low that a standard lab test cannot detect it, this is called having an "undetectable viral load." Taking HIV medicine and getting and keeping an undetectable viral load is the best thing you can do to stay healthy and prevent transmission to your baby.
- If you have HIV and take HIV medicine as prescribed throughout your pregnancy and childbirth and give HIV medicine to your baby for two to six weeks after giving birth, your risk of transmitting HIV to your baby can be less than 1 percent.
- As long as your viral load remains undetectable, you can have a normal delivery.
- Taking HIV medicine reduces the risk of transmitting HIV to your baby through breastfeeding to less than 1 percent. However, the risk is not zero.
- Taking HIV medicine also protects your HIV-negative partner. People with HIV who take HIV medicine as prescribed and get and keep an undetectable viral load can live long and healthy lives and will not transmit HIV to their HIV-negative partners through sex.[2]

HOW DO HUMAN IMMUNODEFICIENCY VIRUS MEDICINES PREVENT PERINATAL TRANSMISSION OF HUMAN IMMUNODEFICIENCY VIRUS?

Pregnant women with HIV should take HIV medicines to reduce the risk of perinatal transmission of HIV. When started early, HIV medicines can be more effective at preventing perinatal transmission of HIV. Women with HIV who are trying to conceive should start HIV medicines before they become pregnant to prevent

---

[2] HIV.gov, "Preventing Perinatal Transmission of HIV," U.S. Department of Health and Human Services (HHS), April 10, 2023. Available online. URL: www.hiv.gov/hiv-basics/hiv-prevention/reducing-mother-to-child-risk/preventing-mother-to-child-transmission-of-hiv. Accessed June 14, 2023.

perinatal transmission of HIV. Pregnant women with HIV should take HIV medicines throughout pregnancy and childbirth to prevent perinatal transmission of HIV. HIV medicines also protect the woman's health.

HIV medicines, when taken as prescribed, prevent HIV from multiplying and reduce the amount of HIV in the body (called the "viral load"). An undetectable viral load is when the level of HIV in the blood is too low to be detected by a viral load test. The risk of perinatal transmission of HIV during pregnancy and childbirth is lowest when a woman with HIV has an undetectable viral load. Maintaining an undetectable viral load also helps keep the mother-to-be healthy.

Some HIV medicines used during pregnancy that pass from the pregnant woman to her unborn baby through cesarean delivery (sometimes called a "C-section") can reduce the risk of perinatal transmission of HIV in women who have a high viral load (more than 1,000 copies/mL) or an unknown viral load near the time of delivery.

After birth, babies born to women with HIV receive HIV medicines to reduce the risk of perinatal transmission of HIV. Several factors determine what HIV medicines babies receive and how long they receive the medicines.

ARE HUMAN IMMUNODEFICIENCY VIRUS MEDICINES SAFE TO USE DURING PREGNANCY?

Most HIV medicines are safe to use during pregnancy. In general, HIV medicines do not increase the risk of birth defects. Health-care providers discuss the benefits and risks of specific HIV medicines when helping women with HIV decide which HIV medicines to use during pregnancy or while they are trying to conceive.[3]

CAN YOU BREASTFEED IF YOU HAVE HUMAN IMMUNODEFICIENCY VIRUS?

The current recommendation in the United States supports shared decision-making between you and your health-care provider

---

[3] See footnote [1].

regarding infant feeding. Taking HIV medicine and keeping an undetectable viral load substantially decreases your risk of transmitting HIV to your baby through breastfeeding to less than 1 percent. However, the risk is not zero. Properly prepared infant formula or banked donor human breast milk are alternative options that eliminate the risk of transmission through breastfeeding. If you are pregnant or thinking of becoming pregnant, talk to your health-care provider as early as possible about what infant feeding choice is right for you.[4]

ARE THERE OTHER WAYS TO PREVENT PERINATAL TRANSMISSION OF HUMAN IMMUNODEFICIENCY VIRUS?

Pregnant women with HIV are encouraged to talk to their medical team about options for feeding their baby after birth. With consistent use of HIV medication and an undetectable viral load during pregnancy and throughout breastfeeding, the risk of transmission to a breastfed baby is low: less than 1 percent, but not zero. Alternatively, properly prepared formula and pasteurized donor human milk from a milk bank are options that eliminate the risk of transmission to a baby after birth. Pregnant women with HIV can speak with their health-care provider to determine what method of feeding their baby is right for them.

Additionally, babies should not eat food that was pre-chewed by a person with HIV.[5]

WHAT SHOULD YOU ASK YOUR HEALTH-CARE PROVIDER ABOUT HAVING A BABY?

You might ask your health-care provider some of these questions:
- What is the safest way to conceive?
- Will HIV cause problems for me during pregnancy or delivery?
- Will my HIV treatment cause problems for my baby?

---

[4] See footnote [2].
[5] See footnote [1].

- What are the pros and cons of taking HIV medicine while I am pregnant?
- What infant feeding option is the best choice for me and my baby?
- Is my viral load undetectable?
- How do I avoid transmitting HIV to my partner(s), surrogate, or baby during conception, pregnancy, and delivery?
- What medical and community programs and support groups can help me and my baby?
- What birth control methods are best for me?

Adopting a baby is also an option for people who want to begin or expand their families. The Americans with Disabilities Act (ADA) does not allow adoption agencies to discriminate against individuals or couples with HIV.[6]

---

[6] See footnote [2].

Chapter 37 | **Pre- and Post-exposure Prophylaxis**

WHAT IS PRE-EXPOSURE PROPHYLAXIS?

The word "prophylaxis" means to prevent or control the spread of an infection or disease.

Pre-exposure prophylaxis (PrEP) is when people who do not have human immunodeficiency virus (HIV) but are at risk of getting HIV take HIV medicine every day to prevent HIV infection. PrEP is used by people without HIV who are at risk of being exposed to HIV through sex or injection drug use.

Two HIV medicines are approved by the U.S. Food and Drug Administration (FDA) for use as PrEP: Truvada and Descovy. Which medicine to use for PrEP depends on a person's individual situation.

If a person is exposed to HIV through sex or injection drug use, having the PrEP medicine in the bloodstream can stop HIV from taking hold and spreading throughout the body. However, if PrEP is not taken every day, there may not be enough medicine in the bloodstream to block the virus.

WHO SHOULD CONSIDER TAKING PRE-EXPOSURE PROPHYLAXIS?

Pre-exposure prophylaxis is for people who do not have HIV but are at risk of getting HIV through sex or injection drug use.

Specifically, the Centers for Disease Control and Prevention (CDC) recommends that PrEP be considered for people who are

HIV-negative and who have had anal or vaginal sex in the past six months and:

- have a sexual partner with HIV (especially if the partner has an unknown or detectable viral load)
- have not consistently used a condom
- have been diagnosed with a sexually transmitted disease (STD) in the past six months

PrEP is also recommended for people without HIV who inject drugs and:

- have an injection partner with HIV
- share needles, syringes, or other equipment to inject drugs

PrEP should also be considered for people without HIV who have been prescribed nonoccupational post-exposure prophylaxis (nPEP) and:

- report continued risk behavior
- have used multiple courses of post-exposure prophylaxis (PEP)

If you think PrEP may be right for you, talk to your health-care provider.

HOW WELL DOES PRE-EXPOSURE PROPHYLAXIS WORK?

Pre-exposure prophylaxis is most effective when taken consistently each day. The CDC reports that studies on PrEP effectiveness have shown that consistent use of PrEP reduces the risk of getting HIV from sex by about 99 percent and from injection drug use by at least 74 percent. Adding other prevention methods, such as condom use, along with PrEP can further reduce a person's risk of getting HIV.

DOES PRE-EXPOSURE PROPHYLAXIS CAUSE SIDE EFFECTS?

In some people, PrEP can cause side effects, such as nausea. These side effects are not serious and generally go away over time. If you are taking PrEP, tell your health-care provider if you have any side effect that bothers you or that does not go away.

WHAT SHOULD A PERSON DO IF THEY THINK THAT PRE-EXPOSURE PROPHYLAXIS CAN HELP THEM?

If you think PrEP may be right for you, see a health-care provider. PrEP can be prescribed only by a health-care provider. If your health-care provider agrees that PrEP may reduce your risk of getting HIV, the next step is an HIV test. You must be HIV-negative to start PrEP.

WHAT HAPPENS ONCE A PERSON STARTS PRE-EXPOSURE PROPHYLAXIS?

Once you start PrEP, you will need to take PrEP every day. PrEP is much less effective when it is not taken every day.

Continue to use condoms while taking PrEP. Even though daily PrEP can greatly reduce your risk of HIV, it does not protect against other STDs, such as gonorrhea and chlamydia. Combining condom use with PrEP will further reduce your risk of HIV, as well as protect you from other STDs.

You must also take an HIV test every three months while taking PrEP, so you will have regular follow-up visits with your health-care provider. If you are having trouble taking PrEP every day or if you want to stop taking PrEP, talk to your health-care provider.[1]

WHAT IS POST-EXPOSURE PROPHYLAXIS?

Post-exposure prophylaxis means taking HIV medicines within 72 hours (three days) after possible exposure to HIV to prevent HIV infection.

PEP should be used only in emergency situations. It is not meant for regular use by people who may be exposed to HIV frequently. PEP is not intended to replace the regular use of other HIV prevention methods, such as the consistent use of condoms during sex or PrEP. PrEP is different from PEP in that people at risk for HIV take a specific HIV medicine daily to prevent getting HIV.

---

[1] HIVinfo, "Pre-exposure Prophylaxis (PrEP)," U.S. Department of Health and Human Services (HHS), August 10, 2021. Available online. URL: https://hivinfo.nih.gov/understanding-hiv/fact-sheets/pre-exposure-prophylaxis-prep. Accessed May 29, 2023.

WHO SHOULD CONSIDER TAKING POST-EXPOSURE PROPHYLAXIS?

Post-exposure prophylaxis may be prescribed for people who are HIV-negative or do not know their HIV status and who in the last 72 hours:

- may have been exposed to HIV during sex
- have shared needles or other equipment (works) to inject drugs
- are sexually assaulted
- may have been exposed to HIV at work

If you think you were recently exposed to HIV, talk to your health-care provider or an emergency room doctor about PEP right away.

A health-care worker who has possible exposure to HIV should seek medical attention immediately.

WHEN SHOULD POST-EXPOSURE PROPHYLAXIS BE STARTED?

Post-exposure prophylaxis must be started within 72 hours (three days) after possible exposure to HIV. The sooner PEP is started after possible HIV exposure, the better. According to research, PEP will most likely not prevent HIV infection if it is started more than 72 hours after a person is exposed to HIV.

If you are prescribed PEP, you will need to take the HIV medicines every day for 28 days.

WHAT HUMAN IMMUNODEFICIENCY VIRUS MEDICINES ARE USED FOR POST-EXPOSURE PROPHYLAXIS?

The Centers for Disease Control and Prevention (CDC) provides guidelines on recommended HIV medicines for PEP. The CDC guidelines include recommendations for specific groups of people, including adults and adolescents, children, pregnant women, and people with kidney problems. The PEP recommendations can be found on the CDC's PEP resources (www.cdc.gov/hiv/risk/pep/).

Your health-care provider or emergency room doctor will work with you to determine which medicines to take for PEP.

HOW WELL DOES POST-EXPOSURE PROPHYLAXIS WORK?

Post-exposure prophylaxis is effective in preventing HIV infection when it is taken correctly, but it is not 100 percent effective. The sooner PEP is started after possible HIV exposure, the better. Every hour counts. While taking PEP, it is important to keep using other HIV prevention methods, such as using condoms with sex partners and using only new, sterile needles when injecting drugs.

DOES POST-EXPOSURE PROPHYLAXIS CAUSE SIDE EFFECTS?

The HIV medicines used for PEP may cause side effects in some people. The side effects can be treated and are not life-threatening. If you are taking PEP, talk to your health-care provider if you have any side effect that bothers you or that does not go away.[2]

---

[2] HIVinfo, "Post-exposure Prophylaxis (PEP)," U.S. Department of Health and Human Services (HHS), August 19, 2021. Available online. URL: https://hivinfo.nih.gov/understanding-hiv/fact-sheets/post-exposure-prophylaxis-pep. Accessed May 29, 2023.

Chapter 38 | Microbicides in Topical Prevention of Sexually Transmitted Diseases

WHAT ARE MICROBICIDES?

Microbicides are experimental products that could be applied to or inserted into the vagina or rectum to safely prevent human immunodeficiency virus (HIV) acquisition. A microbicide would deliver an anti-HIV drug to the mucus membranes lining the surface of the vagina or rectum through materials such as vaginal rings, gels, films, inserts, suppositories, foams, or enemas. A safe, effective, desirable, and affordable microbicide against HIV would expand the number of biomedical HIV prevention options available. That is why researchers are working to develop them. But none are on the market yet.

CAN MICROBICIDES PREVENT HUMAN IMMUNODEFICIENCY VIRUS?

Research studies have shown that some microbicides do offer a modest level of protection against getting HIV.

For example, several large-scale research studies over the past decade have investigated the safety and effectiveness of long-acting vaginal rings that continuously release one or more antiretroviral drugs over time. The ring at the most advanced stage of research is the monthly dapivirine ring, which was tested in two large clinical trials, including A Specialized Platform for Innovative Research Exploration (ASPIRE) study funded by the National Institutes of Health (NIH). This study and another trial called "The Ring Study" found that the dapivirine ring reduced the risk of HIV acquisition by roughly 30 percent overall in women aged 18–45 and was well-tolerated.

The European Medicines Agency (EMA) adopted a positive scientific opinion on the monthly dapivirine vaginal ring in 2020, and the World Health Organization (WHO) subsequently recommended the ring as part of combination prevention approaches for women at substantial risk of acquiring HIV, representing even further progress. If approved by national regulatory agencies, the monthly ring would provide women with a discreet, long-acting HIV prevention option that they can control.

The NIH is also supporting three studies to examine the safety of the monthly dapivirine ring during adolescence and pregnancy when the risk of HIV acquisition is heightened and during periods of breastfeeding when transmission to infants may occur. Researchers are also evaluating a 90-day dapivirine ring.

Other studies are examining potential rectal microbicide gels to reduce the risk of HIV transmission through anal sex. Some of these studies are testing microbicides originally formulated for vaginal use to determine if they are safe, effective, and acceptable when used in the rectum; others focus on the development of products designed specifically for rectal use.

WHY ARE MICROBICIDES IMPORTANT?

The only currently licensed biomedical HIV prevention method is a daily pill taken orally for pre-exposure prophylaxis (PrEP). Oral PrEP is safe and highly effective when taken daily as prescribed. However, a daily pill can be challenging for some people to take, so other forms of biomedical HIV prevention, such as microbicides, are being explored.

For some women, microbicides may offer certain benefits. For example, some women may find microbicides preferable to condoms as an HIV prevention option because women would not have to negotiate their use with a sexual partner. Given that women and girls are at particularly high risk for HIV in many parts of the world, it is especially important to have an effective, desirable, woman-initiated HIV prevention tool. In the future, it may also be possible to formulate products that combine HIV prevention with contraception.

Rectal microbicides would also offer another HIV prevention option for men or women who engage in anal sex.

ARE MICROBICIDES AVAILABLE TO THE PUBLIC?

No microbicide for HIV prevention has received regulatory approval to be marketed yet. However, the International Partnership for Microbicides (IPM), which developed the monthly dapivirine vaginal ring, has applied for regulatory review of the product in countries in eastern and southern Africa, where HIV incidence among women remains high, and in the United States. Meanwhile, research on other formulations and forms of microbicides continues.

For now, available forms of protection against the sexual transmission of HIV continue to be:

- treatment as prevention (a highly effective strategy in which people with HIV take antiretroviral therapy (ART) as prescribed to achieve an undetectable viral load, which prevents the transmission of HIV to their sexual partners)
- daily oral PrEP
- voluntary medical male circumcision
- HIV testing—so that you know your and your partner's HIV status
- using condoms consistently and correctly
- choosing sexual behaviors that have lower risk of HIV transmission
- reducing the number of people you have sex with

The more of these actions you take, the safer you will be.[1]

---

[1] HIV.gov, "Microbicides," U.S. Department of Health and Human Services (HHS), June 16, 2021. Available online. URL: www.hiv.gov/hiv-basics/hiv-prevention/potential-future-options/microbicides. Accessed July 18, 2023.

Chapter 39 |
Effective Sexually Transmitted Diseases Prevention Programs

Chapter Contents

Section 39.1 | Family Interventions

Talk with your teen about how to prevent sexually transmitted diseases (STDs)—even if you do not think your teen is sexually active.

If talking about sex and STDs with your teen makes you nervous, you are not alone. It can be hard to know where to start. But it is important to make sure your teen knows how to stay safe.

HOW DO YOU TALK WITH YOUR TEEN?

Use these tips to help you talk to your teen about preventing STDs:
- think about what you want to say ahead of time
- be honest about how you feel
- try not to give your teen too much information at once
- use examples to start a conversation
- talk while you are doing something together
- get ideas from other parents

You can also ask your child's doctor to talk with your teen about preventing STDs. This is called "STD prevention counscling."

WHY DO YOU NEED TO TALK WITH YOUR TEEN?

All teens can use accurate information about how to prevent STDs. Teens whose parents talk with them about sex and how to prevent STDs are not more likely to have sex. But they are more likely to make healthy choices about sex when they are older.

In fact, teens say that their parents have a bigger influence on their decisions about sex than the media, their siblings, or their friends.

When Young People Are More Likely to Get Sexually Transmitted Diseases

More than half of all STD cases in the United States happen in young people aged 15–24 years. Teens are at a higher risk than adults of getting STDs for several reasons. For example, they may:
- not know they need tests to check for STDs
- not use condoms correctly every time they have sex

- have sexual contact with multiple partners during the same period of time

Some lesbian, gay, bisexual, transgender, queer, and/or questioning (LGBTQ) teens may also be at higher risk for STDs.

WHAT DO YOU NEED TO KNOW ABOUT SEXUALLY TRANSMITTED DISEASES?

Sexually transmitted diseases are diseases that can spread from person to person during vaginal, anal, or oral sex. Some STDs can also spread during any kind of activity that involves skin-to-skin sexual contact.

STDs are sometimes called "sexually transmitted infections" (STIs). Examples of STDs include genital herpes, chlamydia, gonorrhea, and human immunodeficiency virus (HIV).

These diseases are very common. Although many STDs can be cured, they can cause serious health problems if they are not treated. Many STDs do not have any symptoms, so the only way to know for sure if you have an STD is to get tested.

WHAT DO YOU TELL YOUR TEEN ABOUT PREVENTING SEXUALLY TRANSMITTED DISEASES?

Talk to your teen about what STDs are and how to prevent them. Use the following facts and resources to talk with your teen.

It Is Important to Learn about Sexually Transmitted Diseases and How They Spread

Knowing the facts helps teens protect themselves. Check out the following websites together:

- STDs—for Teens (http://kidshealth.org/teen/sexual_health/stds/std.html?tracking=T_RelatedArticle)
- Information for Teens and Young Adults: Staying Healthy and Preventing STDs (www.cdc.gov/std/life-stages-populations/stdfact-teens.htm)

Complete Abstinence Is the Only Sure Way to Prevent Sexually Transmitted Diseases

Complete abstinence means not having any kind of sexual contact. This includes vaginal, anal, or oral sex and skin-to-skin sexual contact. Complete abstinence prevents STDs.

Condoms Can Help Prevent Sexually Transmitted Diseases

Make sure your teen knows how to use condoms—even if you do not think they are sexually active. Offer to help get condoms if your teen does not know where to go. Share the following resources:

- Condoms—for Teens (https://kidshealth.org/en/teens/contraception-condom.html)
- External (sometimes called "Male") Condom Use (www.cdc.gov/condomeffectiveness/external-condom-use.html)
- Internal (sometimes called "Female") Condom Use (www.cdc.gov/condomeffectiveness/internal-condom-use.html)

It Is Important for Teens to Talk with Their Partners about Sexually Transmitted Diseases before Having Sex

Encourage your teen to talk with their partners about STD prevention before having sex. Say that you understand it may not be easy, but it is important for your teen to speak up. The following resources can help:

- Talking to Your Partner About Condoms—for Teens (https://www.kidshealth.org/en/teens/talk-about-condoms.html)
- Talking to Your Partner About STDs—for Teens (https://www.kidshealth.org/en/teens/the-talk.html)
- STD Testing: Conversation Starters (https://health.gov/myhealthfinder/health-conditions/hiv-and-other-stds/std-testing-conversation-starters)

Your Teen May Need to Get Tested for Sexually Transmitted Diseases

Ask your teen to talk honestly with the doctor or nurse about any sexual activity. That way, the doctor can decide which tests your child may need. For example, sexually active teens may need to get tested for:

- chlamydia and gonorrhea
- syphilis
- HIV

It is important to help your teen develop a trusting relationship with the doctor or nurse. Step out of the room to give them a chance to ask about STD testing and prevention in private.

This is an important step in teaching teens to play an active role in their health care.

Keep in mind that your teen can get tested for STDs at the doctor—or go to a clinic. To find an STD clinic near you, do the following:

- Enter your zip code to find a local testing site at https://gettested.cdc.gov/.
- Call 800-CDC-INFO (800-232-4636).

HOW CAN YOU TALK TO YOUR TEEN ABOUT PREVENTING PREGNANCY?

It is also important for all teens to know about preventing pregnancy. Check out the following resources with your teen:

- Choose the Right Birth Control (https://health.gov/myhealthfinder/healthy-living/sexual-health/choose-right-birth-control)
- Contraception Explained: Options for Teens & Adolescents (www.healthychildren.org/English/ages-stages/teen/dating-sex/Pages/Birth-Control-for-Sexually-Active-Teens.aspx)
- About Birth Control—for Teens (www.kidshealth.org/en/teens/contraception.html)

HOW CAN YOU HELP YOUR TEEN BUILD HEALTHY RELATIONSHIPS?

Families have different rules about when it is okay for teens to start dating. Whatever your rules are, the best time to start talking about healthy relationships is before your teen starts dating.

Help your teen develop healthy expectations for relationships.[1]

Section 39.2 | Sexual Health Education at School: An Overview

WHAT IS SEXUAL HEALTH EDUCATION?

Quality sexual health education provides students with the knowledge and skills to help them be healthy and avoid human immunodeficiency virus (HIV), sexually transmitted infections (STIs), and unintended pregnancy.

A quality sexual health education curriculum includes medically accurate, developmentally appropriate, and culturally relevant content and skills that target key behavioral outcomes and promote healthy sexual development.

The curriculum is age-appropriate and planned across grade levels to provide information about health risk behaviors and experiences.

Quality sexual health education programs share many characteristics. These programs:

- are taught by well-qualified and highly trained teachers and school staff
- use strategies that are relevant and engaging for all students
- address the health needs of all students, including the students identifying as lesbian, gay, bisexual, transgender, queer, and questioning (LGBTQ)

---

[1] Office of Disease Prevention and Health Promotion (ODPHP), "Talk with Your Teen about Preventing STDs," U.S. Department of Health and Human Services (HHS), May 31, 2023. Available online. URL: https://health.gov/myhealthfinder/health-conditions/hiv-and-other-stds/talk-your-teen-about-preventing-stds. Accessed June 1, 2023.

- connect students to sexual health and other health services at school or in the community
- engage parents, families, and community partners in school programs
- foster positive relationships between adolescents and important adults

HOW CAN SCHOOLS DELIVER SEXUAL HEALTH EDUCATION?

A school health education program that includes a quality sexual health education curriculum targets the development of functional knowledge and skills needed to promote healthy behaviors and avoid risks. It is important that sexual health education explicitly incorporates and reinforces skill development.

Giving students time to practice, assess, and reflect on skills taught in the curriculum helps move them toward independence, critical thinking, and problem-solving to avoid STIs, HIV, and unintended pregnancy.

Quality sexual health education programs teach students how to:
- analyze family, peer, and media influences that impact health
- access valid and reliable health information, products, and services (e.g., STI/HIV testing)
- communicate with family, peers, and teachers about issues that affect health
- make informed and thoughtful decisions about their health
- take responsibility for themselves and others to improve their health

WHAT ARE THE BENEFITS OF DELIVERING SEXUAL HEALTH EDUCATION TO STUDENTS?

Promoting and implementing well-designed sexual health education positively impacts student health in a variety of ways. Students who participate in these programs are more likely to:
- delay initiation of sexual intercourse
- have fewer sex partners
- have fewer experiences of unprotected sex

- increase their use of protection, specifically condoms
- improve their academic performance

In addition to providing knowledge and skills to address sexual behavior, quality sexual health education can be tailored to include information on high-risk substance use, suicide prevention, and how to keep students from committing or being victims of violence—behaviors and experiences that place youth at risk of poor physical and mental health and poor academic outcomes.

WHAT DOES DELIVERING SEXUAL HEALTH EDUCATION LOOK LIKE IN ACTION?

To successfully put quality sexual health education into practice, schools need supportive policies, appropriate content, trained staff, and engaged parents and communities.

Schools can put the following four elements in place to support sex education:

- Implement policies that foster supportive environments for sexual health education.
- Use health content that is medically accurate, developmentally appropriate, culturally inclusive, and grounded in science.
- Equip staff with the knowledge and skills needed to deliver sexual health education.
- Engage parents and community partners.[2]

Section 39.3 | Syringe Services Programs

Syringe services programs (SSPs) are community-based prevention programs that can provide a range of services, including access to and disposal of sterile syringes and injection equipment,

[2] "What Works in Schools: Sexual Health Education," Centers for Disease Control and Prevention (CDC), March 13, 2023. Available online. URL: www.cdc.gov/healthyyouth/whatworks/what-works-sexual-health-education.htm. Accessed June 2, 2023.

vaccination, testing, and linkage to infectious disease care and substance use treatment. Nearly 30 years of research show these programs are safe, effective, and cost-saving tools that can prevent human immunodeficiency virus (HIV) and high-risk injection behaviors among people who inject drugs.

SSPs help protect communities by preventing infectious disease outbreaks and facilitating safe disposal of used syringes. These programs are not associated with increased drug use, crime, or syringe litter in communities.

The most effective SSPs provide comprehensive services to people who inject drugs, including the distribution of lifesaving medications and referrals to substance use treatment and other health care.

WHAT ARE THE BENEFITS OF SYRINGE SERVICES PROGRAMS?

Syringe services benefit people who inject drugs and their communities in multiple ways.

Sharing and reusing injection equipment is associated with a high risk of transmission of blood-borne diseases—including life-threatening infective endocarditis, HIV, hepatitis B virus (HBV), and hepatitis C virus (HCV)—as well as skin and soft tissue infections. By providing sterile injection equipment, SSPs aim to reduce the transmission of infectious diseases. Syringe services save lives and can significantly reduce HCV transmission and effectively end HIV outbreaks, especially when combined with medications that treat opioid use disorder. In the United States, experts point to these services as especially critical for preventing the community spread of HIV and addressing the intertwined public health crises of HIV and opioid use.

Many SSPs provide additional services such as the distribution of the overdose-reversing medication naloxone, HIV and HCV testing and prevention interventions, vaccination, and referrals for substance use treatment and other health care. These comprehensive approaches result in better substance use outcomes for people who inject drugs and can improve the overall health of communities in which programs operate.

DO SYRINGE SERVICES PROGRAMS INCREASE DRUG USE?

The research funded by the National Institute on Drug Abuse (NIDA) has found that SSPs do not increase drug use. In fact, program participants in these studies were significantly more likely to enter substance use treatment and reduce or stop drug use.

Many SSPs provide additional services, including the distribution of the overdose-reversing medication naloxone, HIV and HCV testing and prevention interventions, vaccination, and referrals for substance use treatment and other health care. These comprehensive approaches result in better substance use outcomes for people who inject drugs and can improve the overall health of communities in which programs operate.

ARE SYRINGE SERVICES PROGRAMS COST-EFFECTIVE?

Syringe services programs have been found to be an effective and cost-effective strategy for preventing and addressing community outbreaks of HIV and HCV. An outbreak in rural Scott County, Indiana, beginning in 2015, led to more than 200 people being diagnosed with both HIV and HCV. The Indiana State Department of Health credited SSPs with halting the increase in transmissions and saving taxpayers an estimated $120 million.[3]

THE SAFETY AND EFFECTIVENESS OF SYRINGE SERVICES PROGRAMS

The nation is currently experiencing an opioid crisis involving the misuse of prescription opioid pain relievers as well as heroin and fentanyl. The increase in substance use, including stimulant use, has resulted in concomitant increases in injection drug use across the country. This has caused not only large increases in overdose deaths but also tens of thousands of viral hepatitis infections annually and is threatening the progress made in HIV prevention. The most effective way for individuals who inject drugs to avoid

---

[3] "Syringe Services Programs (SSPs)," National Institute on Drug Abuse (NIDA), June 7, 2021. Available online. URL: https://nida.nih.gov/research-topics/syringe-services-programs#how-do-syringe. Accessed June 2, 2023.

infections related to unsafe injection drug use is to stop inject-ing. However, many people are unable or unwilling to do so, or they have little or no access to effective treatment. Approximately 3.7 million Americans report having injected a drug in the past year. In 2019, 14.3 percent of high school students reported using opioids without a prescription, and 1.6 percent reported having ever injected drugs.

SSPs are proven and effective community-based prevention pro-grams that can provide a range of services, including access to and disposal of sterile syringes and injection equipment, vaccination, testing, and linkage to infectious disease care and substance use treatment. SSPs reach people who inject drugs, an often hidden and marginalized population. Nearly 30 years of research have shown that comprehensive SSPs are safe, effective, and cost-saving, do not increase illegal drug use or crime, and play an important role in reducing the transmission of viral hepatitis, HIV, and other infec-tions. Research shows that new users of SSPs are five times more likely to enter drug treatment and about three times more likely to stop using drugs than those who do not use the programs. SSPs that provide naloxone also help decrease opioid overdose deaths. SSPs protect the public and first responders by facilitating the safe disposal of used needles and syringes.

Appropriations language from Congress in fiscal years 2016–2018 permits the use of funds from the Department of Health and Human Services (HHS), under certain circumstances, to support SSPs, with the exception that funds may not be used to purchase needles or syringes. State, local, tribal, or territorial health depart-ments must first consult with the Centers for Disease Control and Prevention (CDC) and provide evidence that their jurisdiction is experiencing or at risk for significant increases in hepatitis infec-tions or an HIV outbreak due to injection drug use. The CDC has developed guidance and consults with state, local, tribal, or territorial health departments to determine if they have adequately demonstrated the need according to federal law. Decisions about the use of SSPs to prevent disease transmission and support the health and engagement of people who inject drugs are made at the state and local levels.

Prevention of Infectious Diseases

Viral hepatitis, HIV, and other blood-borne pathogens can spread through injection drug use if people use needles, syringes, or other injection materials that were previously used by someone who had one of these infections. The unsafe injection can also lead to other serious health problems, such as skin infections, abscesses, and endocarditis. The best way to reduce the risk of acquiring and transmitting disease through injection drug use is to stop injecting drugs. For people who do not stop injecting drugs, using sterile injection equipment for each injection can reduce the risk of infection and prevent outbreaks.

During the last decade, the United States has seen an increase in injection drug use—primarily the injection of opioids. Outbreaks of hepatitis C, hepatitis B, and HIV infections have been correlated with these injection patterns and trends. The majority of new HCV infections are due to injection drug use, and the nation has seen a 4.9-fold increase in reported cases of HCV from 2010 to 2019. New HCV infections are increasing most rapidly among young people, with the greatest incidence among individuals aged 20–39.

Until recently, the CDC had observed a steady decline since the mid-1990s in HIV diagnoses attributable to injection drug use. However, recent data show progress has stalled. Notably, new HIV infections among people who inject drugs increased 12 percent from 2014 to 2019. The estimated lifetime cost of treating one person living with HIV is nearly $510,000. Hospitalization in the United States due to substance-use-related infections alone costs over $700 million annually. In the United States, the estimated cost of providing health-care services for people living with chronic HCV infection is $15 billion annually. SSPs can help reduce these health-care costs by preventing viral hepatitis, HIV, endocarditis, and other infections.

SSPs are tools that can help reduce the transmission of viral hepatitis, HIV, and other blood-borne infections. SSPs are associated with an approximately 50 percent reduction in HIV and HCV incidence. When combined with medications that treat opioid dependence (also known as "medications for opioid use disorder" (MOUD) or "medication-assisted treatment" (MAT)), HIV and HCV transmission is reduced by more than two-thirds.

Linkage to Substance Use Treatment, Naloxone, and Other Health-Care Services

SSPs serve as a bridge to other health services, including HCV and HIV diagnosis and treatment and MOUD for substance use. The majority of SSPs offer referrals to MAT, and people who inject drugs who regularly use an SSP are more than five times as likely to enter treatment for a substance use disorder and nearly three times as likely to report reducing or discontinuing injection as those who have never used an SSP. SSPs facilitate entry into treatment for substance use disorders by people who inject drugs. People who use SSPs show high readiness to reduce or stop their drug use. There is also evidence that people who inject drugs and work with a nurse at an SSP or other community-based venue are more likely to access primary care than those who do not, also increasing access to MAT. Many comprehensive community-based SSPs offer a range of preventative services, including vaccination, infectious disease testing, and linkage to health-care services.

SSPs can reduce overdose deaths by teaching people who inject drugs how to prevent and respond to a drug overdose, providing them training on how to use naloxone, a medication used to reverse an overdose, and providing naloxone to them. Many SSPs provide "overdose prevention kits" containing naloxone to people who inject drugs. SSPs have partnered with law enforcement, providing naloxone to local police departments to help them keep their communities safer.

Public Safety

SSPs can benefit communities and public safety by reducing needle-stick injuries and overdose deaths without increasing illegal injection of drugs or criminal activity. Studies show that SSPs protect first responders and the public by providing safe needle disposal and reducing the community presence of needles. As many as one in every three officers may be stuck by a used needle during his or her career. Needlestick injuries are among the most concerning and stressful events experienced by law officers. A study compared the prevalence of improperly disposed of syringes and self-reported disposal practices in a city with SSPs (San Francisco) to a city without SSPs (Miami) and found eight times as many improperly disposed of syringes in Miami, the city without SSPs. People who inject drugs in San Francisco also reported higher rates of safe disposal practices than those in Miami. Data from the CDC's National HIV Behavioral Surveillance System in 2015 showed that the more syringes distributed at SSPs per people who inject drugs in a geographic region, the more likely people who inject drugs in that region were to report safe disposal of used syringes.

Evidence demonstrates that SSPs do not increase illegal drug use or crime. Studies in Baltimore and New York City have found no difference in crime rates between areas with and areas without SSPs. In Baltimore, trends in arrests were examined before and after an SSP was started and found that there was no significant increase in crime rates. The study in New York City assessed whether proximity to an SSP was associated with experiencing violence in an inner-city neighborhood and found no association.

Syringe Services Program Implementation

Not all SSPs are alike. Programs differ in size, scope, geographic location, and delivery venue (e.g., mobile versus fixed sites). Community acceptance and legality also impact program success. Prior to establishing an SSP, it is important for public health agencies (or others) to assess the needs of potential clients, their families, key stakeholders, law enforcement, and the community at large.

The decision to incorporate SSPs as part of a comprehensive prevention program is made at the state and local levels. Laws vary by state and can either increase or reduce access to SSPs. The CDC created a guidance document to aid state and local health departments in managing HIV and hepatitis C outbreaks among people who inject drugs, which provides best practices to consider when establishing an SSP. Conducting a needs assessment prior to the establishment of an SSP, developing evaluation tools, and careful planning of the operational tasks can increase the chances the SSP will be successful in a community.

Emerging Issues

In addition to the concerning increases in hepatitis and HIV rates, The CDC has also identified additional emerging infectious disease risks related to injection drug use, including increases in methicillin-resistant *Staphylococcus aureus* (MRSA) infection rates, which increased 124 percent between 2011 and 2016 among people who inject drugs. In addition, people who inject drugs are 16 times as likely as other people to develop invasive MRSA infections.

Rates of endocarditis, a life-threatening infection of the heart valves that can occur in people who inject drugs, have also increased. For example, in North Carolina alone, the rate of hospital discharge diagnoses for endocarditis related to drug dependence increased more than 12-fold from 2010 to 2015, with unadjusted hospital costs increasing from $1.1 million in 2010 to over $22 million in 2015. Identifying and responding to these emerging infectious disease threats is critical to alleviating the subsequent harms of opioid misuse and abuse. These infections have been linked to the frequency of injecting and syringe sharing. SSPs may help reduce bacterial infections by providing sterile injection equipment and linkage to substance use treatment.[4]

---

[4] "Syringe Services Programs (SSPs)," Centers for Disease Control and Prevention (CDC), January 11, 2023. Available online. URL: www.cdc.gov/ssp/syringe-services-programs-summary.html. Accessed June 2, 2023.

Part 6 | Living with Sexually Transmitted Diseases

Chapter 40 | **Talking about Your Human Immunodeficiency Virus Status**

Chapter Contents

Section 40.1 | Whom to Tell about Your Positive Test Result

It is important to share your human immunodeficiency virus (HIV) status with your sex partner(s) and/or people with whom you inject drugs. Whether you disclose your status to others is your decision.

PARTNERS

It is important to disclose your HIV status to your sex partner(s) and anyone you shared needles with, even if you are not comfortable doing it. Communicating with each other about your HIV status means you can take steps to keep both of you healthy.

If you are nervous about disclosing your test result or you have been threatened or injured by a partner, you can ask your doctor or the local health department to help you tell your partner(s) that they might have been exposed to HIV. This type of assistance is called "partner notification" or "partner services." Health departments do not reveal your name to your partner(s). They will only tell your partner(s) that they have been exposed to HIV and should get tested.

Many states have laws that require you to tell your sexual partners if you are HIV-positive before you have sex (anal, vaginal, or oral) or tell your drug-using partners before you share drugs or needles to inject drugs. In some states, you can be charged with a crime if you do not tell your partner your HIV status, even if you use a condom or another type of protection and the partner does not become infected.

HEALTH-CARE PROVIDERS

Your health-care providers (doctors, clinical workers, dentists, etc.) have to know about your HIV status in order to be able to give you the best possible care. It is also important that health-care providers know your HIV status so that they do not prescribe medication for you that may be harmful when taken with your HIV medications.

Some states require you to disclose your HIV-positive status before you receive any health-care services from a physician or dentist. For this reason, it is important to discuss the laws in your state about disclosure in medical settings with the health-care provider who gave you your HIV test results.

Your HIV test result will become part of your medical records so that your doctor or other health-care providers can give you the best care possible. All medical information, including HIV test results, falls under strict confidentiality laws such as the Privacy Rule of the Health Insurance Portability and Accountability Act (HIPAA) and cannot be released without your permission. There are some limited exceptions to confidentiality. These come into play only when not disclosing the information could result in harm to the other person.

FAMILY AND FRIENDS

In most cases, your family and friends will not know your test results or HIV status unless you tell them yourself. While telling your family that you have HIV may seem hard, you should know that disclosure actually has many benefits—studies have shown that people who disclose their HIV status respond better to treatment than those who do not.

If you are under 18, however, some states allow your health-care provider to tell your parent(s) that you received services for HIV if they think doing so is in your best interest.

EMPLOYERS

In most cases, your employer will not know your HIV status unless you tell them. But your employer does have a right to ask if you have any health conditions that would affect your ability to do your job and that pose a serious risk to others (e.g., they might be a health-care professional, such as a surgeon, who does procedures in which there is a risk of blood or other body fluids being exchanged).

If you have health insurance through your employer, the insurance company cannot legally tell your employer that you have HIV. But it is possible that your employer could find out if the insurance company provides detailed information to your employer about the benefits it pays or the costs of insurance.

All people with HIV are covered under the Americans with Disabilities Act (ADA). This means that your employer cannot discriminate against you because of your HIV status as long as you can do your job.[1]

Section 40.2 | Partner Communication and Agreements

TELLING YOUR SEX PARTNERS

This may be one of the hardest things you have to do. But you need to tell your sex partner(s) that you are living with human immunodeficiency virus (HIV), whether you have a primary partner such as a spouse or girlfriend or boyfriend, have more than one partner, or are casually dating.

What follows are tips for talking to your main partner, other partners, and former partners.

TALKING TO YOUR MAIN PARTNER(S)

If you are in a relationship, one of the first things you will probably think about after learning that you have HIV is telling your partner or partners. For some couples, a positive HIV test may have been expected. For others, the news will be a surprise that can be difficult.

Your partner may not be prepared to offer you support during a time when you need it. Your partner may be worrying about their own HIV status. On the other hand, if you think you may have contracted HIV from your partner, you are probably dealing with your own feelings.

Unless your partner is known to have an HIV infection, they should get an HIV test right away. Do not assume that the results will come back positive, even if you have been having unprotected

---

[1] HIV.gov, "Talking about Your HIV Status," U.S. Department of Health and Human Services (HHS), May 15, 2017. Available online. URL: www.hiv.gov/hiv-basics/hiv-testing/just-diagnosed-whats-next/talking-about-your-hiv-status. Accessed July 5, 2023.

sex or sharing needles. Your partner may assume the worst and may blame you for possibly spreading the disease. It is important that you discuss these feelings with each other in an open and honest way, perhaps with a licensed counselor.

TALKING TO NEW PARTNER(S)

Talking about HIV with someone you are dating casually or someone you met recently may be difficult. You might not know this person very well or know what kind of reaction to expect. When telling a casual partner or someone you are dating, each situation is different, and you might use a different approach each time. Sometimes, you may feel comfortable being direct and saying, "Before we have sex, I want you to know that I have HIV."

Other times, you may want to bring it up by saying something like, "Let's talk about safer sex." Whichever approach you choose, you should tell the person that you have HIV before you have sex for the first time. Otherwise, there may be hurt feelings or mistrust later. Also, be sure to take your HIV medications every day (this is very effective in protecting partners from infection) and practice safer sex.

TALKING TO FORMER PARTNER(S)

With people you had sex with in the past or people you have shared needles with, it can be very difficult to explain that you have HIV. However, it is important that they know so that they can get tested. If you need help telling people that you may have been exposed to HIV, most city or county health departments will tell them for you without using your name. Ask your provider about this service.

REMEMBER

Before telling your partner that you have HIV, take some time to think about how you want to bring it up:
- Decide when and where would be the best time and place to have a conversation. Choose a time when you expect that you will both be comfortable and as relaxed as possible.

Talking about Your Human Immunodeficiency Virus Status

- Think about how your partner may react to stressful situations. If there is a history of violence in your relationship, consider your safety first and make a plan with a social worker or counselor.
- Imagine several ways in which your partner might react to the news. Write down what they might say and then think about what you might say in response.[2]

---

[2] "Sex and Sexuality and HIV: Entire Lesson," U.S. Department of Veterans Affairs (VA), May 28, 2019. Available online. URL: www.hiv.va.gov/patient/daily/sex/single-page.asp. Accessed June 9, 2023.

Chapter 41 | Standing up to Human Immunodeficiency Virus Stigma

WHAT IS HUMAN IMMUNODEFICIENCY VIRUS STIGMA?

Human immunodeficiency virus (HIV) stigma is negative attitudes and beliefs about people with HIV. It is the prejudice that comes with labeling an individual as part of a group that is believed to be socially unacceptable.

Here are a few examples:
- believing that only certain groups of people can get HIV
- making moral judgments about people who take steps to prevent HIV transmission
- feeling that people deserve to get HIV because of their choices

WHAT IS DISCRIMINATION?

While stigma refers to an "attitude" or "belief," discrimination is the behaviors that result from those attitudes or beliefs. HIV discrimination is the act of treating people living with HIV differently than those without HIV.

Here are a few examples:
- a health-care professional refusing to provide care or services to a person living with HIV
- refusing casual contact with someone living with HIV

- socially isolating a member of a community because they are HIV positive
- referring to people as "HIVers" or "Positives"

WHAT CAUSES HUMAN IMMUNODEFICIENCY VIRUS STIGMA?

Human immunodeficiency virus stigma is rooted in a fear of HIV. Many of the ideas about HIV come from the HIV images that first appeared in the early 1980s. There are still misconceptions about how HIV is transmitted and what it means to live with HIV today.

The lack of information and awareness combined with outdated beliefs lead people to fear getting HIV. Additionally, many people think of HIV as a disease that only certain groups get. This leads to negative value judgments about people who are living with HIV.[1]

Human immunodeficiency virus stigma and discrimination can pose complex barriers to prevention, testing, treatment, and support for people living with or at risk for HIV. Some examples of stigma include being shunned by family, peers, and the wider community; receiving poor treatment in health-care and education settings; and experiencing judgmental attitudes, insults, or harassment. Some individuals with HIV have been denied or lost employment, housing, and other services; prevented from receiving health care; denied access to educational and training programs; and have been victims of violence and hate crimes. HIV-related stigma and discrimination prevent individuals from learning their HIV status, disclosing their status even to family members and sexual partners, and/or accessing medical care and treatment, weakening their ability to protect themselves from getting or transmitting HIV and to stay healthy. HIV-related stigma is made more complicated when individuals also experience stigma related to substance use, mental health, sexual orientation, gender identity, race/ethnicity, or sex work.

---

[1] "HIV Stigma and Discrimination," Centers for Disease Control and Prevention (CDC), June 1, 2021. Available online. URL: www.cdc.gov/hiv/basics/hiv-stigma/index.html. Accessed June 9, 2023.

LEGAL PROTECTIONS FOR PEOPLE LIVING WITH HUMAN IMMUNODEFICIENCY VIRUS AND ACQUIRED IMMUNODEFICIENCY SYNDROME

Numerous federal laws protect people living with HIV and AIDS from discrimination. For example, people living with HIV and AIDS are protected from discrimination under the Americans with Disabilities Act (ADA), a federal act that guarantees equal opportunities in employment, housing, public accommodations, telecommunications, and transportation and also applies to all local and state government services. People living with HIV and AIDS are also guaranteed protection from housing discrimination under the federal Fair Housing Act (FHA) and are protected from being excluded from federally funded programs under Section 504 of the Rehabilitation Act of 1973. Furthermore, under the Affordable Care Act (ACA), people with preexisting health conditions, including HIV, can no longer be dropped from, denied, or charged more for health-care coverage, and under the Health Insurance Portability and Accountability Act of 1996 (HIPAA), the privacy and security of individuals' medical records and other health information maintained by HHS-funded programs and services is protected.

ENVISIONING A FUTURE FREE FROM HUMAN IMMUNODEFICIENCY VIRUS-RELATED STIGMA AND DISCRIMINATION

The National HIV/AIDS Strategy: Updated to 2020 (the Strategy) calls for a reduction in stigma and elimination of discrimination associated with HIV status and commits to developing an indicator to measure HIV stigma and track progress toward that target. The Strategy identifies several HIV stigma reduction steps, including mobilizing communities to reduce HIV-related stigma; strengthening the enforcement of civil rights laws; assisting states in protecting people with HIV from violence, retaliation, and discrimination associated with HIV status; and promoting the public leadership of people living with HIV. These actions will help achieve the Strategy's vision, "The United States will become a place where new HIV infections are rare and when they do occur, every person regardless of age, gender, race/ethnicity, sexual orientation, gender identity or socioeconomic circumstance, will have unfettered access to high quality, life-extending care, free from stigma and discrimination."

Across the federal government, multiple agencies play a role in enforcing federal civil rights protections, providing technical assistance for carrying out the mandates of the ADA and other laws, and developing and disseminating information about civil rights and protections. While some departments have the authority to enforce these protections, nearly all have the ability to disseminate relevant information about protecting the rights of persons living with HIV and to take steps to confront and reduce HIV-related stigma.[2]

STIGMA SCENARIOS: SUPPORT IN ACTION

Know what to do when you witness HIV stigma. The first step to stopping HIV is talking openly about it and addressing the stigma head-on. It is important to speak up and take action when you witness others behaving in ways that are stigmatizing.

But it can be hard to know what to say or do. Many of them struggle with how best to address HIV stigma and discrimination when they experience it. Check out the following tips for ways to act against stigma in everyday situations.

Human Immunodeficiency Virus Stigma and Discrimination in Families
SCENARIO

You arrive at a family reunion picnic with your sister, who recently shared with the family that she was diagnosed with HIV. As you make your way around to say hello and offer hugs to family members, your cousin hesitates when greeting your sister, commenting, "I'm not going to get it, am I?"

---

[2] HIV.gov, "Activities Combating HIV Stigma and Discrimination," U.S. Department of Health and Human Services (HHS), May 20, 2017. Available online. URL: www.hiv.gov/federal-response/federal-activities-agencies/activities-combating-hiv-stigma-and-discrimination. Accessed June 9, 2023.

WHAT YOU CAN DO
- Model positive behavior by hugging your sister.
- Share HIV basics, including facts about how HIV is transmitted. "I'm not sure if you know, but HIV is not spread by hugging, shaking hands, or socially kissing someone who has HIV. HIV cannot survive outside the body."
- Offer to have a conversation and answer any other questions she might have about HIV.
- Follow up later with an email or text that links to educational resources.

Human Immunodeficiency Virus Stigma and Discrimination with Partners
SCENARIO
You are dating a new girl, and things are getting more serious. You decide that it is time to share with her that you have HIV. When you tell her, she gets angry and says she does not understand why you did not just date someone who was already sick.

WHAT YOU CAN DO
- Whether you choose to pursue a relationship or not, this is an opportunity to stand up to HIV stigma and raise awareness of how hurtful it can be.
- Acknowledge that you know that learning a partner has HIV can be surprising. But let her know that it was not easy for you to share your status with her because her reaction is not unusual.
- Use the opportunity to correct her stigmatizing language. You can say, "It really is not appropriate to call people with HIV 'sick'. I would appreciate it if you used the phrase 'people with HIV' instead." Let her know that with proper treatment, people with HIV can live long and healthy lives.
- Explain that someone with HIV who takes their HIV medicine as prescribed and gets and keeps an

undetectable viral load will not transmit HIV to their sex partners. Encourage her to learn more about HIV and other prevention strategies used when one member of a couple has HIV and the other does not, including condoms and pre-exposure prophylaxis (PrEP).

Human Immunodeficiency Virus Stigma and Discrimination with Friends
SCENARIO

Your friend gathers you and several other friends to disclose he has HIV. One friend's first reaction is, "How did you get it, and do you know who gave it to you?"

WHAT YOU CAN DO

- Redirect the conversation by showing empathy and saying, "We are just happy you felt comfortable sharing this with us. Do you want to talk more about how you are feeling?"
- Ask your friend if he has sought treatment. If not, offer to go with your friend to visit his doctor to explore his options for treatment.
- Later, talk to your friend who posed the question and explain that asking about transmission is insensitive. This would be a good time to explain what HIV stigma is and how it can be a barrier to treatment for those with HIV. Try not to pass judgment; instead, show empathy as you help them learn more.
- Learning more about HIV is one of the first steps to support your loved one in living a healthy life with HIV. Educate yourself about the basic facts about the virus, how it is transmitted, and treatment options available to those with HIV.

Communicating openly and asking questions about HIV is important to promote learning and understanding of HIV. But remember, we have to do our part in being thoughtful and supportive—rather than stigmatizing or being offensive—in our responses to situations of HIV disclosure or misunderstandings about HIV.

Human Immunodeficiency Virus Stigma and Discrimination in the Community
SCENARIO

During your weekly basketball league game, the subject comes up with a team member sharing on Facebook that he was going to get an HIV test. This individual is absent from the game on this day. Several negative and judgmental comments are expressed by your fellow teammates.

WHAT YOU CAN DO

- Share the last time you were tested for HIV and ask him if he is thinking about getting tested, too. Explain that HIV testing is a normal and routine part of health care and knowing your status is important because it helps keep you healthy.
- Explain to the team that they are contributing to HIV stigma when making judgments about people who take steps to prevent HIV transmission. Let them know that these types of stigmatizing remarks can lead people to be afraid of what people will say and less likely to get tested for HIV.

Human Immunodeficiency Virus Stigma and Discrimination in the Workplace
SCENARIO

A friend at work remarks to you that another coworker should not be participating in the office potluck because he has HIV. How do you respond?

WHAT YOU CAN DO

- Respond to your friend's misconception kindly by explaining the facts. "You do not need to worry. You can't get HIV from eating food handled by a person with HIV."
- Help your friend understand that refusing casual contact with someone with HIV is a form of stigma.

- Model positive behavior by eating the food your coworker with HIV brings to the potluck. Have lunch together regularly and check in with your coworker to ensure he is not feeling isolated.[3]

STIGMA LANGUAGE GUIDE

Know how to talk about HIV to avoid stigma. The words you use matter. Keep the following in mind:

- When talking about HIV, certain words and language may have a negative meaning for people at high risk for HIV or those who have HIV.
- You can do your part to stop HIV stigma by being intentional and thoughtful when choosing your words and choosing to use supportive—rather than stigmatizing—language when talking about HIV.

Consider using the preferred terms as provided in Table 41.1 to avoid promoting stigma and misinformation around HIV.

Table 41.1. Problematic and Preferred Word or Phrase for Describing HIV[4]

Problematic Word or Phrase	Preferred Word or Phrase
AIDS (when referring to the virus, HIV)	HIV HIV and AIDS (when referring to both)
Why: AIDS itself is not a condition. It is a range of conditions or a syndrome that occurs when a person's immune system is weakened by the HIV infection.	
To catch AIDS To catch HIV To pass on HIV	To be diagnosed with HIV To acquire HIV To transmit HIV
Why: AIDS cannot be caught or transmitted. People get HIV. HIV can be transmitted, but it is not hereditary.	

---

[3] "Stigma Scenarios: Support in Action," Centers for Disease Control and Prevention (CDC), November 3, 2022. Available online. URL: www.cdc.gov/stophivtogether/hiv-stigma/stigma-scenarios.html. Accessed June 9, 2023.
[4] "Ways to Stop HIV Stigma and Discrimination," Centers for Disease Control and Prevention (CDC), November 3, 2022. Available online. URL: www.cdc.gov/stophivtogether/hiv-stigma/ways-to-stop.html. Accessed June 9, 2023.

Table 41.1. Continued

Problematic Word or Phrase	Preferred Word or Phrase
Unprotected sex	Sex without a condom or medicines to prevent or treat HIV (such as pre-exposure prophylaxis (PrEP) or antiretroviral therapy (ART))
Why: "Unprotected sex" is often associated with sex without a condom. More precise terms are necessary as today there are numerous ways outside condom use to engage in safe sex to prevent HIV.	
Body fluids	Blood, amniotic fluid, semen, pre-ejaculate, vaginal fluids, rectal fluids, breast milk
Why: Only some body fluids transmit HIV. "Body fluids" covers all fluids coming from the body and not just those involved in HIV transmission. Be specific when possible.	
To battle HIV and/or AIDS war against HIV/AIDS	Response to HIV and AIDS
Why: These terms may be considered militaristic and may lead others to think that people with HIV have to be "fought" or eliminated	
Risk Risky behavior High(er) risk group(s) Groups with high-risk behavior	people with certain risk factors people who engage in behaviors that may increase their chances of getting HIV risk factors: • behaviors that increase the chances of getting or transmitting HIV • communities overrepresented in the HIV epidemic • populations with a high prevalence/incidence of HIV
Why: Some risk-related terms can be stigmatizing and may imply that the condition is inherent to a person or group rather than the actual causal factors.	
Victims Sufferers Contaminated Sick	People/persons with HIV
Why: Some people with HIV feel that these terms imply that they are powerless, with no control over their lives. Other unhelpful terms negatively define people with HIV by the condition. These terms also segregate the people who have HIV.	

Table 41.1. Continued

Problematic Word or Phrase	Preferred Word or Phrase
AIDS patient HIV patient Patient	Person with AIDS Person with HIV
Why: The term "patient" implies a constant state of illness that can be misleading and demoralizing. Outside a clinical context, a person is not a patient.	
Positives HIVers AIDS or HIV carrier(s)	Persons/people with HIV People with HIV (PWH or PWHIV) Persons with HIV (PWH or PWHIV) Persons/people with diagnosed HIV (PWDH or PWDHIV)
Why: A person is not HIV or AIDS. A person lives with HIV once he or she gets the virus or progresses to having an AIDS diagnosis.	
Injection (injecting) drug users (IDUs)	Persons/people who inject drugs (PWID)
Why: Injecting drug use refers to the transmission category and not the people themselves.	
People who have an undetectable viral load have little risk of transmission	**Treatment as prevention** People with HIV who have an undetectable viral load: • do not/don't transmit • will not/won't transmit Undetectable = Untransmittable or U=U People who are undetectable have effectively no risk of transmitting HIV People who are undetectable have negligible risk of transmitting HIV
Why: Research has shown that having an undetectable viral load prevents HIV transmission to others through sex or syringe sharing and during pregnancy, birth, and breastfeeding. This is sometimes referred to as "treatment as prevention" (TasP).	

EDUCATE OTHERS ABOUT HUMAN IMMUNODEFICIENCY VIRUS STIGMA

You can make a difference in stopping HIV stigma by learning more about HIV and sharing that knowledge with others. You can do this in person or on social media. All that matters is that you take action.

Take Action with the Centers for Disease Control and Prevention's Stop HIV Stigma Pledge Cards!

Use the Stop HIV Stigma pledge cards to commit to helping create and sustain communities that promote awareness, understanding, and acceptance of people with HIV.

The Stop HIV Stigma pledge cards will help you lead by example and may help those around you assess and recognize their own attitudes and perceptions.

Download, customize, and share the pledge cards to fight the stigma and raise awareness of HIV misinformation.

Amplify Your Voice Online

Share posts and facts about HIV and HIV stigma to help start conversations among your friends, family, community, and followers!

The following are a few tips and ideas to help you get started in creating your social media posts:

- Remember to keep it positive, show empathy, and tune in to comments on your posts.
- Listen and respond thoughtfully to what others have to say or questions they may have.
- Use CDC's *Let's Stop HIV Together* social media toolkits to get you started.
- Use #StopHIVStigma or #StopHIVTogether in your posts.
- Add CDC's Instagram #StopHIVStigma stickers to your photos and stories.
- Links to *Let's Stop HIV Together* website pages or social media accounts in your posts.
- Double-check statements before posting to make sure they are based on facts.
- Share how HIV has touched your life.[5]

---

[5] "Educate Others about HIV Stigma," Centers for Disease Control and Prevention (CDC), November 3, 2022. Available online. URL: www.cdc.gov/stophivtogether/hiv-stigma/educate-others.html. Accessed June 9, 2023.

Chapter 42 | **Treatment Use of Investigational Drugs**

WHAT IS AN INVESTIGATIONAL HUMAN IMMUNODEFICIENCY VIRUS DRUG?

An investigational human immunodeficiency virus (HIV) drug is an experimental drug that is being studied to see whether it is safe and effective. Investigational HIV drugs are studied in medical research studies called "clinical trials." Once an investigational HIV drug has been proven safe and effective in a clinical trial, the U.S. Food and Drug Administration (FDA) may approve the drug for general use or sale in the United States.

WHAT TYPES OF INVESTIGATIONAL HUMAN IMMUNODEFICIENCY VIRUS DRUGS ARE BEING STUDIED?

Investigational HIV drugs being studied include drugs to treat HIV and prevent HIV. Some types of investigational HIV drugs being studied include microbicides, immune modulators, latency-reversing agents, gp120 attachment inhibitors, and rev inhibitors.

HIV researchers are also studying investigational vaccines to prevent HIV and treat HIV. The goal of a preventive HIV vaccine is to prevent HIV in people who do not have HIV but who may be exposed to the virus. A safe and effective HIV treatment vaccine (also called a "therapeutic HIV vaccine") could prevent HIV from advancing to acquired immunodeficiency syndrome (AIDS), replace the daily use of HIV medicines, and help prevent HIV transmission.

HOW ARE CLINICAL TRIALS OF INVESTIGATIONAL DRUGS CONDUCTED?

Clinical trials are conducted in phases as shown in Figure 42.1. Each phase has a different purpose and helps researchers answer different questions about the investigational drug.

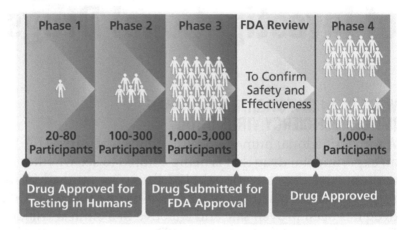

Figure 42.1. The Four Phases of a Clinical Trial

HIVinfo, U.S. Department of Health and Human Services (HHS)

- **Phase 1 trial.** Initial testing in a small group of people (20–80) to evaluate the drug's safety and to identify side effects.
- **Phase 2 trial.** Testing in a larger group of people (100–300) to determine the drug's effectiveness and to further evaluate its safety.
- **Phase 3 trial.** Continued testing in large groups of people (1,000–3,000) to confirm the drug's effectiveness, monitor side effects, compare it with standard or equivalent treatments, and collect information to ensure that the investigational drug can be used safely.

  In most cases, an investigational drug must be proven effective and must show continued safety in a phase 3 clinical trial to be considered for approval by the FDA

for sale in the United States. (However, some drugs go through the FDA's accelerated approval process and are approved before a phase 3 clinical trial is complete.)
- **Phase 4 trial**. Ongoing tracking that occurs after a drug is approved by the FDA for sale in the United States. The purpose of the tracking is to seek more information about the drug's risks, benefits, and optimal use.

HOW CAN A PERSON FIND A CLINICAL TRIAL THAT IS STUDYING AN INVESTIGATIONAL HUMAN IMMUNODEFICIENCY VIRUS DRUG?

- To find an HIV and AIDS clinical trial that is studying an investigational HIV drug, use the find a study search feature on ClinicalTrials.gov (https://clinicaltrials.gov).
- For help with your search, call a Clinicalinfo health information specialist at 800-448-0440 or email to ContactUs@HIVinfo.NIH.gov.
- You can also join ResearchMatch (www.researchmatch.org/about), which is a free, secure online tool that makes it easier for the public to become involved in clinical trials.

ARE INVESTIGATIONAL HUMAN IMMUNODEFICIENCY VIRUS DRUGS AVAILABLE FOR USE OUTSIDE OF A CLINICAL TRIAL?

In some cases, an investigational HIV drug may be available through an expanded access program. Expanded access allows for the use of an investigational drug outside of a clinical trial to treat a person who has a serious or immediate life-threatening disease and who has no FDA-approved treatment options. Drug companies must have permission from the FDA to make an investigational drug available for expanded access.

People seeking expanded access to an investigational HIV drug should talk to their health-care provider to see if they may qualify to take part in an expanded access program.

IS IT SAFE TO USE AN INVESTIGATIONAL HUMAN IMMUNODEFICIENCY VIRUS DRUG?

One goal of HIV research is to identify safer, more effective HIV medicines. Researchers try to make clinical trials as safe as possible. However, taking an investigational HIV drug can involve both benefits and risks. Risks may include unexpected side effects from the drug, which can be unpleasant, serious, or even life-threatening.

The benefits and possible risks of participating in a clinical trial or an expanded access program are explained to people before they decide whether to participate.

HOW CAN A PERSON FIND MORE INFORMATION ON INVESTIGATIONAL HUMAN IMMUNODEFICIENCY VIRUS DRUGS?

To find more information on investigational HIV drugs, use the Clinicalinfo Drug Database (https://clinicalinfo.hiv.gov/en/drugs), which includes up-to-date information on many investigational HIV drugs.[1]

---

[1] HIVinfo, "What Is an Investigational HIV Drug?" U.S. Department of Health and Human Services (HHS), August 20, 2021. Available online. URL: https://hivinfo.nih.gov/understanding-hiv/fact-sheets/what-investigational-hiv-drug. Accessed June 20, 2023.

Chapter 43 | Human Immunodeficiency Virus Medicines Approved by the U.S. Food and Drug Administration

Treatment with human immunodeficiency virus (HIV) medicines is called "antiretroviral therapy" (ART). ART is recommended for everyone with HIV, and people with HIV should start ART as soon as possible. People on ART take a combination of HIV medicines (called an "HIV treatment regimen") every day. A person's initial HIV treatment regimen generally includes three HIV medicines from at least two different HIV drug classes.

Table 43.1 lists HIV medicines recommended for the treatment of HIV infection in the United States, based on the U.S. Department of Health and Human Services (HHS) human immunodeficiency virus/acquired immunodeficiency syndrome (HIV/AIDS) medical practice guidelines. All of these drugs are approved by the U.S. Food and Drug Administration (FDA). The HIV medicines are listed according to drug class and identified by generic and brand names.[1]

---

[1] HIVinfo, "FDA-Approved HIV Medicines," U.S. Department of Health and Human Services (HHS), March 23, 2023. Available online. URL: https://hivinfo.nih.gov/understanding-hiv/fact-sheets/fda-approved-hiv-medicines. Accessed June 9, 2023.

Table 43.1. List of HIV Medicines Approved by the U.S. Food and Drug Administration (FDA)

Drug Class	Generic Name (Other Names and Abbreviations)	Brand Name	FDA Approval Date
Nucleoside Reverse Transcriptase Inhibitors (NRTIs)			
NRTIs block reverse transcriptase, an enzyme HIV needs to make copies of itself.	abacavir (abacavir sulfate, ABC)	Ziagen	December 17, 1998
	emtricitabine (FTC)	Emtriva	July 2, 2003
	lamivudine (3TC)	Epivir	November 17, 1995
	tenofovir disoproxil fumarate (tenofovir DF, TDF)	Viread	October 26, 2001
	zidovudine (azidothymidine, AZT, ZDV)	Retrovir	March 19, 1987
Non-Nucleoside Reverse Transcriptase Inhibitors (NNRTIs)			
NNRTIs bind to and later alter reverse transcriptase, an enzyme HIV needs to make copies of itself.	doravirine (DOR)	Pifeltro	August 30, 2018
	efavirenz (EFV)	Sustiva	September 17, 1998
	etravirine (ETR)	Intelence	January 18, 2008
	nevirapine (extended-release nevirapine, NVP)	Viramune	June 21, 1996
		Viramune XR (extended release)	March 25, 2011
	rilpivirine (rilpivirine hydrochloride, RPV)	Edurant	May 20, 2011

Table 43.1. Continued

Drug Class	Generic Name (Other Names and Abbreviations)	Brand Name	FDA Approval Date
Protease Inhibitors (PIs)			
PIs block HIV protease, an enzyme HIV needs to make copies of itself.	atazanavir (atazanavir sulfate, ATV)	Reyataz	June 20, 2003
	darunavir (darunavir ethanolate, DRV)	Prezista	June 23, 2006
	fosamprenavir (fosamprenavir calcium, FOS-APV, FPV)	Lexiva	October 20, 2003
	ritonavir (RTV)*	Norvir	March 1, 1996
	tipranavir (TPV)	Aptivus	June 22, 2005
Fusion Inhibitors			
Fusion inhibitors block HIV from entering the CD4 T lymphocyte (CD4 cells) of the immune system.	enfuvirtide (T-20)	Fuzeon	March 13, 2003
CCR5 Antagonists			
CCR5 antagonists block CCR5 coreceptors on the surface of certain immune cells that HIV needs to enter the cells.	maraviroc (MVC)	Selzentry	August 6, 2007

Table 43.1. Continued

Drug Class	Generic Name (Other Names and Abbreviations)	Brand Name	FDA Approval Date
Integrase Strand Transfer Inhibitor (INSTIs)			
Integrase inhibitors block HIV integrase, an enzyme HIV needs to make copies of itself.	cabotegravir (cabotegravir sodium, CAB)	Vocabria	January 22, 2021
	dolutegravir (dolutegravir sodium, DTG)	Tivicay	August 12, 2013
		Tivicay PD	June 12, 2020
	raltegravir (raltegravir potassium, RAL)	Isentress	October 12, 2007
		Isentress HD	May 26, 2017
Attachment Inhibitors			
Attachment inhibitors bind to the gp120 protein on the outer surface of HIV, preventing HIV from entering CD4 cells.	fostemsavir (fostemsavir tromethamine, FTR)	Rukobia	July 2, 2020
Post-Attachment Inhibitors			
Post-attachment inhibitors block CD4 receptors on the surface of certain immune cells that HIV needs to enter the cells.	ibalizumab-uiyk (Hu5A8, IBA, Ibalizumab, TMB-355, TNX-355)	Trogarzo	March 6, 2018

Table 43.1. Continued

Drug Class	Generic Name (Other Names and Abbreviations)	Brand Name	FDA Approval Date
Capsid Inhibitors			
Capsid inhibitors interfere with the HIV capsid, a protein shell that protects HIV's genetic material and enzymes needed for replication.	lenacapavir (GS-6207, GS-HIV, GS-CA2, GS-CA1)	Sunlenca	December 22, 2022
Pharmacokinetic Enhancers			
Pharmacokinetic enhancers are used in HIV treatment to increase the effectiveness of an HIV medicine included in an HIV treatment regimen.	cobicistat (COBI, c)	Tybost	September 24, 2014
Combination HIV Medicines			
Combination HIV medicines contain two or more HIV medicines from one or more drug classes.	abacavir and lamivudine (abacavir sulfate/lamivudine, ABC/3TC)	Epzicom	August 2, 2004
	abacavir, dolutegravir, and lamivudine (abacavir sulfate/dolutegravir sodium/lamivudine, ABC/DTG/3TC)	Triumeq	August 22, 2014
		Triumeq PD	March 30, 2022

Table 43.1. Continued

Drug Class	Generic Name (Other Names and Abbreviations)	Brand Name	FDA Approval Date
Combination HIV medicines contain two or more HIV medicines from one or more drug classes.	abacavir, lamivudine, and zidovudine (abacavir sulfate/lamivudine/zidovudine, ABC/3TC/ZDV)	Trizivir	November 14, 2000
	atazanavir and cobicistat (atazanavir sulfate/cobicistat, ATV/COBI)	Evotaz	January 29, 2015
	bictegravir, emtricitabine, and tenofovir alafenamide (bictegravir sodium/emtricitabine/tenofovir alafenamide fumarate, BIC/FTC/TAF)	Biktarvy	February 7, 2018
	cabotegravir and rilpivirine (CAB and RPV, CAB plus RPV, Cabenuva kit, cabotegravir extended-release injectable suspension and rilpivirine extended-release injectable suspension)	Cabenuva	January 22, 2021
	darunavir and cobicistat (darunavir ethanolate/cobicistat, DRV/COBI)	Prezcobix	January 29, 2015
	darunavir, cobicistat, emtricitabine, and tenofovir alafenamide (darunavir ethanolate/cobicistat/emtricitabine/tenofovir AF, darunavir ethanolate/cobicistat/emtricitabine/tenofovir alafenamide, darunavir/cobicistat/emtricitabine/tenofovir AF, darunavir/cobicistat/emtricitabine/tenofovir alafenamide fumarate, DRV/COBI/FTC/TAF)	Symtuza	July 17, 2018

Table 43.1. Continued

Drug Class	Generic Name (Other Names and Abbreviations)	Brand Name	FDA Approval Date
Combination HIV medicines contain two or more HIV medicines from one or more drug classes.	dolutegravir and lamivudine (dolutegravir sodium/lamivudine, DTG/3TC)	Dovato	April 8, 2019
	dolutegravir and rilpivirine (dolutegravir sodium/rilpivirine hydrochloride, DTG/RPV)	Juluca	November 21, 2017
	doravirine, lamivudine, and tenofovir disoproxil fumarate (doravirine/lamivudine/TDF, doravirine/lamivudine/tenofovir DF, DOR/3TC/TDF)	Delstrigo	August 30, 2018
	efavirenz, emtricitabine, and tenofovir disoproxil fumarate (efavirenz/emtricitabine/tenofovir DF, EFV/FTC/TDF)	Atripla	July 12, 2006
	efavirenz, lamivudine, and tenofovir disoproxil fumarate (EFV/3TC/TDF)	Symfi	March 22, 2018
	efavirenz, lamivudine, and tenofovir disoproxil fumarate (EFV/3TC/TDF)	Symfi Lo	February 5, 2018
	elvitegravir, cobicistat, emtricitabine, and tenofovir alafenamide (elvitegravir/cobicistat/emtricitabine/tenofovir alafenamide fumarate, EVG/COBI/FTC/TAF)	Genvoya	November 5, 2015

Table 43.1. Continued

Drug Class	Generic Name (Other Names and Abbreviations)	Brand Name	FDA Approval Date
Combination HIV medicines contain two or more HIV medicines from one or more drug classes.	elvitegravir, cobicistat, emtricitabine, and tenofovir disoproxil fumarate (QUAD, EVG/COBI/FTC/TDF)	Stribild	August 27, 2012
	emtricitabine, rilpivirine, and tenofovir alafenamide (emtricitabine/rilpivirine/tenofovir AF, emtricitabine/rilpivirine/tenofovir alafenamide fumarate, emtricitabine/rilpivirine hydrochloride/tenofovir AF, emtricitabine/rilpivirine hydrochloride/tenofovir alafenamide, emtricitabine/rilpivirine hydrochloride/tenofovir alafenamide fumarate, FTC/RPV/TAF)	Odefsey	March 1, 2016
	emtricitabine, rilpivirine, and tenofovir disoproxil fumarate (emtricitabine/rilpivirine hydrochloride/tenofovir disoproxil fumarate, emtricitabine/rilpivirine/tenofovir, FTC/RPV/TDF)	Complera	August 10, 2011
	emtricitabine and tenofovir alafenamide (emtricitabine/tenofovir AF, emtricitabine/tenofovir alafenamide fumarate, FTC/TAF)	Descovy	April 4, 2016
	emtricitabine and tenofovir disoproxil fumarate (emtricitabine/tenofovir DF, FTC/TDF)	Truvada	August 2, 2004

Table 43.1. Continued

Drug Class	Generic Name (Other Names and Abbreviations)	Brand Name	FDA Approval Date
Combination HIV medicines contain two or more HIV medicines from one or more drug classes.	lamivudine and tenofovir disoproxil fumarate (3TC/TDF)	Cimduo	February 28, 2018
	lamivudine and zidovudine (3TC/ZDV)	Combivir	September 27, 1997
	lopinavir and ritonavir (ritonavir-boosted lopinavir, LPV/r, LPV/RTV)	Kaletra	September 15, 2000

*Although ritonavir is a PI, it is generally used as a pharmacokinetic enhancer as recommended in the Guidelines for the Use of Antiretroviral Agents in Adults and Adolescents with HIV and the Guidelines for the Use of Antiretroviral Agents in Pediatric HIV Infection.

Chapter 44 | Starting Human Immunodeficiency Virus Care

Chapter Contents

HOW DO YOU FIND A HUMAN IMMUNODEFICIENCY VIRUS HEALTH-CARE PROVIDER?

You can find a human immunodeficiency virus (HIV) health-care provider by using the HIV Testing Sites and Care Services Locator (https://locator.hiv.gov) of HIV.gov. Just enter your zip code to be connected to HIV medical care and other services, such as HIV testing locations, housing assistance, substance abuse, and mental health services.

The following are the other ways to find HIV providers and services:

- **Ask your primary care provider.** If you have a primary care provider (someone who manages your regular medical care), that person may have the medical knowledge to treat your HIV. If not, he or she can refer you to a provider who specializes in providing HIV care and treatment.
- **Call your state human immunodeficiency virus/ acquired immunodeficiency syndrome (HIV/AIDS) hotline.** State HIV/AIDS toll-free hotlines are available to help connect you to agencies that can help determine what services you are eligible for and help you get them.
- **Search the Referral Link directory.** The Referral Link of the American Academy of HIV Medicine (AAHIVM; https://providers.aahivm.org/referral-link-search?reload=timezone) is a directory of health-care providers specializing in HIV management and prevention across the country. The doctors and clinicians represented in this database practice in a variety of care settings, including health centers, Ryan White clinics, and private practices.
- **Use your home HIV test hotline.** If you received an HIV diagnosis by using an HIV home test kit, it is important that you take the next steps to make sure your test result is correct. Home test manufacturers

provide confidential counseling to answer questions and provide local referrals for follow-up testing and care.

WHY DO YOU NEED TO FIND A HUMAN IMMUNODEFICIENCY VIRUS HEALTH-CARE PROVIDER?

After you are diagnosed with HIV, it is important to see a health-care provider who can help you start HIV medicine (called "antiretroviral therapy" (ART)) as soon as possible. Treatment with HIV medicine is recommended for all people with HIV, regardless of how long they have had the virus or how healthy they are.

HIV medicine can reduce the amount of HIV in your blood (also called "your viral load") to an undetectable level—a level so low that a standard lab test cannot detect it. People with HIV who take HIV medicine as prescribed and get and keep an undetectable viral load can live long and healthy lives and will not transmit HIV to their HIV-negative partners through sex. This is sometimes referred to as "treatment as prevention" or "undetectable=untransmittable" (U=U).

HOW SOON DO YOU NEED TO FIND A HUMAN IMMUNODEFICIENCY VIRUS HEALTH-CARE PROVIDER?

The U.S. Department of Health and Human Services (HHS) guidelines on the use of HIV medicines in adults and adolescents recommend that people with HIV start medical care and begin HIV treatment as soon as possible after diagnosis. If you have the following conditions, it is especially important to start ART right away: pregnancy, AIDS, certain HIV-related illnesses and coinfections, and early HIV infection. (Early HIV infection is the period up to six months after infection with HIV.)[1]

---

[1] HIV.gov, "Locate an HIV Care Provider," U.S. Department of Health and Human Services (HHS), June 15, 2022. Available online. URL: www.hiv.gov/hiv-basics/starting-hiv-care/find-a-provider/locate-a-hiv-care-provider. Accessed June 9, 2023.

Section 44.2 | What to Expect at Your First Human Immunodeficiency Virus Care Visit

WHAT CAN YOU EXPECT AT YOUR FIRST HUMAN IMMUNODEFICIENCY VIRUS MEDICAL VISIT?

Just like with many other chronic health conditions, seeing a health-care provider for the first time about human immunodeficiency virus (HIV) might make you a bit nervous. But you are on the right path: By taking HIV medicine (called "antiretroviral therapy" (ART)) as prescribed and staying in ongoing medical care, you can live a long, healthy life and will not transmit HIV to your sexual partners.

During your first appointment, your health-care provider will talk to you about HIV and answer any questions you may have. They will help you understand how HIV works in your body, your treatment options, how to prevent passing HIV to others, and the importance of getting and keeping an undetectable viral load. They will also take a complete medical history, conduct a physical exam and mental health assessment, and run some lab tests. You and your provider will also discuss starting HIV medicine if you have not already.

Medical History

When taking your medical history, your health-care provider may ask questions about your:

- HIV-related history (e.g., your approximate date of diagnosis, approximate date of HIV acquisition)
- medical, surgical, and psychiatric (mental health) history
- medication and allergy history
- sexual health history, including any previous diagnosis of other sexually transmitted infections (STIs)
- substance use history
- social, family, and travel history
- immunization status

Your provider will also ask about any recent or new symptoms that you have been experiencing that may be related to HIV.

Physical Exam

During your physical exam, your provider will check your height and weight, measure your vital signs (pulse rate, temperature, blood pressure, etc.), and examine your general body appearance.

They will also examine your skin; eyes, ears, and throat; heart and lungs; genitals/rectum; and other parts of your body.

Mental Health Assessment

Your provider will also assess your mental and emotional health. They may also assess your need for supportive services and make referrals to assist you with any mental health or substance use issues, transportation, or housing needs.

After these assessments, your provider may:

- give you any vaccines you may need or prescribe medicine to prevent opportunistic infections
- refer you to specialty care (e.g., gynecology, colorectal care) if you need it

Lab Tests

Your health-care provider will review the results from any lab tests that have already been completed and run some new lab tests to find out what stage of HIV you are in, screen for other diseases, and assist in the selection of your HIV medicines. These lab tests include the following:

- **Clusters of differentiation 4 (CD4) cell count**. It measures how many CD4 cells are in your blood. CD4 cells are infection-fighting cells in your immune system. HIV attacks and destroys them. If too many CD4 cells are lost, your immune system will have trouble fighting off infections. A CD4 cell count is a good measure of how well your immune system is working and your risk of opportunistic infections. You want your CD4 cell count to be high.

- **An HIV viral load test**. It measures the amount of HIV in your blood. When your viral load is high, you have more HIV in your body. This means your immune system is not fighting HIV very well. HIV viral load tests are used to diagnose recent HIV infections and guide your treatment choices. In follow-up visits, viral load tests will help monitor how well your treatment is working. Once you start HIV medicine, you want your viral load to decrease and stay low.
- **HIV resistance testing**. It helps you and your provider better understand which HIV medications will work best for your HIV infection.

Your lab test results, along with your medical history, physical exam, mental health assessment, and other information you provide, will help you and your provider work together to manage your HIV care.

Your health-care provider will repeat some of these lab tests as part of your ongoing HIV care to see how well your HIV medicine is working so that you can get the virus under control, protect your health, and prevent transmitting the virus to others.

Starting Human Immunodeficiency Virus Treatment as Soon as Possible

If you started HIV treatment immediately upon your diagnosis and are now seeing your health-care provider for the first time for a full assessment, talk about your experience with taking the medicine so far and any side effects you may be experiencing.

If you are not already on HIV treatment, you and your health-care provider will discuss starting treatment. It is recommended that you start it as soon as you possibly can. The sooner you start to take HIV treatment, the sooner you can benefit from it. Research shows that people who start treatment earlier are less likely to get ill or pass HIV on to other people.

While starting HIV treatment as soon as possible after diagnosis is recommended, the decision to start treatment rests with you. Before starting treatment, talk with your health-care provider about how you are feeling. Discuss your readiness to start HIV treatment, the benefits of starting now, and what drug regimens are recommended for you. Also, ask your provider about how to take the HIV medicine and what side effects you may experience.

Scheduling Follow-Up Appointments

Talk to your provider about when you should return for follow-up visits and where you can learn more about HIV. Staying informed about your HIV care and treatment and partnering with your health-care provider are important steps in managing your health and HIV care.[2]

---

[2] HIV.gov, "What to Expect at Your First HIV Care Visit," U.S. Department of Health and Human Services (HHS), December 16, 2022. Available online. URL: www.hiv.gov/hiv-basics/starting-hiv-care/getting-ready-for-your-first-visit/what-to-expect-at-your-first-hiv-care-visit. Accessed June 9, 2023.

Chapter 45 | Taking Care of Yourself

Chapter Contents

SHOULD PEOPLE WITH HUMAN IMMUNODEFICIENCY VIRUS EXERCISE?

Yes. Being human immunodeficiency virus (HIV) positive is no different from being HIV-negative when it comes to exercise. Regular physical activity and exercise are part of a healthy lifestyle for everyone, including people with HIV.

WHAT ARE THE BENEFITS OF PHYSICAL ACTIVITY?

Physical activity has many important benefits. It can:
- boost your mood
- sharpen your focus
- reduce your stress
- improve your sleep

Physical activity can also help you reduce your risk of developing cardiovascular disease (CVD), high blood pressure (HBP), type 2 diabetes, and several types of cancer. These are all health conditions that can affect people living with HIV.

HOW MUCH ACTIVITY SHOULD YOU DO?

According to the evidence-based Physical Activity Guidelines (https://health.gov/our-work/nutrition-physical-activity/physical-activity-guidelines/current-guidelines) adults need at least 150–300 minutes per week of moderate-intensity aerobic activity, such as biking, brisk walking, or fast dancing. Adults also need muscle-strengthening activities, such as lifting weights or doing push-ups, at least two days per week.

If you are living with HIV or have another chronic health condition, talk to your health-care provider or a physical activity specialist to make sure these guidelines are right for you.

WHAT TYPES OF ACTIVITY ARE RIGHT FOR PEOPLE LIVING WITH HUMAN IMMUNODEFICIENCY VIRUS?

People living with HIV can do the same types of physical activities and exercises as individuals who do not have HIV.

577

Physical activity is any body movement that works your muscles and requires more energy than resting. Brisk walking, running, biking, dancing, jumping rope, and swimming are a few examples of physical activity.

Exercise is a type of physical activity that is planned and structured with the goal of improving your health or fitness. Taking an aerobics class and playing on a sports team are examples of exercise.

Both are part of living healthy.

Take time to find a fitness routine that you enjoy. You may consider taking part in a group activity that allows you to engage with others. Make it fun and commit to being physically active regularly.[1]

TRAVELING WITH HUMAN IMMUNODEFICIENCY VIRUS

Traveling outside the United States can be risky for anyone. However, it may require special precautions for people with HIV. For example, travel to some developing countries can increase the risk of getting an opportunistic infection. For some destinations, you may need certain vaccines. Your health-care provider can review your medical record to ensure the vaccines are safe for you.

Before You Travel

- Talk to your health-care provider at least four to six weeks before you travel:
  - Discuss medicine, such as antibiotics to treat traveler's diarrhea, and vaccines you may need.
  - Learn about the health risks in the places you plan to visit.
  - Learn about specific measures you need to take to stay healthy.
  - Gather the names of HIV health-care providers or clinics in the area you plan to visit.

---

[1] HIV.gov, "Exercise and Physical Activity," U.S. Department of Health and Human Services (HHS), April 28, 2022. Available online. URL: www.hiv.gov/hiv-basics/living-well-with-hiv/taking-care-of-yourself/exercise-and-physical-activity. Accessed June 9, 2023.

- Learn about your insurance:
  - Review your medical insurance to see what travel coverage it provides.
  - Take proof of insurance. (Copy or scan your policy and send the image to an email address you can access when traveling.)
  - Leave a copy of your insurance at home and tell your friends or family where you left it.
  - Consider purchasing additional travel insurance if your insurance does not cover emergency transportation to a health-care facility or the cost of care received in other countries.
  - Learn about your destination.
- Find out if the countries you plan to visit have special health rules for visitors, especially visitors with HIV.

During Travel

- Stick to safe eating and drinking habits:
  - Food and water in some developing countries may contain germs that could make you sick.
  - Eat only hot foods.
  - Drink bottled water or drinks, hot coffee or tea, wine, beer, or other alcoholic beverages.
  - Avoid raw fruit or vegetables that you do not peel yourself.
  - Avoid eating raw or undercooked seafood or meat or unpasteurized dairy products.
  - Tap water and drinks or ice made with tap water could make you sick.
- Take care of yourself and protect others:
  - Take all your medications on schedule.
  - Stick to your special diet if you are on one.
  - Take the same precautions you take at home to prevent transmitting HIV to others.
- Avoid direct contact with animal waste:
  - Animal waste (stool) in soil or on sidewalks can be harmful to people with HIV.

- Wear shoes to protect yourself from direct contact with animal waste.
- Use towels to protect yourself from animal waste when lying on a beach or in parks.
- Wash your hands with soap and water after physical contact with animals.
- Avoid hospitals and clinics where coughing tuberculosis (TB) patients are treated:
  - TB is very common worldwide and can be severe in people with HIV.
  - See your health-care provider when you return to discuss whether you should be tested for TB.[2]

Stay Up-to-Date on Your Sexual Health Care

Whether you are traveling or staying close to home for events, the Centers for Disease Control and Prevention (CDC) recommends the following:

- Visit your health-care provider or find a health clinic to stay up to date with your sexual health care. Discuss the types of sex you have so that your provider can offer testing and prevention services, including vaccines, that are right for you.
- Know your HIV status. If you do not know your HIV status, get tested near where you live, work, or play, including options for ordering free self-testing kits. No matter your results, there are steps you can take to stay healthy. If you do not have HIV, you have options to prevent HIV, including finding a pre-exposure prophylaxis (PrEP) provider to see if PrEP is right for you. If you test positive, you can find a care provider and live well with HIV. HIV treatment will keep you healthy and prevent you from transmitting HIV to your sex partners.
- If you are sexually active, get tested for other sexually transmitted infections (STIs), such as gonorrhea and syphilis. This is one of the most important things you can

[2] "Traveling with HIV," Centers for Disease Control and Prevention (CDC), May 20, 2021. Available online. URL: www.cdc.gov/hiv/basics/livingwithhiv/travel.html. Accessed June 9, 2023.

do to protect your health. You can also find STI testing sites near you and learn more about how to prevent STIs.
- Learn more about mpox and be sure to get your two-dose mpox vaccine. Mpox cases in the United States are becoming increasingly rare, but unvaccinated and under-vaccinated people who could benefit from the vaccine may still be at risk. The best protection against mpox occurs two weeks after the second shot, so plan ahead and use other strategies to prevent mpox.
- Get tested for viral hepatitis and consider vaccinations for hepatitis A and B. Be knowledgeable of other infections, such as shigella and meningococcal disease and how to prevent them.

Are There Restrictions on Traveling Abroad?

Some countries restrict visitors with HIV from entering their borders or staying for long periods of time. Others permit discrimination on the basis of sexual orientation or gender identification. According to the State Department, more than 70 countries consider consensual same-sex relations a crime, sometimes carrying severe punishment. Before you travel internationally, be aware of the laws, policies, and practices in the country or countries you plan to visit. This information is usually available from the consular offices of each country (www.usembassy.gov) or in the State Department's country information summaries (https://travel.state.gov/content/travel/en/international-travel/International-Travel-Country-Information-Pages.html), along with information about entry and exit requirements.

Traveling to the United States from Other Countries

As of January 2010, travelers with HIV or acquired immunodeficiency syndrome (AIDS) are allowed entrance into the United States.[3]

---

[3] HIV.gov, "Traveling Outside the U.S." U.S. Department of Health and Human Services (HHS), April 25, 2023. Available online. URL: www.hiv.gov/hiv-basics/living-well-with-hiv/taking-care-of-yourself/traveling-outside-the-us. Accessed June 9, 2023.

Section 45.2 | **Coping Mentally**

Mental health refers to the overall well-being of a person, including a person's mood, emotions, cognition, and behavior.

Many people have strong reactions when they find out they have human immunodeficiency virus (HIV), including feelings such as fear, anger, and a sense of being overwhelmed. Often people may feel helpless, sad, and anxious about the illness despite knowing that HIV can be effectively treated. People might also have negative thoughts related to the stigma of an HIV diagnosis. These feelings and thoughts are normal. With time, hopefully, these will fade.

There are many things you can do to deal with the mental health aspects of living with HIV. What follows are some of the most common challenges associated with a diagnosis of HIV and suggestions on how to cope with them. You may experience some, all, or none of these symptoms, and you may experience them at different times.

Some things to keep in mind about your feelings are as follows:
- No matter what you are feeling, you have a right to feel that way.
- There are no "wrong" or "right" feelings: feelings just are.
- You have choices about how you respond to your feelings.

DENIAL

When diagnosed with HIV, people sometimes deal with the news by denying that it is true. You may believe that the HIV test was wrong or that there was a mix-up of test results. This is a natural and normal first reaction.

If not dealt with, denial can be dangerous. You may fail to take certain precautions or start HIV medications right away or reach out for necessary help and medical support.

It is important that you talk about your feelings with your health-care provider or someone you trust. It is important to do this so that you can begin to receive the care and support you need.

ANGER

Anger is another common and natural feeling related to being diagnosed with HIV. Many people are upset about how they got the virus or angry that they did not know they had the virus. Many of these feelings and thoughts are often related to feelings of helplessness and being overwhelmed with the new diagnosis.

Ways to deal with feelings of anger and other challenges include the following:

- Talk about your feelings with others, such as people in a support group, or with a psychologist, social worker, or friend.
- Try to get some exercise—such as gardening, walking, or dancing—to relieve some of the tension and angry feelings you may be experiencing.
- Avoid situations—involving certain people, places, and events—that cause you to feel angry or stressed out.

SADNESS OR DEPRESSION

It is also normal to feel sad when you learn you have HIV. If, over time, you find that the sadness does not go away or is getting worse, talk with your provider. You may need treatment for depression.

Symptoms of depression can include the following, especially if they last for more than two weeks:

- feeling sad, anxious, irritable, or hopeless
- gaining or losing weight
- sleeping more or less than usual
- moving slower than usual or finding it hard to sit still
- losing interest in the things you usually enjoy
- feeling tired all the time
- feeling worthless or guilty
- having a hard time concentrating
- thinking about death or giving up

To deal with these symptoms, you may want to:
- talk with your provider about treatments for depression, such as therapy or medications

- start HIV treatment if you have not done so already.
  Taking this positive step for your own health may help
  with depression
- join a support group
- spend time with supportive people, such as family
  members and friends

If your mood swings or depression get very severe or if you ever
think about suicide, call your provider or the Veterans Crisis Line
(800-273-8255 or text 838255) right away. No matter what you are
experiencing, there is support for getting your life back on track.

Finding the right treatment for depression takes time—so does
recovery. If you think you may be depressed, talk to your health-
care provider and seek help for depression.

FEAR AND ANXIETY

Fear and anxiety may be caused by not knowing what to expect
now that you have been diagnosed with HIV or not knowing how
others will treat you after they find out you have HIV. You also
may also be afraid of telling people—friends, family members, and
others—that you have HIV.

Fear can make your heart beat faster or make it hard for you to
sleep. Anxiety can also make you feel nervous or agitated. Fear and
anxiety might make you sweat, feel dizzy, or feel short of breath.
Others experience anxiety and fear by avoidance behavior or feeling
paralyzed and overwhelmed.

Ways to manage your feelings of fear and anxiety include the
following:

- Talk to your provider about treatments for anxiety if
  the feelings do not lessen with time or if they get worse.
- Learn as much as you can about HIV.
- Start HIV treatment ("antiretroviral therapy" (ART)).
  Taking action to control HIV will protect your health
  and the health of your sex partners, and this in turn
  may lessen your fears about the future.
- Get your questions answered by your health-care
  provider.

- Talk with your friends, family members, and health-care providers.
- Join a support group.
- Help others who are in the same situation, such as by volunteering at an HIV service organization. This may empower you and lessen your feelings of fear.

STRESS

If you have HIV, you and your loved ones may have to deal with more stress than usual. Stress is unique and personal to each of us. When stress does occur, it is important to recognize and deal with it. The following are a few ways to handle stress. As you gain more understanding about how stress affects you, you will come up with your own ideas for coping with stress.

- **Take care of yourself**. Be sure you get enough rest and eat well. If you are irritable from lack of sleep or if you are not eating right, you will have less energy to deal with stressful situations. If stress keeps you from sleeping, you should ask your provider for help.
- **Try physical activity**. When you are nervous, angry, or upset, try exercise or some other kind of physical activity. Walking, yoga, and gardening are just some of the activities you might try to release your tension.
- **Talk about it**. It helps to talk to someone about your concerns and worries. You can talk to a friend, family member, counselor, or health-care provider.
- **Let it out**. A good cry can bring relief to your anxiety, and it might even prevent a headache or other physical problems. Taking some deep breaths also releases tension.

NEUROCOGNITIVE DISORDERS ASSOCIATED WITH HUMAN IMMUNODEFICIENCY VIRUS

Human immunodeficiency virus or acquired immunodeficiency syndrome (AIDS) and some medications for treating HIV may affect your brain. When HIV itself infects the brain, it can sometimes cause problems with thinking, emotions, and movement. Symptoms of HIV-associated neurocognitive disorders (HAND) can include the following:

- forgetfulness
- confusion
- difficulty paying attention
- sudden shifts in mood or behavior
- muscle weakness
- clumsiness

If you think you may have HAND:

- do not be afraid to tell your health-care provider that you think something is wrong
- keep a notepad with you and write down your symptoms whenever they occur (This information can help your doctor help you.)
- build as much support as possible, including friends, family, and health-care providers (Although it is possible to treat HAND successfully, it may take a while for some symptoms to go away.)

COPING TIPS

It is completely normal to have a negative reaction when you are diagnosed with HIV. These reactions do not last forever. There are many things that you can do to help take care of your mental health needs. Here are just a few ideas:

- Start HIV medications (ART) right away—an effective ART regimen will improve and protect your health and protect your sex partners, and the knowledge you are taking this positive step may improve your feelings about yourself and the future.
- Talk about your feelings with your providers, friends, family members, or other supportive people.
- Try to find activities that relieve your stress, such as exercise or hobbies.
- Try to get enough sleep each night to help you feel rested.

Taking Care of Yourself

- Learn relaxation methods such as meditation, yoga, or deep breathing.
- Limit the amount of caffeine and nicotine you use.
- Eat small, healthy meals throughout the day.
- Join a support group.

There are many kinds of support groups that provide a place where you can talk about your feelings, help others, and get the latest information about HIV. Check with your health-care provider for a listing of local or virtual support groups. Some medical centers have support groups available at the clinic or hospital.

More specific ways to care for your emotional well-being include various forms of therapy and medication. Used by themselves or in combination, these may help you deal with the symptoms you are experiencing. Therapy can help you better express your feelings, negative thoughts, and unhelpful behaviors and find ways to cope with your experiences. Medications may help with managing these symptoms.

You should always talk with your provider about your options. There are many ways to care for your emotional health, but treatments must be carefully chosen by your health-care provider based on your specific circumstances and needs.

The most important thing to remember is that you are not alone; there are support systems in place to help you, including doctors, psychologists, social workers, family members, friends, support groups, and other services.[4]

[4] "Mental Health and HIV: Entire Lesson," U.S. Department of Veterans Affairs (VA), December 2, 2020. Available online. URL: www.hiv.va.gov/patient/daily/mental/single-page.asp. Accessed June 9, 2023.

Section 45.3 | Housing and Employment: Know Your Rights and Find Support

HOUSING AND HEALTH
Why Do People with HIV Need Stable Housing?

Stable housing is closely linked to successful HIV outcomes. With safe, decent, and affordable housing, people with HIV are better able to access medical care and supportive services, get on HIV treatment, take their HIV medication consistently, and see their health-care provider regularly. In short: The more stable your living situation, the better you do in care.

Individuals with HIV who are homeless or lack stable housing, on the other hand, are more likely to delay HIV care and less likely to access care consistently or to adhere to their HIV treatment.

Throughout many communities, people with HIV risk losing their housing due to factors such as stigma and discrimination, increased medical costs and limited incomes, or reduced ability to keep working due to HIV-related illnesses.

What Federal Housing Assistance Programs Are Available for People with HIV?

To help take care of the housing needs of low-income people with HIV and their families, the Office of HIV/AIDS of the U.S. Department of Housing and Urban Development (HUD) manages the Housing Opportunities for Persons With AIDS (HOPWA) program. The HOPWA program is the only federal program dedicated to addressing the housing needs of people with HIV. Under the HOPWA program, HUD makes grants to local communities, states, and nonprofit organizations to provide housing assistance and supportive services for low-income people with HIV and their families.

Many local HOPWA programs and projects provide short- and long-term rental assistance, operate community residences, or provide other supportive housing facilities that have been created to address the needs of people with HIV.

Are People with HIV Eligible for Other HUD Programs?

In addition to the HOPWA program, people with HIV are eligible for any HUD program for which they might otherwise qualify (such as by being low-income or homeless). Programs include public housing, the Section 8 Housing Choice Voucher Program (HCVP), housing opportunities supported by Community Development Block Grants (CDBGs), the HOME Investment Partnerships Program (HOME), and the Continuum of Care (CoC) Homeless Assistance Program.[5]

EMPLOYMENT AND HEALTH
Working with HIV

With proper care and treatment, many people living with HIV lead normal, healthy lives, including having a job. Most people living with HIV can continue working at their current jobs or look for a new job in their chosen field. Your overall well-being and financial health can be more stable when you are gainfully employed.

Getting a New Job or Returning to Work

Working will affect a lot of your life: your medical status, your finances, your social life, the way you spend your time, and perhaps even your housing or transportation needs. Before taking action on getting a new job or returning to work, you may want to get information and perspectives from:

- your HIV case manager or counselor, if you have one
- benefits counselors at an HIV service organization or other community organization
- the Social Security Administrations (SSA) Work Incentives Planning and Assistance Program (WIPA)
- other people living with HIV who are working or have returned to work
- providers of any of your housing, medical, or financial benefits

---

[5] HIV.gov, "Housing and Health," U.S. Department of Health and Human Services (HHS), January 5, 2023. Available online. URL: www.hiv.gov/hiv-basics/living-well-with-hiv/taking-care-of-yourself/housing-and-health. Accessed June 9, 2023.

- public and nonprofit employment and training service providers

Here are some questions to discuss with them:
- What are my goals for employment?
- What kind of work do I want to do?
- What are the resources that can help me set and achieve a new career goal?
- Are there state or local laws that further strengthen antidiscrimination protections in the American Disabilities Act (ADA)?
- How do I access training or education that will help me achieve my goals?
- How can I plan to take care of my health if I go to work?
- How will my going to work impact the benefits I am receiving?

Requesting Reasonable Accommodations

Qualified individuals with disabilities, including people living with HIV, have the right to request reasonable accommodations in the workplace. A reasonable accommodation is any modification or adjustment to a job or work environment that enables a qualified person with a disability to apply for or perform a job. An accommodation may be tangible (e.g., a certain type of chair) or non-tangible (e.g., a modified work schedule for someone with a medical condition requiring regular appointments with a health-care provider). You are qualified if you are able to perform the essential functions of the job, with or without reasonable accommodation.

Your supervisor may not be trained in reasonable accommodations or know how to negotiate them. For that reason, often, it is best to go directly to the person responsible for human resources at your employer, even if that person works in a different location. In a small business, that person may well be the owner.

When you request an accommodation, state clearly what you need (e.g., time off for a clinic visit every third Tuesday of the month, a certain type of chair, or a change in your work hours) and be ready to supply a doctor's note supporting your request. The initial note need not contain your diagnosis, but it should verify that you are under that doctor's care and that he/she believes you need the accommodation to maintain your health or to be able to fulfill essential functions of your job.

Many people living with HIV do not want to give a lot of details about their health. If you prefer not to provide a lot of information, you may want to limit the medical information you initially give to your employer. However, if your need for accommodation is not obvious, your employer may require that you provide medical documentation to establish that you have a disability as defined by the ADA, to show that the employee needs the requested accommodation, and to help determine effective accommodation options. This can, but often does not, include disclosing your specific medical condition.

Be aware that not all people with HIV or AIDS will need accommodations to perform their jobs and many others may only need a few or simple accommodations. The U.S. Department of Labor (DOL) Job Accommodation Network (JAN) provides free, expert, and confidential technical assistance to both employees and employers on workplace accommodations and disability employment issues, which includes resources for employees living with HIV or AIDS.[6]

---

[6] HIV.gov, "Employment and Health," U.S. Department of Health and Human Services (HHS), May 15, 2017. Available online. URL: www.hiv.gov/hiv-basics/living-well-with-hiv/taking-care-of-yourself/employment-and-health. Accessed June 9, 2023.

Chapter 46 | Antidiscrimination Law: Know Your Civil Rights

WHAT LAWS PROTECT PEOPLE WITH HUMAN IMMUNODEFICIENCY VIRUS OR ACQUIRED IMMUNODEFICIENCY SYNDROME FROM DISCRIMINATION?

If you have human immunodeficiency virus (HIV) or acquired immunodeficiency syndrome (AIDS), you are protected against discrimination based on your HIV status under Section 504 of the Rehabilitation Act of 1973, the Americans with Disabilities Act of 1990 (ADA), and Section 1557 of the Affordable Care Act (ACA). Under these laws, discrimination means that you are not allowed to participate in a service that is offered to others or you are denied a benefit because you have HIV.

HOW DO THESE LAWS PROTECT AGAINST DISCRIMINATION?

Section 504, the ADA, and Section 1557 prohibit discrimination against qualified persons, including those with HIV or AIDS.

The ADA prohibits discrimination by employers, places of public accommodation, and state and local government entities. Section 504 prohibits health and human service providers or organizations that get federal funds or assistance from discriminating against you because you have HIV or AIDS. Section 1557 prohibits discrimination based on race, color, national origin, age, sex (including pregnancy, sexual orientation, or gender identity), or disability (including HIV or AIDS) in certain health programs or activities.

593

Examples of entities that may be covered by the ADA and/or Section 504 include hospitals, clinics, social services agencies, drug treatment centers, nursing homes, doctors' offices, dentists' offices, day cares, public pools, and fitness gyms. Again, under these laws, discrimination means that you are not allowed to participate in a service that is offered to others or you are denied a benefit because you have HIV. The ADA also protects your family and friends from discrimination because of your HIV status, based on their association with you.

HOW DO YOU FILE A CIVIL RIGHTS COMPLAINT?

Your complaint must:
- be filed in writing by mail, fax, email, or via the Office for Civil Rights (OCR) Complaint Portal
- name the health-care or social service provider involved and describe the acts or omissions you believe violated civil rights laws or regulations
- be filed within 180 days of when you knew that the act or omission complained of occurred (The OCR may extend the 180-day period if you can show "good cause.")

Language assistance services for OCR matters are available and provided free of charge. OCR services are accessible to persons with disabilities. For assistance, call toll-free 800-368-1019 or TDD toll-free 800-537-7697.[1]

HUMAN IMMUNODEFICIENCY VIRUS, EMPLOYMENT DISCRIMINATION, AND THE LAW

- The ADA prohibits employment discrimination on the basis of disability. The ADA, which covers employers of 15 or more people, applies to employment decisions at all stages. Court decisions have found that an individual with even asymptomatic HIV is protected under this law.

---

[1] HIV.gov, "Civil Rights," U.S. Department of Health and Human Services (HHS), April 17, 2023. Available online. URL: www.hiv.gov/hiv-basics/living-well-with-hiv/your-legal-rights/civil-rights. Accessed June 9, 2023.

- The Health Insurance Portability and Accountability Act of 1996 (HIPAA) addresses some of the barriers to health care facing people with HIV, as well as other vulnerable populations. The HIPAA gives people with group coverage new protections from discriminatory treatment, makes it easier for small groups (such as businesses with a small number of employees) to obtain and keep health insurance coverage, and gives those losing/leaving group coverage new options for obtaining individual coverage.
- The Family Medical Leave Act of 1993 (FMLA) applies to private sector employers with 50 or more employees within 75 miles of the work site. Eligible employees may take leave for serious medical conditions or to provide care for an immediate family member with a serious medical condition, including HIV/AIDS. Eligible employees are entitled to a total of 12 weeks of job-protected, unpaid leave during any 12-month period.
- The Consolidated Omnibus Budget Reconciliation Act of 1986 (COBRA) allows employees to continue their health insurance coverage at their own expense for a period of time after their employment ends. For most employees ceasing work for health reasons, the period of time to which benefits may be extended ranges from 18 to 36 months.

FILING A CHARGE OF EMPLOYMENT DISCRIMINATION

Any individual who believes that his or her employment rights have been violated may file a charge of discrimination with the Federal Equal Employment Opportunity Commission (EEOC). In addition, an individual, an organization, or an agency may file a charge on behalf of another person in order to protect the aggrieved person's identity.[2]

---

[2] HIV.gov, "Workplace Rights," U.S. Department of Health and Human Services (HHS), May 15, 2017. Available online. URL: www.hiv.gov/hiv-basics/living-well-with-hiv/your-legal-rights/workplace-rights. Accessed June 9, 2023.

Part 7 | Additional Help and Information

Chapter 47 | Glossary of Terms Related to Sexually Transmitted Diseases

abstinence: Not having sexual intercourse.

acquired immunodeficiency syndrome (AIDS): A disease of the immune system due to infection with human immunodeficiency virus (HIV). HIV destroys the CD4 T lymphocytes (CD4 cells) of the immune system, leaving the body vulnerable to life-threatening infections and cancers. AIDS is the most advanced stage of HIV infection.

adherence: Taking medications exactly as prescribed. Poor adherence to an HIV treatment regimen increases the risk of developing drug-resistant HIV and virologic failure.

antiretroviral therapy (ART): The recommended treatment for HIV infection. ART involves using a combination of three or more antiretroviral (ARV) drugs from at least two different HIV drug classes to prevent HIV from replicating.

bacteria: Microorganisms that can cause infections.

bacterial vaginosis (BV): A vaginal infection that develops when there is an increase in harmful bacteria and a decrease in good bacteria in the vagina.

biopsy: Removal of tissue, cells, or fluid from the body for examination under a microscope. Biopsies are used to diagnose disease.

CD4 cell count: A laboratory test that measures the number of CD4 T lymphocytes (CD4 cells) in a sample of blood. In people with HIV, the CD4 count is the most important laboratory indicator of immune function and the strongest predictor of HIV progression. The CD4 count is one of the factors used to determine when to start ART. The CD4 count is also used to monitor response to ART.

cervical cancer: A type of cancer that develops in the cervix. Cervical cancer is almost always caused by the human papillomavirus (HPV), which is spread through sexual contact.

chancroid: A sexually transmitted disease (STD) caused by the bacterium *Haemophilus ducreyi*. Chancroid causes genital ulcers (sores).

chlamydia: A common sexually transmitted disease caused by the bacterium *Chlamydia trachomatis*. Chlamydia often has mild or no symptoms, but if left untreated, it can lead to serious complications, including infertility.

coinfection: When a person has two or more infections at the same time. For example, a person infected with HIV may be coinfected with hepatitis or tuberculosis (TB) or both.

condom: A device used during sexual intercourse to block semen from coming in contact with the inside of the vagina. Condoms are used to reduce the likelihood of pregnancy and to prevent the transmission of sexually transmitted diseases (STDs), including human immunodeficiency virus (HIV). The male condom is a thin rubber cover that fits over an erect penis. The female condom is a polyurethane pouch that fits inside the vagina.

dental dam: A thin, rectangular sheet, usually latex rubber, used as a barrier to prevent the transmission of sexually transmitted infections (STIs) during oral sex.

drug resistance: When a bacteria, virus, or other microorganism mutates (changes form) and becomes insensitive to (resistant to) a drug that was previously effective.

fallopian tubes: Tubes on each side of the ovaries to the uterus.

genital warts: A sexually transmitted disease caused by HPV. Genital warts appear as raised pink or flesh-colored bumps on the surface of the vagina, cervix, tip of the penis, or anus.

gonorrhea: A sexually transmitted disease caused by the bacterium *Neisseria gonorrhoeae*. Gonorrhea can also be transmitted from an infected mother to her child during delivery. Gonorrhea often has mild or no symptoms. However, if left untreated, gonorrhea can lead to infertility, spread into the bloodstream, and affect the joints, heart valves, and brain.

Glossary of Terms Related to Sexually Transmitted Diseases

hepatitis B virus (HBV) infection: Infection with the HBV. HBV can be transmitted through blood, semen, or other body fluids during sex or injection drug use. Because HIV and HBV share the same modes of transmission, people infected with HIV are often also coinfected with HBV.

hepatitis C virus (HCV) infection: Infection with the HCV. HCV is usually transmitted through blood and rarely through other body fluids, such as semen. HCV infection progresses more rapidly in people coinfected with HIV than in people infected with HCV alone.

herpes simplex virus 2 (HSV-2) infection: An infection caused by HSV-2 and usually associated with lesions in the genital or anal area. HSV-2 is very contagious and is transmitted by sexual contact with someone who is infected (even if lesions are not visible).

human immunodeficiency virus (HIV): The virus that causes acquired immunodeficiency syndrome (AIDS), which is the most advanced stage of HIV infection. HIV is a retrovirus that occurs in two types: HIV-1 and HIV-2. Both types are transmitted through direct contact with HIV-infected body fluids, such as blood, semen, and genital secretions, or from an HIV-infected mother to her child during pregnancy, birth, or breastfeeding (through breast milk).

human papillomavirus (HPV): The virus that causes HPV infection, the most common STI. There are two groups of HPV types that can cause genital warts and types that can cause cancer. HPV is the most frequent cause of cervical cancer.

immune system: A complex network of cells, tissues, organs, and the substances they make that helps the body fight infections and other diseases. The immune system includes white blood cells and organs and tissues of the lymph system, such as the thymus, spleen, tonsils, lymph nodes, lymph vessels, and bone marrow.

immunosuppression: A state of the body in which the immune system is damaged and does not perform its normal functions. Immunosuppression may be induced by drugs (e.g., in chemotherapy) or result from certain disease processes, such as HIV infection.

injection drug use: A method of illicit drug use. The drugs are injected directly into the body into a vein, into a muscle, or under the skin with a needle and syringe. Bloodborne viruses, including HIV and hepatitis, can be transmitted via shared needles or other drug injection equipment.

molluscum contagiosum: A common, usually mild skin disease caused by the virus molluscum contagiosum and characterized by small white, pink, or flesh-colored bumps with a dimple in the center. Molluscum contagiosum is spread by touching the affected skin of an infected person or by touching a surface with the virus on it. The bumps can easily spread to other parts of the body if someone touches or scratches a bump and then touches another part of the body.

mother-to-child transmission (MTCT): When a mother infected with human immunodeficiency virus (HIV) passes the virus to her infant during pregnancy, labor and delivery, or breastfeeding (through breast milk). Antiretroviral (ARV) drugs are given to HIV-infected women during pregnancy and to their infants after birth to reduce the risk of MTCT of HIV.

opportunistic infection: An infection that occurs more frequently or is more severe in people with weakened immune systems, such as people with HIV or people receiving chemotherapy, than in people with healthy immune systems.

Papanicolaou (Pap) test: A procedure in which cells and secretions are collected from inside and around the cervix for examination under a microscope. Pap test also refers to the laboratory test used to detect any infected, potentially precancerous, or cancerous cells in the cervical cells obtained from a Pap test.

pelvic inflammatory disease (PID): Infection and inflammation of the female upper genital tract, including the uterus and fallopian tubes. PID is usually due to bacterial infection, including some sexually transmitted diseases, such as chlamydia and gonorrhea. Symptoms, if any, include pain in the lower abdomen, fever, smelly vaginal discharge, irregular bleeding, or pain during intercourse. PID can lead to serious complications, including infertility, ectopic pregnancy (a pregnancy in the fallopian tube or elsewhere outside of the womb), and chronic pelvic pain.

post-exposure prophylaxis (PEP): Short-term treatment started as soon as possible after high-risk exposure to an infectious agent, such as HIV, hepatitis B virus (HBV), or hepatitis C virus (HCV). The purpose of PEP is to reduce the risk of infection. An example of high-risk exposure is exposure to an infectious agent as the result of unprotected sex.

pubic lice: Also called "crab lice" or "crabs," pubic lice are parasitic insects found primarily in the pubic or genital area of humans.

Glossary of Terms Related to Sexually Transmitted Diseases

rapid HIV test: A screening test for detecting antibodies to HIV that produces very quick results, usually in 5–30 minutes. For diagnosis of HIV infection, a positive rapid test is confirmed with a second rapid test made by a different manufacturer.

scabies: An infestation of the skin by the human itch mite (*Sarcoptes scabiei* var. *hominis*). The microscopic scabies mite burrows into the upper layer of the skin where it lives and lays its eggs. The most common symptoms of scabies are intense itching and a pimple-like skin rash. The scabies mite is usually spread by direct, prolonged, skin-to-skin contact with a person who has scabies.

semen: A thick, whitish fluid that is discharged from the male penis during ejaculation. Semen contains sperm and various secretions. HIV can be transmitted through the semen of a man with HIV.

sexually transmitted disease (STD): An infectious disease that spreads from person to person during sexual contact. STDs, such as syphilis, HIV infection, and gonorrhea, are caused by bacteria, parasites, and viruses.

syphilis: An infectious disease caused by the bacterium *Treponema pallidum*, which is typically transmitted through direct contact with a syphilis sore, usually during vaginal or oral sex. Syphilis can also be transmitted from an infected mother to her child during pregnancy. Syphilis sores occur mainly on the genitals, anus, and rectum but also on the lips and mouth.

transmission: The spread of disease from one person to another.

trichomoniasis: A sexually transmitted disease caused by a parasite.

ulcer: An open lesion on the surface of the skin or a mucosal surface caused by superficial loss of tissue, usually with inflammation.

vaccination: Giving a vaccine to stimulate a person's immune response. Vaccination can be intended either to prevent a disease (a preventive vaccine) or to treat a disease (a therapeutic vaccine).

vaginal fluid: The natural liquids produced inside a woman's vagina. In an infected person, sexually transmitted diseases can be passed when vaginal fluids come in contact with the genital area of a woman's sex partner.

vesicle: A small, fluid-filled bubble, usually superficial, and less than 0.5 cm.

viral load: The amount of HIV in a sample of blood. Viral load is reported as the number of HIV RNA copies per milliliter of blood.

virus: A microscopic infectious agent that requires a living host cell in order to replicate. Viruses often cause diseases in humans, including measles, mumps, rubella, polio, influenza, and the common cold. HIV is the virus that causes acquired immunodeficiency syndrome (AIDS).

window period: The time period from infection with HIV until the body produces enough HIV antibodies to be detected by standard HIV antibody tests. The length of the window period varies depending on the antibody test used. During the window period, a person can have a negative result on an HIV antibody test despite being infected with HIV.

yeast infection: A fungal infection caused by overgrowth of the yeast Candida (usually *Candida albicans*) in moist areas of the body. Candidiasis can affect the mucous membranes of the mouth, vagina, and anus.

Chapter 48 | Directory of Organizations That Provide Information about Sexually Transmitted Diseases

GOVERNMENT AGENCIES

Agency for Healthcare Research and Quality (AHRQ)
5600 Fishers Ln.
7th Fl.
Rockville, MD 20857
Phone: 301-427-1364
Website: www.ahrq.gov

Centers for Disease Control and Prevention (CDC)
1600 Clifton Rd.
Atlanta, GA 30329-4027
Toll-Free: 800-CDC-INFO
(800-232-4636)
Toll-Free TTY: 888-232-6348
Website: www.cdc.gov

Federal Trade Commission (FTC)
600 Pennsylvania Ave., N.W.
Washington, DC 20580
Phone: 202-326-2222
Website: www.ftc.gov

National Cancer Institute (NCI)
9609 Medical Center Dr.
Rockville, MD 20850
Toll-Free: 800-4-CANCER
(800-422-6237)
Website: www.cancer.gov
Email: NCIinfo@nih.gov

Resources in this chapter were compiled from several sources deemed reliable; all contact information was verified and updated in July 2023.

National Center for Complementary and Integrative Health (NCCIH)
9000 Rockville Pike
Bethesda, MD 20892
Toll-Free: 888-644-6226
Website: www.nccih.nih.gov
Email: info@nccih.nih.gov

National Center for Health Statistics (NCHS)
3311 Toledo Rd.
Metro 4 Bldg.
Hyattsville, MD 20782-2064
Phone: 301-458-4000
Website: www.cdc.gov/nchs
Email: nhis@cdc.gov

National Institute of Allergy and Infectious Diseases (NIAID)
5601 Fishers Ln.
MSC 9806
Bethesda, MD 20892-9806
Toll-Free: 866-284-4107
Phone: 301-496-5717
Toll-Free TDD: 800-877-8339
Fax: 301-402-3573
Website: www.niaid.nih.gov
Email: ocpostoffice@niaid.nih.gov

National Institute of Mental Health (NIMH)
6001 Executive Blvd., Rm. 6200
MSC 9663
Bethesda, MD 20892-9663
Toll-Free: 866-615-6464
Phone: 301-443-4513
TTY: 301-443-8431
Toll-Free TTY: 866-415-8051
Fax: 301-443-4279
Website: www.nimh.nih.gov
Email: nimhinfo@nih.gov

National Institute of Neurological Disorders and Stroke (NINDS)
P.O. Box 5801
Bethesda, MD 20824
Toll-Free: 800-352-9424
Website: www.ninds.nih.gov

National Institute on Aging (NIA)
P.O. Box 8057
Gaithersburg, MD 20898
Toll-Free: 800-222-2225
Toll-Free TTY: 800-222-4225
Website: www.nia.nih.gov
Email: niaic@nia.nih.gov

National Institutes of Health (NIH)
9000 Rockville Pike
Bethesda, MD 20892
Phone: 301-496-4000
TTY: 301-402-9612
Website: www.nih.gov
Email: olib@od.nih.gov

National Prevention Information Network (NPIN)

Website: https://npin.cdc.gov
Email: NPIN-Info@cdc.gov

Office of Disease Prevention and Health Promotion (ODPHP)

1101 Wootton Pkwy., Ste. 420
Rockville, MD 20852
Website: https://health.gov/about-odphp

Office of Minority Health Resource Center (OMHRC)

1101 Wootton Pkwy., Ste. 100
Tower Oaks Bldg.
Rockville, MD 20852
Toll-Free: 800-444-6472
TDD: 301-251-1432
Fax: 301-251-2160
Website: www.minorityhealth.hhs.gov
Email: info@minorityhealth.hhs.gov

Substance Abuse and Mental Health Services Administration (SAMHSA)

5600 Fishers Ln.
Rockville, MD 20857
Toll-Free:
877-SAMHSA-7(877-726-4727)
Toll-Free TTY: 800-487-4889
Website: www.samhsa.gov
Email: SAMHSAInfo@samhsa.hhs.gov

U.S. Department of Health and Human Services (HHS)

200 Independence Ave., S.W.
Hubert H. Humphrey Bldg.
Washington, DC 20201
Toll-Free: 877-696-6775
Website: www.hhs.gov

U.S. Food and Drug Administration (FDA)

10903 New Hampshire Ave.
Silver Spring, MD 20993-0002
Toll-Free: 888-INFO-FDA
(888-463-6332)
Website: www.fda.gov

U.S. National Library of Medicine (NLM)

8600 Rockville Pike
Bethesda, MD 20894
Toll-Free: 888-FIND-NLM
(888-346-3656)
Phone: 301-594-5983
Website: www.nlm.nih.gov
Email: custserv@nlm.nih.gov

PRIVATE AGENCIES

Advocates for Youth
1325 G St., N.W., Ste. 980
Washington, DC 20005
Phone: 202-419-3420
Fax: 202-419-1448
Website: www.advocatesforyouth.org
Email: info@advocatesforyouth.org

AIDS Healthcare Foundation (AHF)
6255 Sunset Blvd.
21st Fl.
Los Angeles, CA 90028
Phone: 323-860-5200
Website: www.aidshealth.org

AIDS.org
Website: www.aids.org

American Cancer Society (ACS)
3380 Chastain Meadows Pkwy.,
N.W., Ste. 200
Kennesaw, GA 30144
Toll-Free: 800-227-2345
Website: www.cancer.org

American Foundation for AIDS Research (amfAR)
120 Wall St.
13th Fl.
New York, NY 10005-3908
Phone: 212-806-1600
Fax: 212-806-1601
Website: www.amfar.org
Email: information@amfar.org

American Medical Association (AMA)
AMA Plz., 330 N. Wabash Ave.,
Ste. 39300
Chicago, IL 60611-5885
Toll-Free: 800-621-8335
Phone: 312-464-4782
Website: www.ama-assn.org

American Sexual Health Association (ASHA)
P.O. Box 13827
Research Triangle Park, NC 27709
Phone: 919-361-8400
Fax: 919-361-8425
Website: www.ashasexualhealth.org
Email: info@ashasexualhealth.org

American Society for Colposcopy and Cervical Pathology (ASCCP)
23219 Stringtown Rd., Ste. 210
Clarksburg, MD 20871
Phone: 301-857-7877
Website: www.asccp.org
Email: info@asccp.org

American Society of Reproductive Medicine (ASRM)
726 Seventh St., S.E.
Washington, DC 20003
Phone: 202-863-4985
Website: www.asrm.org
Email: asrm@asrm.org

The Body

461 Fifth Ave.
14th Fl.
New York, NY 10017
Phone: 212-695-2223
Fax: 212-695-2936
Website: www.thebody.com

Children and AIDS

Website: www.childrenandaids.org

Cleveland Clinic

9500 Euclid Ave.
Cleveland, OH 44195
Toll-Free: 800-223-CARE
(800-223-2273)
Phone: 216-444-2200
Website: my.clevelandclinic.org

Elizabeth Glaser Pediatric AIDS Foundation (EGPAF)

1350 Eye St., N.W., Ste. 400
Washington, DC 20036
Toll-Free: 888-499-HOPE
(888-499-4673)
Phone: 202-296-9165
Website: www.pedaids.org
Email: info@pedaids.org

Engender Health

505 Ninth St., N.W., Ste. 601
Washington, DC 20004
Phone: 202-902-2000
Website: www.engenderhealth.org
Email: info@engenderhealth.org

Foundation for Women's Cancer (FWC)

230 W. Monroe St., Ste. 710
Chicago, IL 60606
Phone: 312-578-1439
Website: www.
foundationforwomenscancer.org
Email: FWCinfo@sgo.org

Gay and Lesbian Medical Association (GLMA)

1629 K St., N.W., Ste. 300
Washington, DC 20006
Toll-Free: 833-456-2202
Website: www.glma.org
Email: info@glma.org

Gay Men's Health Crisis (GMHC)

307 W. 38th St.
New York, NY 10018
Toll-Free: 800-243-7692
Phone: 212-367-1000
Website: www.gmhc.org
Email: info@gmhc.org

Go Ask Alice!

Website: goaskalice.columbia.edu

Guttmacher Institute

125 Maiden Ln.
7th Fl.
New York, NY 10038
Toll-Free: 800-355-0244
Phone: 212-248-1111
Fax: 212-248-1951
Website: www.guttmacher.org
Email: info@guttmacher.org

Hepatitis B Foundation
3805 Old Easton Rd.
Doylestown, PA 18902
Phone: 215-489-4900
Fax: 215-489-4920
Website: www.hepb.org
Email: info@hepb.org

Hepatitis Foundation International (HFI)
504 Blick Dr.
Silver Spring, MD 20904
Toll-Free: 800-891-0707
Phone: 301-879-6891
Fax: 301-879-6890
Website: https://
hepatitisfoundation.org
Email: info@hepatitisfoundation.
org

HIV Medicine Association
4040 Wilson Blvd., Ste. 300
Arlington, VA 22203
Phone: 703-299-1215
Fax: 703-299-8766
Website: www.hivma.org
Email: info@hivma.org

I Want the Kit (IWTK)
Website: www.iwantthekit.org
Email: iwantthekit@jhmi.edu

Immunize.org
2136 Ford Pkwy., Ste. 5011
Saint Paul, MN 55116
Phone: 651-647-9009
Fax: 651-647-9131
Website: www.immunize.org
Email: admin@immunize.org

Kaiser Family Foundation (KFF)
185 Berry St., Ste. 2000
San Francisco, CA 94107
Phone: 650-854-9400
Fax: 650-854-4800
Website: www.kff.org

National Cervical Cancer Coalition (NCCC)
P.O. Box 13827
Research Triangle Park, NC 27709
Toll-Free: 800-685-5531
Fax: 919-361-8425
Website: www.nccc-online.org
Email: nccc@ashasexualhealth.org

National Coalition for LGBTQ Health
1630 Connecticut Ave., N.W.
Ste. 500
Washington, DC 20009
Phone: 202-232-6749
Website: https://healthlgbtq.org
Email: info@healthlgbt.org

Pan American Health Organization
525 23rd St., N.W.
Washington, DC 20037
Phone: 202-974-3000
Fax: 202-974-3663
Website: www.paho.org

Planned Parenthood Action Fund, Inc.
123 William St.
10th Fl.
New York, NY 10038
Toll-Free: 800-430-4907
Phone: 212-541-7800
Fax: 212-245-1845
Website: www.
plannedparenthoodaction.org

Sexuality Information and Education Council of the United States (SIECUS)
1012 14th St., N.W., Ste. 1108
Washington, DC 20005
Phone: 202-265-2405
Website: www.siecus.org
Email: info@siecus.org

The Well Project
P.O. Box 220410
Brooklyn, NY 11222
Toll-Free: 888-616-WELL
(888-616-9355)
Website: www.thewellproject.org
Email: info@thewellproject.org

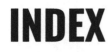

INDEX

INDEX

Page numbers followed by "n" refer to citation information; by "t" indicate tables; and by "f" indicate figures.

A

abdominal cramps
  opportunistic infections (OIs) 186
  proctocolitis 291
abdominal pain
  chlamydia 136
  gonorrhea 75
  opportunistic infections (OIs) 186
  sexually transmitted infections
    (STIs) 24
  Shigella infections 283
  viral hepatitis 209
acquired immunodeficiency syndrome
  (AIDS)
  antidiscrimination law 593
  cervical cancer 62
  cryptosporidiosis 279
  gonorrhea 147
  hepatitis 216
  HIV stigma 543, 550t
  HIV vaccine 491
  HIV viral load 441
  HIV-associated neurocognitive
    disorders (HAND) 585
  molluscum contagiosum 288
  neurocognitive disorders 585
  neurosyphilis 320

overview 163–168
public health challenges 38
sexually transmitted infections
  (STIs) 23, 67, 363
vaginal douching 457
Acquired Immunodeficiency
  Syndrome (AIDS) Drug Assistance
  Program (ADAP), Affordable Care
  Act (ACA) 203
ADAP *see* Acquired
  Immunodeficiency Syndrome
  (AIDS) Drug Assistance Program
Advocates for Youth, contact
  information 608
aerobics, living with HIV 578
Agency for Healthcare Research
  and Quality (AHRQ), contact
  information 605
AIDS *see* acquired immunodeficiency
  syndrome
AIDS Healthcare Foundation (AHF),
  contact information 608
AIDS.org, contact information 608
alcohol
  genital herpes 159
  gonorrhea 152
  high-risk sexual behavior 430
  human immunodeficiency virus
    (HIV) 182, 356
  human papillomavirus (HPV) 233
  pelvic inflammatory disease
    (PID) 327

Index

Index

Index

Index

625

Index

Index